MODERN MEDICINE FOR NURSES

Modern Medicine for Nurses

JOHN GIBSON, M.D., F.R.C.Psych., D.P.M.

THIRD EDITION

BLACKWELL SCIENTIFIC PUBLICATIONS

OXFORD LONDON EDINBURGH MELBOURNE

© 1970, 1972, 1975 Blackwell Scientific Publications
Osney Mead, Oxford
85 Marylebone High Street, London W1
9 Forrest Road, Edinburgh
P.O. Box 9, North Balwyn, Victoria, Australia

ISBN 0 632 08860 5

First published 1970
Second edition 1972
Third edition 1975

Distributed in the U.S.A. by
J. B. Lippincott Company, Philadelphia
and in Canada by
J. B. Lippincott Company of Canada, Ltd, Toronto

Printed in Great Britain at the Alden Press, Oxford
and bound
by Webb, Son & Co Ltd, Ferndale

Contents

Abbreviations

BP	blood-pressure
CSF	cerebrospinal fluid
ECF	extracellular fluid
ECG	electrocardiogram
EEG	electroencephalogram
ESR	erythrocyte sedimentation rate
ICF	intracellular fluid
g	gram
Hb	haemoglobin
K	potassium
kilo	kilogram
mcg	microgram
mg	milligram
ml	millilitre
mm	millimetre
Na	sodium
RBC	red blood cell
SG	specific gravity
WBC	white blood cell
WR	Wassermann reaction

Preface to the third edition

This book has been revised and brought up to date throughout. New sections have been added on acute myocarditis, cytomegalovirus infection, giant cell arteritis, epidemic neuromyasthenia, and the irritable bowel syndrome. Sections which have been extensively rewritten include those on herpes simplex, ulcerative colitis, migraine, Bell's palsy, and infective and serum hepatitis.

1 Introduction to Medicine

Medicine is the name given to the study of all kinds of diseases — of how they are caused, where they occur, the frequency of their occurrence, the way they affect the patient, how they are treated, what happens to the patient, the whole of the healing art.

The term medicine is also used in a more limited sense — as it is in this book — to describe those diseases that are particularly 'medical', the illnesses that are in the main treated by drugs, by psychotherapy, by methods of treatment other than operation or manipulation, the methods of treating 'surgical' illnesses. But the reader should understand that this division is not an absolute one: the physician (who treats medical illnesses) may perform minor operations and must know when surgical treatment is advisable, and the surgeon must have a knowledge of medical methods of care.

THE NATURE OF DISEASES

Diseases can be due to many causes. The causes of some are unknown. Basically the factors are heredity and environment, heredity being what a person inherits from his parents and environment what happens to him after the moment of his conception. Those whose causes have been discovered are classified.

HEREDITY

Every person inherits genes from his parents (see Chapter 11). Abnormalities in these genes can cause a person to inherit a disease or a liability to be affected in a particular way in certain circumstances. Examples of inherited diseases are haemophilia and Huntington's chorea.

INJURY

Injuries by damaging cells, tissues and organs — are common causes of disease and disability. Most injuries are the province of a surgeon. Tissues can be injured by extremes of heat and cold, by radio-activity, and by chemical substances.

DEGENERATION

All cells need nourishment, must respire (taking in oxygen and giving out carbon dioxide), and must be protected from harm. In adverse conditions cells degenerate, function badly or not at all. If the adverse conditions are not continued for too long,

1   *Introduction to Medicine*

the cell may recover and start to function normally again. If the adverse conditions continue for too long the cell dies. Some cells are more sensitive than others: fibrous tissue can survive a long time without oxygen, but brain-cells without it die in 5 minutes. *Necrosis* is death of cells. Common causes of degeneration and necrosis are:

(a)   lack of oxygen, due to cutting off or reducing the blood-supply

(b)   anaemia and a failure of the blood to transport adequate amounts of oxygen,

(c)   lack of an essential food-factor or hormones,

(d)   poison, e.g. an excessive consumption of alcohol.

It is not known whether the degeneration of many tissues that can set in in old age is due to a natural ageing process or to the action of several adverse factors, such as lack of essential factors in the diet and infections.

DISEASES OF BLOOD-VESSELS

An adequate supply of blood is necessary for all tissues. Some, especially the brain and heart, require more than the others. If the supply becomes inadequate, the tissues suffer and degenerate and may die. Diseases of the blood-vessels are a common cause of disease in other organs. *Athero-sclerosis* is a degeneration of the inner lining of the arteries, reducing the size of the tube through which blood has to pass. *Thrombosis* is clotting of blood in a blood-vessel; it is due to athero-sclerosis, to slowing of the circulation, or to a tendency of the blood in certain conditions to

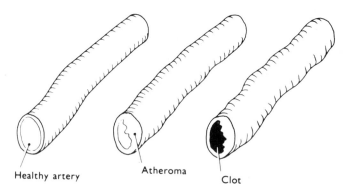

Fig. 1. The formation of an atheromatous patch and then a clot in an artery.

Healthy artery   Atheroma   Clot

clot. An *embolus* is a piece of clot or of tissue that is carried along in the blood-stream until it sticks in a blood-vessel and blocks it, cutting off the blood-supply to the tissue supplied by that particular vessel. *Haemorrhage* is a bleeding, large or small, from a blood-vessel. An *infarct* (infarction) is an area of tissue that degenerates and dies as a result of a sudden cutting-off of its blood-supply.

INFLAMMATION

Inflammation is the process in which fluid and cells accumulate in an irritated tissue to protect the tissue from further irritation and damage. The causes of the irritation can be micro-organisms, fungi, protozoa[1], poisons and injury.

[1] *protozoa:* small uni-cellular organisms, some of which are harmful

Irritation by harmful micro-organisms is a common cause of inflammation.

Some micro-organisms are normally present in some parts of the body — on the skin, in the throat, in the mouth, in the large intestine. Most of them are harmless

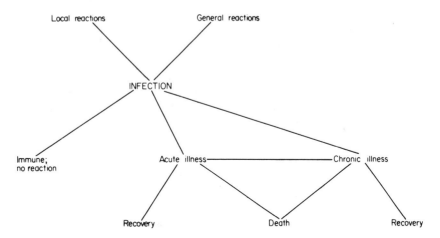

Fig. 2. Reactions of the body to infection.

if they stay in their normal position, but can be harmful if they move elsewhere. The organism called *E.coli* lives in the large intestine and is an essential part of the micro-biological life going on there, but if it moves into the urinary tract it causes inflammation.

Inflammation due to micro-organisms is (a) *acute,* when there is a sudden sharp reaction to them, (b) *chronic,* when the reactions are slower and last longer, and (c) *subacute,* when the inflammation is somewhere between acute and chronic.

In *acute inflammation* the changes that take place in the tissues are: (a) after a slight preliminary constriction of the arterioles, there is a dilatation of arterioles, veins and capillaries, (b) a liberation of *histamine,* a chemical substance that causes a further dilation of blood-vessels, (c) an invasion of the tissues by *polymorphonuclear white blood-cells* (probably attracted by some chemical factor), which pass through the walls of the capillaries and attack and attempt to destroy the invading micro-organisms, (d) an out-pouring of *fluid.* As a result of all these reactions, the signs of inflammation appear: heat, swelling, redness, pain and loss of function. Suppuration is the process by which with the death of cells and micro-organisms a greenish-yellow fluid called *pus* is formed; an *abscess* is a collection of pus. Many inflammations clear up before the development of suppuration and with recovery the tissues resume their normal appearance.

In *chronic inflammation* the reaction to invasion is less sharp but prolonged over a longer period. Such an inflammation is likely to show at the same time degenerating processes in one place and healing processes in another. Attempts at healing produce fibrous tissue and scar-formation. Chronic inflammation is called granulomatous when there is an accumulation of fibrous tissue and other cells, often with giant cells, large cells with many nuclei. Tuberculosis and sarcoidosis are two examples of granulomatous inflammation.

Introduction to Medicine

INFECTION An *infection* is the disease-process produced by the invasion of the body by harmful micro-organisms. An *infectious disease* is one transmitted directly or indirectly from man to man, from animal to animal, or from animal to man, by a transference of the micro-organisms from one to the other.

Such a transfer can be:

(a) by *direct contact,* person to person, e.g. smallpox, syphilis.

(b) by *droplet infection:* a fine mist of tiny drops containing the micro-organisms is sprayed into the air by coughing, sneezing, etc.; a person can be infected directly or by infected dust from floors, carpets, curtains, bedclothes, handkerchiefs, etc. on which the spray has fallen; e.g. pulmonary tuberculosis, measles, whooping cough.

(c) by *eating or drinking infected food, water, milk;* e.g. food poisoning, typhoid fever, undulant fever.

(d) *from mother to unborn child* through the placenta; e.g. congenital syphilis.

(e) *by infected soil getting into a wound or cut,* e.g. tetanus.

(f) *from infected insects or animals*; e.g. yellow fever, rabies.

The *incubation period* is the period between infection by micro-organisms and the appearance of the first symptoms. It varies with different infections from hours to months, but it is usually fairly constant for a particular infection.

A *carrier* is a person who carries the micro-organisms on or in his body and while not harmed by them himself can infect other people; usually, but not always, he has had previously an attack of the particular infection the organisms cause. People can become carriers of diphtheria, typhoid fever, streptococci, staphylococci, and other organisms.

Cross-infection is the acquisition by a person of an infection when he is being treated in hospital for some other condition.

Infections can be:

(a) *sporadic:* cases occurring here and there;

(b) *endemic:* cases occurring all the time in a place;

(c) *epidemic:* many cases occurring in one place at one time;

(d) *pandemic:* many cases occurring all over the world at about the same time.

Resistance to infection The body has defence-mechanisms against attack by micro-organisms. These defences are local and general.

Local defences are:

(a) the *skin:* with its constantly shedding surface and its sweat, the skin can cope with most or all micro-organisms that land on it; it cannot so readily cope with organisms that land on a cut or scratch or get admission with the bite of an insect or animal;

(b) the *tears,* which can deal with most organisms that land on the conjunctiva of the eye, by washing them away and killing them;

(c) the *mucus* and *cilia* of cells in the respiratory tract, which prevent organisms from reaching the cells and waft them away from the lungs and other internal structures;

(d) the *gastric juice*, whose acidity destroys many swallowed organisms.

(e) the *vaginal secretions,* whose acidity destroys many organisms.

General reactions come into action if the local defences of the body are breached and the tissues attacked by harmful micro-organisms. A large number of factors, some of them complex, determine whether the organisms die or live to produce disease:

(a)   a *large number* of organisms is more likely to cause disease, by mass attack, than a small number, for the defences can often cope with a small number and be overwhelmed by a large number.

(b)   some *strains* of organisms are more dangerous than others. A strain is a type of a particular organism varying in slight degree from other organisms of the same kind.

(c)   the *patient* may be debilitated by some other disease, by lack of food, by cold, and so more likely to be affected; he may have a natural or acquired *immunity* to that particular organism (see next section). Previous exposure to radio-activity makes tissues more vulnerable.

(d)   *Polymorphonuclear white blood-cells* (polymorphs) and cells of the reticulo-endothelial and lymph systems can destroy micro-organisms.

(e)   *damaged tissues* and *red blood cells* liberate substances that kill micro-organisms.

If the micro-organisms get a foothold in the body, they invade and multiply, causing inflammation and damage. Some of them (e.g. those that cause tetanus, diphtheria) produce an *exotoxin*, a poisonous substance that can cause damage in tissues (such as those of the heart) not directly invaded by the organism.

IMMUNITY   Immunity is the degree of resistance.that a body can put up to a type of invading micro-organism. It can be the result (a) of inheritance, (b) of having an attack of that particular infection, (c) of vaccination or some other artificial means of preventing a disease.

Immunity is due to the presence of antibodies. *Antibodies* are proteins present in the serum of blood. *Antigens* are any substances that stimulate the production of antibodies or react with them.

Antibodies can occur naturally or be acquired by vaccination, etc. Harmful micro-organisms, invading the body, act as antigens and stimulate the production of antibodies, which oppose their activities. Antibodies are specific, reacting only against a particular kind of micro-organism or even a particular strain of it. When the organism invades the body, antibodies to it may be already there, and if they are in adequate amounts the organisms are overcome and the person infected does not develop the disease. If the micro-organism does invade the tissue, antibodies to it are produced in about 10 days. Once antibodies have been produced, they are likely to remain indefinitely in the blood and may prevent a person getting a second attack of that particular infection. It is thus unusual for a person to have a second attack of mumps because there is a large antibody reaction, but very common for him to have many attacks of the common cold, to which the antibody reaction is slight.

A child acquires some antibodies from his mother when she has had a particular

Introduction to Medicine

infection and can transmit them to the child *in utero*. These antibodies can usually prevent a newly born child from getting the particular infection, but they disappear within a few weeks, leaving the child open to attack.

The production of antibodies can be stimulated in various ways, especially by vaccination. The word *vaccination* was originally used for vaccination against smallpox, but the word has been extended to include similar techniques directed against other infections. A vaccine is a preparation of dead organisms or of organisms whose power to harm has been weakened by growing them in adverse conditions. When injected into the body the vaccine has the power to stimulate the formation of antibodies against that particular organism, and these antibodies will then prevent the person from getting that particular infection. Another way of stimulating antibody-production is by injecting a *toxoid* (which is a toxin treated to make it less harmful).

In *auto-immune diseases* it is thought that some antigen within the body stimulates the production of the antibodies that can act upon the cells of the same body.

The antigen-antibody reaction is important in the transplanting of tissues or organs from one person to another. Except where it is possible to transplant from an identical twin, when a tissue is transplanted it acts as an antigen and stimulates the production in the body of certain antibodies which then attack the cells of the transplant and destroy them. This is a major problem in transplant surgery. To prevent antibody formation, the person to whom the transplant is made may be given total irradiation or a course of cortico-steroid drugs; but both these methods have dangers.

HYPERSENSITIVITY

Some people are hypersensitive to small amounts of certain proteins and if exposed to them react sharply in a way that a person who is not so sensitive does not. Hypersensitivity can be (a) an allergy, (b) anaphylaxis, (c) hypersensitivity to a particular organism. The substance that provokes a reaction is called an *allergen*. Allergens can produce a reaction by being breathed in, eaten, coming into contact with the skin or being injected.

All these reactions are of the antigen-antibody type (see p. 5) and the person must have previously been 'sensitized' by earlier experience of the particular allergen.

In allergy patients are sensitive to proteins of various kinds — in pollen of grass and flowers, dust of various kinds, some foods (milk, chocolate, fish, shellfish, strawberries, etc.) drugs, chemicals. Common reactions are vasomotor rhinitis, asthma, hay-fever, dermatitis.

In *anaphylaxis* there is an acute reaction with spasm of involuntary muscle (especially in the bronchi), collapse and sometimes death. It can be caused by a second injection of a protein-containing substance 10 days after the first injection. Some proteins are in certain 'antitoxins' used in the treatment of some infections (diphtheria, tetanus) and come from the animal which has been used for the preparation of the antitoxin. Serum sickness is a milder reaction (with fever, weals in the skin, and swellings of joints) due to injections of serum.

In *hypersensitivity to micro-organisms* the hypersensitivity has developed in the course of an infection. This can happen in tuberculosis, and the test called a tuberculin test (an example of this hypersensitivity) is used to decide whether a patient has had an attack of tuberculosis previously.

DEFICIENCY DISEASES
There are due to the absence from the diet of substances necessary for normal health, growth and replacement of tissues. There may be a general shortage of food (as is common in many parts of the world) and in particular a shortage of protein, or there may be a shortage of a vitamin or a salt. Other diseases are due to a reduction of the hormones secreted by endocrine glands.

Examples of deficiency diseases are:
kwashiorkor: due to protein deficiency
scurvy: due to shortage of vitamin C
rickets: due to shortage of vitamin D
beri-beri: due to a shortage of vitamin B (thiamine).

DISEASES PRODUCED BY PSYCHOLOGICAL FACTORS
The number of diseases that can be shown to be due to psychological factors is small. Many mental diseases (so-called because mental symptoms are prominent) are due to physical conditions (e.g. the dementias) and some of the others (e.g. manic-depressive psychosis, schizophrenia) are probably due to some biochemical abnormality in the brain. The neuroses are generally attributed to psychological factors; and the psycho-somatic diseases are those in which psychological factors are thought – sometimes on not very strong evidence – to be responsible for the physical changes. However, psychological factors can be important in the production of symptoms, in aggravating a condition; stress, anxiety, grief, disappointment, fear, can all contribute to the symptoms and prolongation of an illness.

TUMOURS
Tumours (new growths, neoplasms). These are overgrowths of cells which have undergone some change that make them multiply themselves. Tumours can arise in any cells, but they arise more commonly in some cells than others. They can be divided into benign and malignant growths.

(a) *Benign tumours* (simple, non-malignant) are tumours that grow slowly; their cells resembly closely the cells they grow from and do not show abnormal forms; they are usually surrounded by a capsule of fibrous tissue and are easily distinguished from the tissues around them; they may not produce any symptoms, but can cause trouble if they press on important structures (a benign tumour of the meninges can press on the brain) or if they are composed of secreting cells (a tumour of the pancreas can produce too much insulin); and they do not spread to any other part of the body.

(b) *Malignant tumours* (cancers, carcinomas; or sarcomas - a rare form starting in certain cells) have cells that are changed fundamentally from the cells

7

Introduction to Medicine

they start in, show an abnormal appearance of a more primitive kind, and are of irregular sizes and shapes; spread rapidly and in a disorderly manner; do not have a capsule and spread between normal cells so that it is usually impossible to say, by naked examination, what is healthy and what is cancerous; and usually, in addition to spreading where they arise, can invade other parts of the body. This invasion is: (a) by growing along lymph-vessels into lymph-nodes and from one group of lymph-nodes to another; (b) by invading a capillary or vein, getting into the blood-stream and being carried with it into other parts of the body, near or far, (c) by spreading across the surface of the peritoneum or pleural cavity. A metastasis or secondary growth is any growth of malignant cells in some part other than that in which they started; the cells of the secondary growth resemble those of the primary they have come from. If the malignant cells are not destroyed or removed they cause *cachexia* — malaise, loss of weight, weakness, anaemia — and eventually death.

The causes of many malignant growths are unknown. Viruses have been suspect for some growths but without proof. Among the identified causes of cancer are:

(a)   tobacco: cancer of the bronchus (lung), possibly cancer of the larynx and bladder;

(b)   ionizing radiations from X-rays and radio-active salts: cancer of the skin and internal organs;

(c)   schistosomiasis (a parasite): cancer of the bladder and rectum;

(d)   aniline dyes in industry: cancer of the bladder.

(e)   soot, oil: cancer of the skin.

PARASITES These are creatures that live on the skin or inside the body or bowels of other creatures and do them harm. They are a common cause of illness in tropical countries.

TERMS USED IN MEDICINE

Pathology: the study of disease-processes in tissues and organs.

Chemical pathology: the study of chemical abnormalities in the cells and fluids of the body.

Micro-biology: the study of micro-organisms — viruses, bacilli, cocci, spirochaetes, etc. (formerly called bacteriology).

Aetiology: the study of the causes of disease.

Epidemiology: the study of epidemics.

Clinical Features: the symptoms (what is appreciated by the patient) and the signs (the evidence found by doctor and nurse) of a disease.

Complication: any abnormality that occurs during or after an illness, but is not bound to occur always.

Sequelae: clinical features that may occur when the illness is apparently over.

Diagnosis: the discovery of the kind of illness the patient is suffering from. Differential diagnosis: the consideration of what diseases the patient may be suffering from, a preliminary to making a diagnosis.

Syndrome: name given to a collection of clinical features before it is dignified with the name of 'disease'.

Prognosis: the expected outcome of a disease.

2 Infections

Infections are produced by the invasion of the body by harmful micro-organisms. The effects of infection are discussed in Chapter 1. Micro-organisms are organisms too small to be seen with the naked eye. The larger micro-organisms can be seen with a light microscope, the smaller micro-organisms with an electron microscope. Micro-organisms are classified as follows.

1. Viruses [2]

These are the smallest of micro-organisms. A virus is composed of either ribonucleic acid (RNA) or deoxyribonucleic acid (DNA) within a protein capsule. Such is their composition that viruses can be regarded as large chemical molecules. A virus can multiply only within a living cell. Having invaded such a cell, the virus compels the chemical activities going on inside the cell to turn out viruses of the same sort as the invading one.

Among the diseases caused by viruses are:

common cold	influenza	acute poliomyelitis
mumps	German measles	chickenpox
smallpox	infective hepatitis	

2. Bacteria [3]

These are larger than viruses and appear in several forms.

(a) *Cocci: Staphylococci* [4] are small, rounded or ovoid, and grow in clumps, Among the diseases caused by staphylococci are:

boils	carbuncles	osteomyelitis
styes	impetigo	one kind of food-poisoning

Streptococci [5] are small, rounded or ovoid, and grow in chains. Among the diseases caused by streptococci are:

tonsillitis	pharyngitis	scarlet fever
erysipelas	subacute bacterial endocarditis	

Diplococci are short, sometimes kidney-shaped, and grow in pairs. Among the diseases caused by diplococci are:

pneumonia	gonorrhoea	meningococcal meningitis

[2] *virus:* Latin: *virus* – poison
[3] *bacterium:* Greek: *bacterium* – little stick
[4] *staphylococcus:* from Greek: *staphyule* – grape; *coccus* – berry
[5] *streptococcus:* from Greek: *streptos* – twisted

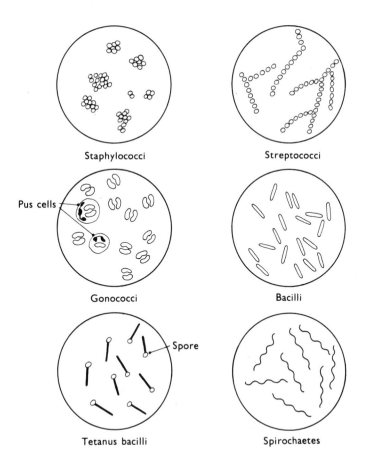

Fig. 3. Some micro-
organisms.

Staphylococci

Streptococci

Pus cells

Gonococci

Bacilli

Spore

Tetanus bacilli

Spirochaetes

(b)   *Bacilli* [6] These are larger and rod-shaped; curved ones are called vibrios. Among the diseases caused by bacilli are:

tuberculosis	typhoid fever	tetanus
whooping cough	diphtheria	anthrax

(c)   *Spirochaetes* [7] These are thin and have a cork-screw spiral. Among the diseases caused by spirochaetes are:

syphilis	Vincent's angina	infective spirochaetal jaundice

3. Rickettsiae [8]   These are organisms intermediate in size between viruses and bacteria with some of the properties of each. They are commonly parasites of fleas and other insects. Among the diseases caused by rickettsiae is:

typhus fever

4. Fungi.   These are larger than bacilli, form filaments and networks, and reproduce both sexually and asexually. Among the diseases caused by fungi are:

ringworm	thrush

[6] *bacillus:* Latin: *bacillus* – a little stick
[7] *spirochaete:* from Greek: *spiros* – coil; *chaete* – bristle
[8] *rickettsia:* named after H.T.Ricketts (1871 - 1910) who died of typhus fever while studying it.

Infections

5. Protozoa. These are large uni-cellular organisms with a complex life-history. Among the diseases caused by protozoa are:

malaria amoebic dysentery trichomonas infections

SCHEDULE OF IMMUNIZATIONS

Vaccines are available for the immunization of children against:

diphtheria measles whooping cough tetanus
smallpox poliomyelitis tuberculosis German me...

In order to reduce the number of injections necessary while providing maximum benefit for as many children as possible, it is usual to combine some of the injections. Table 1 shows one scheme.

Table 1

Age	Vaccine	Number
3–6 months	(a) combined diphtheria, tetanus, whooping cough; (b) oral poliomyelitis	3 at intervals of 4–8 weeks
1–2 years	(a) & (b) booster doses (c) measles	1 of each
5 years	(a) & (b) booster doses	1 of each
8–12 years	(a) & (b) booster doses	1 of each
11–14 years	girls: German measles	1
12 years (earlier if exposed to infection)	BCG for children who are tuberculin-negative	1

MEASLES

This is a very infectious disease with a characteristic rash and catarrhal inflammation of the upper respiratory tract. It is caused by a virus and spread by droplet infection or by handkerchiefs and bedclothes. It occurs in endemic form with epidemics every 2-3 years. It is a disease of children; infants under 6 months have usually acquired a temporary trans-placental immunity from the mother. One attack usually confers lifelong immunity. Incubation period: about 11 days.

Clinical features

Onset. Sudden, with fever, malaise, headache, querulousness; muscular pains; coughing, sneezing, nasal discharge; conjunctival inflammation, photophobia; diarrhoea.

1. *Koplik's spots:* occur during the first 4 days; they are small white spots on an erythematous background occurring on the mucous membrane of the mouth, often on the inner side of the cheek opposite the molar teeth; they are diagnostic, but not always present.

2. *Rash:* usually appears 2-7 days after onset; begins on face, forehead, behind the ears; spreads over face, neck trunk and limbs; usually not on hands and feet; is a

macular or maculo-papular reddish brown rash on a blotchy erythematous base; fades in the order it has occurred, leaving a fine desquamation[9].

Course. The fever may rise sharply with the outbreak of the rash, up to about 39.5°C (103°F) and then falls by lysis. The patient may develop bronchiolitis[1] a cough. Abdominal pain (sometimes mimicking acute appendicitis) may occur, due to enlargement of lymph-nodes and tissue within the abdomen.

Complete recovery is usual within 18 days. Measles may be fatal for poorly nourished young children in poor health.

Complications

Bronchopneumonia, laryngitis, acute otitis media, bronchiectasis.

Secondary infection with streptococci, pneumococci, *B. influenzae.* React-ivation of a pre-existing pulmonary tuberculosis.

Acute haemorrhagic lesions, with haemorrhages into the skin and mucous membrane, and death.

Encephalo-myelitis (rare) with fever, vomiting, stiff neck, stupor, fits; about 10 per cent of affected patients die; about half the survivors show permanent post-encephalitic effects.

Prevention

Vaccine: a measles vaccine, composed of a live attenuated virus, should be given before the age of 3 to children who have not had measles. A slight measles-like reaction and non-infectious illness may develop about a week after vaccination and last a day or two.

Immuno-globulin: for temporary immunity a dose of 250 - 750 mg intra-muscularly can be given to young children who have been exposed to infection and are in poor health; given within the first 5 days after exposure it will prevent infection; given during 6 - 9th day it will weaken the attack.

Treatment

1. Bed; isolation for 14 days; fluids; sponging if necessary; darkened room to relieve photophobia. [2]
2. Penicillin if there is a secondary infection.

GERMAN MEASLES

Other name: rubella

This is an acute infectious disease caused by a virus. It is endemic, with epidemics occurring in the spring and early summer in the northern hemisphere. It usually affects older children, adolescents and young adults. It is spread by droplet infection. One attack usually confers immunity. Incubation period: 17-18 days.

[9] *desquamation:* scaling
[1] *bronchiolitis:* inflammation of small bronchi
[2] *photophobia:* dislike of light

Infections

Clinical features   The onset is with malaise, slight fever, sore throat, stiffness of neck and sometimes conjunctivitis. The rash begins on 1st day and may be first sign of the disease; it begins on the face and spreads rapidly to trunk and limbs and consists of raised pink spots, which are separate at first and then run together; it fades progressively and has gone by 3rd day.

Lymph-nodes in neck become enlarged, and are firm and distinct. The knees, ankles and other joints are occasionally sore and painful.

Course: the disease is usually mild. The fever and rash subside on the 3rd day.

Complications   Encephalitis can occur. A child *in utero* can become infected, via the placenta, if the mother develops German measles, and when this occurs during the first 3 months of pregnancy the child has about a 1 in 10 chance of being abnormal. The abnormality may be mental retardation, microcephaly, cataracts, unequal eyeballs, deafness, abnormally shaped ears, cleft palate, hare-lip, talipes, eruption of teeth and cardiac malformations.

Prevention   Girls should be encouraged to contract the disease before they reach child-bearing age. A live vaccine is given to girls of 11-14 years. An interval of 3-4 weeks should elapse between giving this vaccine and any other vaccine, whichever is given first. It is not given to an adult woman unless she is sero-negative; about 80 per cent of women in western countries are sero-positive.

Treatment   A few days in bed is all that is necessary. Isolation is not necessary, but a woman who might be pregnant should — even if she has had an attack of German measles herself — not come into contact with the patient.

MUMPS [3]   *Other name:* epidemic parotitis [4]

This acute infectious disease is caused by a virus and characterized by enlargement of the salivary glands and sometimes other tissues. Spread is by droplet infection or direct contact. It occurs usually in children of 5-15 years, but as it is not very infectious many reach adult life without having had it. One attack usually gives immunity for life. Incubation period: 14-21 days; can be 1 month or longer.

Clinical features   1. *Onset:* fever, malaise, loss of appetite, nausea.

2. *Salivary glands:* about the 2nd day, swelling of one or both parotid glands occur, filling up the space behind the angle of the jaw, pushing the lobe of the ear upwards and outwards, making eating difficult and painful. The opening of the parotid duct on the inside of the mouth may be reddened. The swelling is at its greatest 2-3 days later. Sometimes enlargement of the submandibular and sublingual glands occurs.

Course. The fever starts to subside about the 3rd-4th day, and thereafter the patient usually improves rapidly. The glands take a week or more to subside to normal size.

[3] *mumps:* Old English — to sulk, mope.
[4] *parotitis:* inflammation of parotid gland

Complications	*Orchitis*[5] is more common in adult life than in childhood. Usually one testicle only is affected; it becomes swollen, painful and extremely tender. Orchitis usually occurs when the other symptoms and signs are disappearing and produces a second rise of temperature. Fibrosis of the gland has followed, and when this affects both testicles the patient may cease to develop male hormones.
Mastitis (inflammation of the breast) and *oophoritis* (inflammation of the ovaries) can occur.
Pancreatitis causes epigastric pain, nausea, vomiting and tenderness of the pancreas to deep palpation.
Aseptic meningitis. Deafness.
Prevention	Mumps virus vaccine can be given to children over one year and to adults. No important local or general side-effects occur. It is not known yet whether immunity is permanent.
Treatment	The patient should be isolated in bed for about 14 days. Food may have to be minced for ease of swallowing and drinks sucked through a straw. Cleanliness of the mouth is important. Acetylsalicylic acid is given to relieve pain. The testicles should be supported by cotton wool; prednisolone 15 mg 6-hourly relieves orchitis.
CHICKENPOX	*Other name:* varicella (from Latin: *variola* – pustule)
This is usually a mild infection of childhood. Infection by a virus occurs via the respiratory tract. One attack usually confers immunity. The same virus causes herpes zoster. Incubation period: 14-16 days.
Clinical features	1. Slight fever and malaise for a few days.
2. Rash: starts as a crop of papules, which change into vesicles; the vesicles crust, some become pustular. Other crops occur during the next few days. The rash is more extensive and prominent on the trunk than the limbs, and at one time papules, vesicles and crust can be seen; both these points help to distinguish the condition from smallpox. Boils and impetigo can occur if the spots are scratched.
3. Enlarged lymph-nodes may occur, especially in the suboccipital and posterior cervical regions.
Complications	These are unusual, but the following can occur:
glomerulo-nephritis   pneumonitis   encephalitis
neuritis of cranial nerves; temporary blindness.
Treatment	The patient should be confined to bed until the rash has disappeared. Itching can be relieved by a dusting powder or lotion of calamine and phenol. The finger nails should be cut short to prevent scratching.

[5] *orchitis:* inflammation of the testicle
[6] *herpes zoster:* from Greek: *herpo* – creep; *zoster* – girdle

HERPES ZOSTER [6]   *Other name:* shingles [7]

This is an infection of the nervous system due to the same virus that causes chicken-pox. It usually occurs in middle- or old age, and is thought to be an attack by the virus which has been dormant in the body since the original attack of chickenpox. The virus attacks the posterior root ganglion of a spinal nerve or the corresponding ganglion of a sensory cranial nerve, causing inflammation and death of nerve cells and fibres. Attacks become more severe with advancing age.

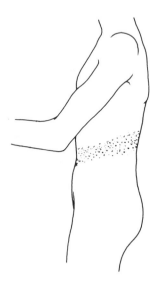

Fig. 4. Attack of herpes zoster involving the left tenth thoracic segment.

Clinical features   1. There is sometimes a prodromal period of 3-4 days of malaise, fever and pain.
2. An erythematous and vesicular rash appears in the cutaneous distribution of a spinal or cranial nerve, most commonly on the chest, neck or face and usually on one side only. The vesicles start to dry up in about a week and the scabs fall off about a week later. In some cases no vesicles appear.
3. Severe irritation or pain occurs in the region of the distribution of the affected nerves before, with or after the appearance of the rash.
4. Lymph-nodes of the area involved become slightly enlarged.

Complications   Persistent post-herpetic pain in the affected region, especially in old people who have no interests to take their mind off the pain.

Infection of the skin from scratching.

If the first or second division of the trigeminal nerve is involved, the cornea can become affected and severly ulcerated.

Treatment   Bed for the first few days is advisable. Idoxuridine dissolved in dimethyl sulphoxide (DMSO) is applied on lint continuously for 3-4 days. Cytarabine is given in a single daily intravenous injection of 2-3 mg per kilo body-weight. Pain is relieved by anal-

[7] *shingles:* from Latin: *cingulum* – belt

gesics; morphine may be necessary. Post-herpetic neuralgia can be difficult to relieve and has driven patients to suicide. Prolonged self-administered transcutaneous electric stimulation from a special stimulator relieves pain in many patients and can produce a cure. If other methods fail, posterior root section or ganglionectomy [8] may be necessary.

HERPES SIMPLEX

This infection is caused by a virus which establishes itself in the body and remains there in a latent form, emerging to produce an attack of herpes at various times — during a fever, menstruation, exposure to strong sunlight, trauma, emotional crises, smoking cannabis. Severe and sometimes fatal attacks can occur in patients whose immunity mechanisms are upset, e.g. after undergoing a transplantation or receiving large doses of steroids, immuno-suppressive drugs or anti-cancer drugs.

Clinical features

In primitive societies the primary infection occurs in early childhood, producing a mild illness of which stomatitis is usually a feature.

In more highly developed societies the primary infection is more likely to occur in adolescence or early adult life. The typical feature is a crop of vesicles around the mouth, inside the mouth, on the fingers, or elsewhere. The genital organs can be infected by sexual intercourse. Pyrexia, malaise, and enlargement of the liver, spleen or lymph-nodes can occur. A painful whitlow can occur on one or more fingers or on the toes.

Complications

Impairment of vision following involvement of the eye.
Encephalitis is a serious complication, producing death in about half of those who develop it and severe neurological damage in another quarter. Only about half the survivors take up useful work again.

Treatment

Idoxuride dissolved in dimethyl sulphoxide (DMSO) is applied locally. Cytabarine is given in a single daily dose of 3 mg per kilo body-weight.

INFECTIVE MONONUCLEOSIS

Other name: glandular fever
This is an acute infectious disease probably due to a virus. It occurs as single cases or in small epidemics. It can occur at any age, but is most common at 10-35 years. Incubation period: not definitely known.

Clinical features

1. *Onset:* sudden, with fever, sore throat, pain on swallowing, stiff neck, general aching, loss of appetite.
2. *Adenitis:* within the next 2-3 days the cervical lymph-nodes on the one side become enlarged and tender; the nodes on the other side become enlarged and then axillary, inguinal, mediastinal and mesenteric glands. The nodes remain discrete and do not suppurate.

[8] *ganglionectomy:* surgical removal of a posterior-root ganglion.

Infections

3. *Liver and Spleen:* become slightly enlarged; jaundice can occur; rupture of the spleen has caused death.

4. *Skin:* erythematous, macular, maculo-papular or urticarial rashes can appear.

5. *Neurological symptoms:* can occur, indicating involvement of brain, meninges, spinal cord and cranial and spinal nerves. Neurological complications have caused death.

Course: variable. Recovery within 3-6 weeks is usual. The fever can last from a few days to several weeks. The nodes do not return to normal for several weeks. Fever can be prolonged for several weeks; relapses of fever and adenitis can occur; convalescence is slow and it is often a long time before the patient regains his normal vitality. Depression can occur.

Special Tests

1. Blood count: after an initial decrease, there is a lymphocytosis, many of the cells being abnormal.

2. Paul-Bunnell test (for certain agglutinins which clump red blood cells of sheep): diagnostic when positive, but is not always positive.

Treatment

There is no specific treatment. If the patient is jaundiced, he is given a high carbo-hydrate and protein diet. He should stay in bed for at least a week after the fever has subsided and not get up until he feels quite well.

INFLUENZA [9]

This is an acute infectious disease which may appear in several forms, usually characterized by a sudden onset, muscular pain and prostration; a gastro-intestinal type can occur. It is due to a virus of the influenza group, found in the upper respiratory tract during an attack. There are 3 distinct types of the virus: *influenza A, influenza B, influenza C.* A is more common that B; C is rare.

The disease is notorious for its unpredictability, for its variations from year to year. It commonly occurs in epidemics and there is almost every year an epidemic occurring somewhere in the world. The World Health Organization is in constant touch with international influenza centres, which provide it with information about the incidence and spread of epidemics and the type of virus. Pandemics occur rarely, many years apart. In highly populated areas epidemics tend to occur suddenly, last a few weeks and then stop. People of all ages are susceptible. An attack by one type may give an immunity to it for several months only and not to infection by another type. Spread is by droplet infection. Incubation period: 1-2 days.

Clinical features

Onset: sudden, with chill, fever, malaise, loss of appetite; epistaxis; headache, muscular pains, sore throat, injected fauces; flushed face, sneezing, nasal discharge; prostration; a dry cough and retrosternal pain, due to tracheitis.

Course: the course and severity vary from epidemic to epidemic. An acute illness of 3-4 days is common. The temperature falls gradually. The patient often feels weak and depressed for several days afterwards; suicide may be precipitated. The outlook for previously healthy people is good. The disease may be fatal for

[9] *influenza:* Italian: *influssio* – discharge or *influenze* – influence, i.e. by the stars etc.

patients with chronic cardiac or pulmonary disease or alcoholism for they are particularly liable to develop bronchopneumonia, oedema of the lungs and myocarditis.

The *gastro-intestinal type* is characterized by fever, abdominal pain, vomiting, diarrhoea, muscular pains and prostration.

Complications
Bronchitis, bronchopneumonia, oedema of the lungs.
Acute myocarditis, pericarditis.
Sinusitis, acute otitis media, mastoiditis.
Involvement of nervous system: encephalo-myelitis, cranial and spinal nerve paralysis.

Prevention
Mass immunization (e.g. of hospital staff) is recommended when a new virus A subtype appears (which happens about every 10 years) and for 2-3 years afterwards. In intervening years only people at risk need be vaccinated — the old, the chronic sick, and people with chronic heart or lung disease.

Treatment
The patient should be isolated in bed and stay there for at least a week. He will require the usual nursing care for an acute fever. Acetylsalicyclic acid or codeine is given to relieve pain. Secondary infections require treatment by antibiotics or sulpha drugs.

INFECTIVE HEPATITIS and SERUM HEPATITIS
These diseases are thought to be produced by similar hepatic viruses, virus A producing infective hepatitis and virus B serum hepatitis. The viruses have different incubation periods, are usually spread in different ways, but produce similar effects on the liver and have similar clinical features.

Virus A is spread by faecal contamination of food or water. The incubation period is 15-40 days. The virus is present in blood and faeces during an attack, and patients may be carriers of it for months. Small epidemics can occur.

Virus B is spread usually by contamination by infected blood and to a much lesser extent by contaminated faeces or water. Common sources of infection are: contact with infected blood, contaminated needles and syringes, transfusion of contaminated blood, plasma or blood-products. It is a serious risk to the staff of artificial kidney units. The incubation period is 40-150 days.

Clinical features
The patient feels ill and loses his appetite and any desire to smoke or drink. Severe nausea, brought on by food or by the smell or sight of it, is typical. Vomiting, headache and constipation are common. There is pyrexia, which can be slight, moderate or in acute attacks very severe, rising to 40.5°C (105°F).

Jaundice develops a few days after the onset, and persists for 1-2 weeks. The liver becomes enlarged, sometimes to the umbilicus, and tender. In 20 per cent of cases the spleen can be felt.

Some patients have gastro-enteritis only and no jaundice. Such cases are not likely to be diagnosed except during an epidemic. It is possible that children may have gastro-enteritis only; and as one attack of the illness gives a life-long immunity, it is likely that adults who develop the disease are those who have not acquired this immunity in childhood.

The acute stage of the illness lasts for 2-4 weeks. Recovery is usual; a relapse can occur. Some patients develop cirrhosis of the liver. Death is uncommon.

Convalescence is often a slow affair, for depression and fatigue can persist for long after the acute phase is over and it may be months before the patient feels he is himself again.

Special tests   Liver function tests show evidence of liver damage.

Treatment   There is no specific treatment. If the illness is believed to be due to virus A, strict care must be taken in nursing the patient to avoid any faecal contamination.

The patient should stay in bed for at least a fortnight, and longer if the acute stage is persisting. Diet can be unrestricted, unless the patient has a dislike for fatty foods which should then be omitted. If the jaundice does not clear up in a few weeks, cortico-steroid treatment is given.

The patient should be warned to abstain from alcohol for at least 3 months after an attack, for he is he is likely to have an intolerance for it and to become drunk on a very slight amount; moreover, alcohol can precipitate a relapse.

Australian antigen   This antigen (HbAg) is present in the blood of some people who have had serum hepatitis and indicates that they are potential carriers of virus B. They can infect other people who come into contact with their blood. They are not a danger if their skin is intact and they are not bleeding from a mucous membrane.

Likely carriers of Australian antigen are:

(a)   patients with acute or chronic liver disease
(b)   patients with mongolism
(c)   patients living in long stay institutions, psychiatric hospitals, prisoners
(d)   patients from tropical countries (where the incidence is usually higher than in temperate countries)
(e)   drug-addicts who inject themselves, tattooed persons, male homosexuals, sexually promiscuous people
(f)   patients who have had a blood-transfusion within the last 6 months, because of the risk that they might have had an untested transfusion
(g)   professional blood-donors.

Precautions to be taken with an Australian antigen positive patient in hospital
1. Laboratory tests are reduced to the absolute minimum. Blood is taken only when absolutely necessary.
2. Blood, urine and faeces are regarded as dangerous.
3. Staff should wear protective clothing and gloves when taking blood. A plastic sheet is placed under the patient's arm.
4. Blood is transferred gently into the container. None is sprayed into the air or put on the outside or rim of the container. The container must be perfect and have a screw cap.
5. The container is placed in an individual plastic bag. The bag is heat-sealed and marked with a self-adhesive label, which is marked "HIGH RISK SPECIMEN

AUSTRALIAN ANTIGEN POSITIVE". The label must not be licked. The laboratory request form is not put inside the bag.

6. Spilt blood is diluted at once with strong hydrochlorite solution before being wiped up.

7. Needle and syringe are sent in a rigid container for destruction.

8. Porters and drivers are requested to take special care and report at once if a container is broken or leaks.

Prevention of Virus A infection

The spread of virus A is prevented by scrupulous attention to personal hygiene, by the provision of adequate sanitation, and by the destruction of flies.

SMALLPOX

Other name: variola

This is an acute, frequently severe and always very infectious disease with a characteristic rash which affects people of all ages, even the fetus of an infected mother. It is caused by a virus, which is spread by droplet infection from the skin lesions and from dust and clothing. The virus appears to vary in intensity and there is great variety in the severity of epidemics. One attack appears to confer immunity. Vaccination, performed successfully and repeated at the right intervals, confers immunity. Incubation period: 10-14 days, but can be shorter or longer.

Clinical features

Onset: sudden, with fever up to 39·5-40°C (103°-104°F) shivering, vomiting, frontal headache, pain in back, sore throat, cough, prostration; fits in children.

Rash: various rashes — erythematous, petechial, haemorrhagic, urticarial — may appear on the 2nd day, usually on the lower abdomen and inner surfaces of the thighs — and then fade.

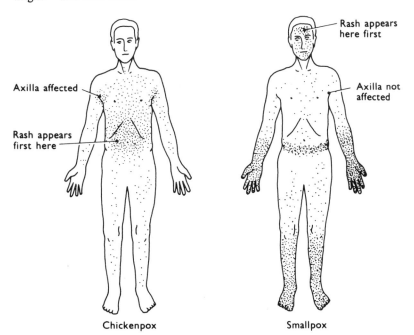

Axilla affected

Rash appears first here

Rash appears here first

Axilla not affected

Chickenpox

Smallpox

Fig. 5. Distribution of the rash in chickenpox and smallpox.

Infections

The characteristic rash appears on the 3rd day. It begins on the face and spreads rapidly over the neck, arms, trunk and legs. It is worse on the face, hands and feet than on the trunk, the arms and legs. It begins as reddish-brown papules, which turn to vesicles (6th day); the vesicles turn to pustules (8th day); the pustules turn to scabs. Only one kind of lesion is present at one time. When the scab falls off a scar may be left (hence the term a 'pock-marked' face). The vesicles are 'umbilicated' (depressed at the centre). On the mucous membranes ulcers may form at the same time as the rash on the skin. Scabs on the scalp take a long time to drop off.

The rash can be distinguished from that of chickenpox by:
1. The distribution on the skin; in chickenpox it is worse on the trunk than on the limbs, and worse on the arms and legs than on the hands and feet.
2. In chickenpox, papules, vesicles and pustules and scabs can all be present at the same time.
3. In chickenpox the vesicles do not become umbilicated.

Course: The temperature, after remaining high for 3-4 days, falls, but there may be a secondary rise at the time the pustules are forming. The cervical lymph-nodes, the liver and the spleen can become enlarged. In severe attacks there is prostration, severe toxaemia, delirium, and death. Respiratory complications are serious. The mortality is greatest in young children and the old.

Special tests
1. Electron microscope studies of cells.
2. Culture in eggs.

Varieties
1. *Modified smallpox:* slight fever and a mild rash can occur in people who have a partial immunity.
2. *Variola minor:* a similarly mild disease due to a weakened virus.
3. *Haemorrhagic smallpox:* a very serious kind with haemorrhages into the skin and from the mucous membranes.

Complications
Conjunctivitis, corneal ulcers.
Laryngitis, bronchitis, bronchopneumonia, myocarditis.
Boils, abscesses, erysipelas, impetigo.
Encephalo-myelitis, hemiplegia, polyneuritis.
Diarrhoea, and acute otitis media in children.

Prevention
Vaccination. Vaccination is carried out with glycerinated calf lymph, which contains the virus of vaccinia (a disease of cows), a virus which is believed to be a weakened form of the virus of smallpox. By developing an attack of vaccinia a person develops an immunity to smallpox.

Vaccination is recommended for people likely to come into contact with smallpox or living in or travelling to countries where it occurs. Vaccination is carried out by (a) cleaning an area of skin with soap and water — not with antiseptics, which can inactivate the virus, (b) squeezing lymph on to the skin from the capsule container; (c) using either a multiple-pressure technique with the point of a needle by pressing 15-30 times on to the skin without drawing blood, or making a scratch 0.5 cm long through the lymph. A papule appears on the 3rd day, turns to a vesicle on the 5th-6th day, and to a pustule about 8th day; a scab is then formed and drops off about 3 weeks later. The patient may feel slight malaise and develop adenitis of the lymph-nodes draining the vaccinated area. Immunity to smallpox develops about 9 days after vaccination.

Contra-indications to routine vaccination include infantile dermatitis, exposure to infectious disease, fits, any intercurrent illness, treatment by cortico-steroids.

Complications of vaccination are (a) local sepsis, which can be prevented by keeping the vaccination part dry and clean; (b) generalized vaccinia (rare), with lesions all over the body and an acute infection; (c) encephalitis (rare) usually only in people who have not been vaccinated in infancy and early childhood.

Methisazone (Marboran) is an anti-viral drug; it appears to be effective in preventing smallpox, but how it acts, is not known. It is given to unvaccinated people who have been exposed to smallpox and for whom there is no time for vaccination to act. An initial dose of 200 mg per kilo of body-weight is followed by 8 doses of 50 mg per kilo at 6-hourly intervals. An anti-emetic drug should be given at the same time. Methisazone is of no use in the treatment of smallpox.

Treatment

Anti-viral drugs (cytarabine, vidarabine) are given. The patient must be isolated for at least 14 days in an isolation hospital. The patient should be regarded as infectious so long as there are any scabs or unhealed lesion of the skin. His room and clothing must be disinfected by the local Health Authority. He is nursed in bed. Any person attending him must have been vaccinated. He requires full nursing care, with particular attention to the skin, mouth, eyes and nose. Warm alkaline lotions may be applied to the skin to allay irritation or potassium permanganate 1: 4,000 to prevent infection. Dehydration is treated with fluids given intravenously, sub-cutaneously or rectally. Penicillin or a sulpha drug is given for secondary infections. Prolonged convalescence is necessary.

ACUTE
POLIOMYELITIS [1]

Other name: infantile paralysis

This is an acute infectious disease caused by a virus, which acts on the anterior horn cells of the spinal cord and similar cells in the bulbar part of the brain. An acute inflammation is produced which can cause degeneration and death of these nerve-cells and their fibres.

Acute poliomyelitis occurs both sporadically and epidemically among people who have not been rendered immune by vaccination or by having had a previous mild 'abortive' attack of the disease. It is a disease of children and young adults; pregnant women are particularly liable. Epidemics (for no clear reason) usually occur at the end of a hot summer.

The virus is thought to enter the nervous system via the blood. It is spread by direct contact, by faeces, by infected water and food, and by flies and cockroaches. It is present in the faeces of a patient during an attack and for several weeks after-wards. One attack renders the patient immune for life; many adults are immune probably because of having had an abortive attack in childhood. Tonsillectomy and

[1] *poliomyelitis:* Greek: *polio* – grey; *muetos* – marrow.

Infections

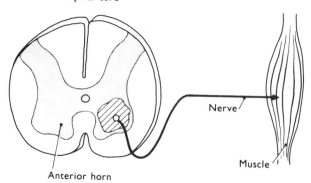

Transverse section of spinal cord

Nerve

Muscle

Anterior horn

Fig. 6. Acute poliomyelitis affects the anterior horn of grey matter in the spinal cord and by destroying the cells of the motor nerves produces a 'lower motor neurone lesion' with paralysis, muscle-wasting and loss of tendon reflexes.

inoculations are precipitating factors. Severe exercise taken at the beginning of an attack can produce extensive paralysis.

Incubation period: usually 7-12 days; can be shorter or longer.

Clinical features

Onset (pre-paralytic stage): sudden, with fever (up to 40°C-104°F); malaise, listlessness; sore throat; vomiting; stiffness and pain in back; headache; tremors; hypersensitivity to touch; agitation and apprehension.

Abortive attacks — with pyrexia, malaise, sore throat and headache lasting for up to 48 hours — occur and are recognizable only by the development of the full illness in a member of the family.

Paralytic stage: begins within 2-3 days of onset of illness. Patient finds that some part of him is paralysed. The paralysis varies from slight weakness of a muscle to complete paralysis of one or more limbs. The legs, arms, back, chest, face, intercostal muscles and diaphragm are affected most commonly in that order. The paralysis, at its worst from the beginning, is due to the damage to the cells of the motor-nerves and is therefore of the lower motor neurone type with flaccidity, loss of tendon reflexes and subsequent wasting of the muscles.

In the *bulbar form* of the disease, paralysis of the respiratory centre may occur, causing death from respiratory paralysis if the patient is not promptly treated with a respirator. Paralysis of other centres can produce paralysis of the pharynx (with difficulty in swallowing), of the larynx (with difficulty in speaking), of the eye muscles and the facial muscles.

Course: the fever subsides with the onset of paralysis. The patient may (a) die, (b) recover completely or (c) be left with some degree of paralysis and wasting; recovery of function may go on for several weeks and it is not until 2-4 months have passed that any further improvement can be discounted.

Complications

During acute stage: acute retention of urine, oedema of lungs, bronchopneumonia.

Subsequently: muscle wasting; contractures; deformities; poor circulation through affected part, diminution or cessation of growth in affected part; renal calculi.

Prevention   *Immunization:* in childhood or early adult life with an oral vaccine of live attenuated strain of poliomyelitis vaccine (Sabin type). Dose: 3 doses of 3 drops each at intervals of 4-8 weeks. It is safe to immunize during an epidemic and at any season of the year. No other immunizing procedure should be performed within 3 weeks. Any 'cold' surgery should be postponed during the course. The vaccine should not be given if the person has diarrhoea or is in poor health.

Measures during an epidemic: any child or young adult who feels ill or runs a temperature should be isolated in bed. No violent exercise should be taken or strenuous games played. Children's parties and unnecessary travelling and visiting are cancelled. Dental extractions and ear, nose and throat operations are if possible postponed.

Treatment   The patient is isolated as soon as the disease is suspected and put to bed with complete rest. Full precautions against the spread of infection are taken. Nurses attending him wear gown and mask. Discharges from nose and throat are burnt, faeces and urine disinfected before being disposed of.

If paralysis develops, any paralysed muscle is put in the best position to relieve it of any stretching or weight-bearing. If, for example, the deltoid is paralysed, the arm is kept abducted to a right-angle by a sandbag.

If the respiratory muscles are paralysed, artificial respiration must be begun at once. A mechanical respirator will be required; but if the pharyngeal muscles are also paralysed, artificial respiration can cause the secretions of the pharynx to be sucked into the lungs, and for this paralysis a tracheostomy must be performed, sucking and intermittent positive-pressure respiration carried out.

Physiotherapy of the appropriate kind is undertaken by the physiotherapist at the direction of the physician and orthopaedic surgeon. Subsequent care includes: physiotherapy; occupational therapy; orthopaedic operations; the provision of any necessary surgical shoe, walking aid or wheel-chair; and the re-training of an adult to new work if he cannot carry out his old.

EPIDEMIC
ENCEPHALITIS

Other names: encephalitis lethargica

This acute infectious disease is probably due to a virus. The description 'epidemic' is unfortunate as, after a pandemic in 1916-26, the disease has tended to occur sporadically and there are other forms of encephalitis that occur in epidemic form. The infecting organism produces an acute inflammation and degeneration of the central nervous system, especially of the basal ganglia and medulla oblongata and to a lesser extent of the cerebral cortex. Incubation period: uncertain, probably up to 21 days.

Clinical features   It occurs in many forms, of varying degrees of severity, and mimics other diseases of the nervous system.

Onset: sudden or gradual. Fever may be high, slight or absent. Evidence of cerebral involvement is seen in : (a) sleepiness, (b) excitement, acute mania, delirium, (c) paralysis of a cranial nerve, usually one to the muscles of the eye with the production of a squint or ptosis.

Course: very variable. In fulminating cases death can occur within a few hours. Mental disturbances, irritability, headache, dizziness and insomnia may persist for years. A *post encephalitic state* is likely to develop in 3 out of 4 cases who recover from the acute state. Parkinsonism (due to degeneration of the basal ganglia) develops: these patients show signs of paralysis agitans, rigidity, tremor, stoop, small steps, mask-like face; but excessive sweating and production of saliva are common. Some patients have occulo-gyric crises in which the eyeballs are skewed into one direction or another and fixed there for long periods. Sleep-rhythm is sometimes inverted, the patient sleeping by day and being awake at night. Various tics and muscular spasms of many kinds can occur. Mental deterioration and personality changes for the worse can occur.

Treatment   There is no specific treatment. During the acute stage the patient has to be isolated and given full nursing care. Sedation may be required to check excitement. Parkinsonism is treated like paralysis agitans. Patients with antisocial conduct present serious problems. Tranquillisers may be needed, with heavier sedation from time to time; some patients have to be looked after indefinitely in a psychiatric hospital.

EPIDEMIC MYALGIA

Other names: Bornholm[2] disease, epidemic pleurodynia[3]
This acute infection, in which the characteristic feature is pain in the region of the attachment of the diaphragm, is due to viruses of the Coxsackie group and is liable to occur in small epidemics. Other muscles can be affected.

Clinical features   The onset is acute, the pain very severe, the patient acutely distressed and often thought to be suffering an acute thoracic or abdominal emergency, such as a perforated ulcer. Fever fluctuates from 38°-40°C (101-104°F), and there is malaise, headache, sore throat, nausea, vomiting, and tenderness of the affected areas. An attack lasts usually 2-4 days, but it can last up to 3 weeks. Recovery is the rule, but relapses can occur.

Complications   Orchitis. Pleurisy. Aseptic meningitis. Pericarditis.

Treatment   Rest in bed; analgesics and antipyretics such as acetyl-salicyclic acid (aspirin).

BENIGN LYMPHOCYTIC MENINGITIS

This is a mild meningitis with fever, headache and a stiff neck due to Coxsackie and ECHO virus group. Small epidemics occur among families. The CSF shows an increase in lympocytes. It has to be distinguished from other kinds of meningitis. No special treatment is indicated.

ECHO VIRUSES [4]

The ECHO viruses are a group of viruses found in the throat and faeces; they can cause upper respiratory tract infections and gastro-intestinal upsets. Incubation period: 7-10 days.

Clinical features   Some ECHO viruses are associated with mild common-cold or influenza-like illnesses in some patients and with attacks of nausea, vomiting, diarrhoea and abdominal discomfort in others. The illness is usually mild and clears up in a few days.

Complication   Encephalitis.

Treatment   There is no specific treatment.

EPIDEMIC VOMITING

This is a common virus infection, often affecting several members of a family about the same time. The onset is sudden with nausea, vomiting, slight fever and sometimes diarrhoea. It clears up in two days. It has to be distinguished from other illnesses starting with nausea and vomiting; the mildness of the illness and the family incidence are the clues to the diagnosis. Bed for a couple of days is all the necessary treatment.

[2] *Bornholm:* Danish island where first recorded epidemic took place
[3] *pleurodynia:* from Greek: *pleura* – rib, *odune* – pain; pain in the chest
[4] *ECHO:* abbreviation for **E**nteric (bowel), **C**ytopathogenic (harmful to cells), **H**uman **O**rphan (originally and erroneously thought not to have a human host).

EPIDEMIC POLYARTHRITIS	Epidemics of this have occurred in Australia and elsewhere. It is thought to be due to a new virus. The disease is a mild one, with pain in the joints of the hands and feet, slight pyrexia and a rash. No special treatment is required.
ADENO-VIRUS INFECTION	This is a virus infection of the upper respiratory tract, with symptoms varying from those of the common cold to a severer infection with fever, sore throat and sometimes lymph-node enlargement, pneumonic consolidation and conjunctivitis. It lasts about 10 days. No special treatment is indicated.
CAT-SCRATCH FEVER	This is an infection produced by the scratch of a cat, the cat itself being apparently healthy. It is probably due to virus, but the actual organism has not been identified. The family pet may produce a household epidemic. Incubation period: a few days.
Clinical features	A papule or ulcer appears at the site of the scratch; 1-3 weeks later there is slight fever and the local lymph-nodes enlarge and may suppurate. The length of the illness is very variable – extremes of 2 weeks and 2 years have been described. The lymph-nodes are likely to remain enlarged long after the fever has subsided.
Treatment	Tetracycline 250 mg 6-hourly is given for 5 days in the hope of preventing suppuration in the nodes.
PSITTACOSIS [5]	*other name:* ornithosis[6] This infection of birds (occurring in pigeons, canaries etc.) and cats can be transmitted from bird to man or from man to man by droplet infection. The cause is a virus-like organism. Incubation period: 7-15 days.
Clinical features	In man an atypical pneumonia occurs. The condition, which should be considered a possibility whenever chest symptoms develop in a bird-fancier, differs from ordinary pneumonia in several ways: the respiratory rate and pulse-rate may not be raised, the X-ray shows a patchy consolidation, the white cell count may not be raised. Headache, giddiness and confusion can occur. The condition may be mistaken for typhoid fever. Death sometimes occurs.
Treatment	Treatment is by penicillin or tetracycline. The patient should be barrier-nursed.
STREPTOCOCCAL INFECTIONS	Streptococci commonly infect man causing a number of diseases. Some streptococci live normally in the upper respiratory tract and cause disease only if they get into other tissues, producing for instance bacterial endocarditis and some cases of sinusitis. Some streptococci are called haemolytic[7] streptococci because when they are grown on blood-containing agar they dissolve the blood around them. The diseases caused by streptococci are:

(a)   acute pharyngitis and tonsillitis
(b)   quinsy
(c)   scarlet fever
(d)   erysipelas
(e)   streptococcal pneumonia

[5] *psittacosis:* from Greek *psittakos* – parrot
[6] *ornithosis:* from Greek *ornis* – bird
[7] *haemolytic:* from Greek, *haima* – blood; *lysis* – dissolving

27

(f)   streptococcal puerperal fever

(g)   rheumatic fever.

There is considerable variation in the actions of these streptococci; any one of them can in different people cause any one of these diseases and any one of these diseases can be caused by a haemolytic streptococcus. The degree of illness varies from the very mild to the very severe.

Infection is common in children, among whom carriers abound.

Reaction to infection varies very much with (a) the age of the person infected and (b) the particular type of streptococcus.

Spread is by droplet infection. Incubation period: 2-4 days.

Treatment of any Streptococcal Infection

Whatever the disease produced, the treatment is basically the same.

1. Bed; isolation, liquid or light diet.

Acetylsalicyclic acid (aspirin): 300-900 mg 3-4 hourly to relieve sore throat.

2. Penicillin.

3. Suppurating lymph-nodes are incised.

Acute Pharyngitis and Tonsillitis in children under 4

Onset sudden, with slight fever, malaise, sore throat, a running nose and swollen anterior cervical lymph-nodes. Suppurative complications are particularly likely to occur: sinusitis, acute otitis media, mastoiditis, suppurating cervical nodes, impetigo.

In older children and adults

Onset sudden, with high fever, sore throat, tonsillitis and pharyngitis; the tonsils become enlarged and covered with a creamy exudate; if tonsils have been removed the tonsillar bed is injected. Suppurative conditions are not so likely to develop as are certain other conditions: rheumatic fever, nephritis, mesenteric adenitis[8].

The rash of a streptococcal infection may occur, and when this happens the disease is called scarlet fever.

Quinsy [9]

Other name: peritonsillar abscess

This is an abscess in the tonsillar bed, behind the tonsil, and is often the result of haemolytic streptococcal infection. After an acute tonsillitis and pharyngitis, there

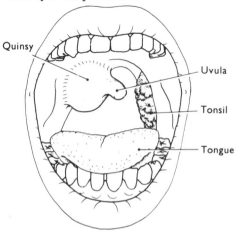

Fig. 7. Quinsy.

[8] *mesenteric adenitis:* enlargement of the lymph-nodes in the mesentery of the abdomen

[9] *quinsy* from Latin: *quinancia,* from Greek: *kynanche* – dog-throttling

28

Chapter 2

is a rise in temperature and malaise and an increase in pain in the throat and swallowing becomes difficult or impossible. There is a swelling at the side of the neck, and the tonsil is pushed forward by the abscess behind it. The abscess has to be opened and tonsillectomy performed later or a quinsy-tonsillectomy performed.

Scarlet fever

Scarlet fever is a haemolytic streptococcal infection in which a rash appears. Why a rash should appear in some cases and not in others is obscure.

The patient has the usual malaise, sore throat and pyrexia. The *rash* is a punctate erythema — tiny red spots on a pink flush. It appears on 1st-2nd day on the chest and quickly spreads over face, trunk, and limbs. On the face there is erythema only; the part round the lips is not usually affected, producing a circum-oral pallor [1]. The rash lasts a few days before fading. Where it has been worst (e.g. in the flexure of the elbow and on the abdomen) a slight pigmentation may persist.

The tongue is usually coated and shows prominent red papillae.

The disease follows the usual course of a streptococcal infection and has the usual complications. It was formerly a very serious disease with serious complications; it is now a mild disease, probably as a result of some change in the infecting organism.

Erysipelas [2]

This is an acute haemolytic streptococcal infection. Patients with erysipelas commonly have the streptococci in their nasopharynx and probably infect themselves through tiny abrasions in the skin. Wounds and surgical incisions can become infected in this way or from the infected nasopharynx of a doctor or nurse. The disease is most common in the middle-aged and elderly. Treatment with penicillin has reduced the mortality enormously, but it can be a serious and sometimes fatal disease in infants, in chronic alcoholics, and in the very old. Recurrences are common. Incubation period: 2-7 days.

Clinical features

1. *Onset:* sudden, with fever, a rigor, headache and vomiting.
2. *Skin:* becomes reddened and oedematous. The inflamed area spreads rapidly, with a characteristically definite and sometimes raised edge. Vesicles form on the reddened area. The face is a common site; if the eyelids are involved they become very swollen. On trunk and limbs, erysipelas can advance very rapidly.
3. *Toxaemia:* varies with severity and site of infection, and with the age of the patient. Recovery within a few days is now usual.

Complications

Local abscesses (in 5-10 per cent of patients).
Glomerulo-nephritis (uncommon). Rheumatic fever (rare).

Streptoccal pneumonia

Streptococci cause pneumonia only rarely, usually as a complication of influenza.

Streptococcal puerperal fever

Streptococci are responsible for about 40 per cent of all cases of puerperal fever (a fever occurring after childbirth). The site from which the placenta has become

[1] *circum-oral:* around the mouth
[2] *erysipelas* – probably from Greek, *erythros* – red; *pella* – skin

detached is the usual site of entry, but it can be through a wound. Infection may be by droplet infection from the infected throat of a doctor, nurse or visitor, or from an infected instrument, and is common after prolonged labour and instrumental delivery. Infection produces an endometritis (infection of the endometrium of the uterus), thrombo-phlebitis and general septicaemia and pyaemia. A rash similar to that of scarlet fever may appear. The treatment is that of a very acute and dangerous infection by large doses of penicillin. The patient's sensitivity to penicillin should be tested first.

Rheumatic fever

Other name: acute rheumatism

This acute infection — with fever, arthritis and heart disease — follows and is associated with infection by a haemolytic streptococcus. Its precise nature and cause are obscure: it has been thought to be an auto-immune disease (see Chapter 10). The usual history is one of sore throat or an attack of tonsillitis followed about 3 weeks later by rheumatic fever. It is rare in young children, being a disease of older children, adolescents and young adults. One attack does not confer immunity and is frequently followed by others.

Clinical features

The onset is sudden, with malaise, chill, stiffness and pain in the joints. The course is then one of fever, sweating, arthritis, anaemia and involvement of the heart.

Arthritis develops quickly, involving many of the medium-sized joints, which become inflamed, painful, swollen, red at first and then dead-white. Typically the arthritis flits from joint to joint — affecting one and then subsiding in it as it affects another.

Fever: can rise to 39.5°C (103°F), is irregular, falling as the arthritis subsides and rising if it recurs. Severe pyrexia — up to 41.5°C (107°F) can occur and is of serious import, provoking delirium, coma and sometimes death. Rigors do not occur.

Anaemia: severe. There is an increase in white cells (up to 30,0000 per mm^3).

Heart: usually affected. Endocarditis, myocarditis and pericarditis occur, being involved in a mild inflammation of the whole organ. Areas of degeneration appear in the myocardium. The valves are inflamed and swollen; when the inflammation settles down they may become fibrosed, stiff and mis-shapen with vegetations forming on them; rheumatic fever is therefore one of the causes of chronic valvular disease of the heart. A pericardial effusion can occur. Evidence of carditis is seen in an increased pulse rate, abnormal heart sounds and enlargement of the heart.

Rheumatic nodules sometimes appear; they are small white nodules in the skin, usually around a joint.

Complications

Pleurisy

Petechial haemorrhages, purpura

Erythema multiforme

Chorea

MENINGOCOCCAL MENINGITIS

Other names: cerebrospinal meningitis

It is an acute specific fever caused by infection by the meningococcus. Children and young adults are usually affected. Individual cases occur or small epidemics where there is over-crowding, cold and fatigue, as in refugee or military camps. The organism enters the body through the upper part of the naso-pharynx. The organism can persist in the naso-pharynx, turning the host into a carrier. Infection is airborne by direct or close contact, or can be spread by handkerchiefs.

From the naso-pharynx the organism invades the bloodstream to be distributed throughout the body. It affects in particular the meninges, causing an acute purulent meningitis. In chronic cases fibrosis of the meninges occurs, and blocking of the foramina of Luschka and Magendie can cause hydrocephalus. Sinusitis, arthritis, broncho-pneumonia and purpura can also occur during the acute phase.

Incubation period: 1-3 days.

Clinical features

1. *Onset:* sudden, with nasal infection, headache, fever, rigor, convulsions, pains in the neck and limbs, nausea and vomiting.
2. *Signs of meningitis* (2nd-4th day): headache, vomiting, dizziness, rigidity of neck, restlessness, photophobia, confusion, delirium, unconsciousness. The pupils may be dilated and sluggish; Kernig's sign[3] may be present; the tendon reflexes may be brisk or diminished. Cranial nerves may be paralysed.
3. *Signs of generalized infection:* irregular pyrexia, purpura or a petechial rash; arthritis; herpes on the lips; loss of weight.
4. *Signs of meningeal fibrosis:* cranial nerve paralysis, deafness, blindness, hydrocephalus.

Death may be due to encephalitis or to a massive haemorrhage into an adrenal gland. A chronic meningococcal septicaemia may persist for weeks.

Special tests

Cerebrospinal fluid: under increased pressure; turbid or purulent; meningococci may be present inside or outside cells; very large increase in number of polymorphs; protein content increased; chloride and sugar content decreased.

Blood: polymorph increase up to 40,000 per mm^3; culture may reveal meningococci.

Treatment

Strict isolation is essential at first, but can be relaxed after 24 hours treatment. Nurses should at first wear masks.

Full nursing care is necessary; the patient should be nursed on a ripple-bed or other precautions are taken to prevent bedsores.

Treatment is by penicillin. Ampicillin is sometimes given, but is no more effective than penicillin.

TUBERCULOSIS

This is an infection caused by the *Mycobacterium tuberculosis* (commonly called the tuberculosis bacillus) and is so-called because of the little 'tubercles' or lumps that it causes. The two types of the organism that affect man are: (1) the human type and (2) the bovine type.

The *human type* causes tuberculosis in man, monkeys, pigs and sometimes dogs

[3] *Kernig's sign:* resistance or pain produced by attempting to extend the leg completely at the knee with the thigh flexed to a right angle

Infections

and parrots. It is the cause of pulmonary tuberculosis, which in Britain and other countries from which bovine tuberculosis has been eradicated is the only common type of tuberculosis. Infection is by droplet infection or indirectly by infected dust. The organism is killed by sunlight or by ordinary washing processes, but it can persist for months on clothes, bedclothes and carpets, surviving best in dank dark places.

The *bovine type* occurs in man, cattle, horses and pigs. It is the usual cause of abdominal tuberculosis and tuberculous adenitis, and a common cause of bone and genito-urinary infection. It is spread by drinking infected untreated milk from infected cows and has ceased to exist in countries where tuberculosis in cows has been eliminated.

Tuberculosis occurs most where there are poverty, malnutrition and over-crowding; it is common in backward countries and becomes less common as standards of living improve. It is estimated that 3 million people die of tuberculosis in the world every year. In advanced communities the incidence of the disease and the death-rate from it have fallen sharply as a result of:

(a)   better social conditions and housing,
(b)   better food,
(c)   the eradication of bovine tuberculosis,
(d)   the discovery of early and symptom-free cases by mass-radiography,
(e)   immunization by BCG vaccine,
(f)   treatment by streptomycin, para-amino-salicyclic acid, isoniazid etc.

Mass-radiography findings show, however, that there are in Britain today several thousand unrecognized cases of pulmonary tuberculosis, many of them infectious. In Britain tuberculosis is becoming increasingly a disease of older people, nearly half the patients notified being over the age of 60. In England 1375 people died of tuberculosis in 1972.

Infants are born with little or no resistance to the disease, developing it within a few months. The highest incidence of the disease usually occurs in adolescence and early adult life, but in some areas pulmonary tuberculosis is now more common in middle-aged and old people than in the young. In urban communities many people, exposed to repeated infection, developed infection in one lung, a mild infection that might not produce any symptoms, was likely to heal, and would in this way promote resistance to the disease, preventing it from developing unless the person happened to be in poor health or was exposed to a massive, overwhelming infection. With a reduction of the number of cases, this early infection is not now so common. In primitive communities tuberculosis is likely to spread in epidemic form as an acute illness with a high mortality and with the development in the survivors of a chronic form of the illness; in impoverished countries and the tropics the infection affects millions of young people in an active form.

Having invaded the body the tubercle bacilli settle in one or more places and multiply. In these places the blood-vessels become congested, fluid is exuded, leucocytes accumulate. A *tubercle* forms. The tubercle may: (a) heal; fibrous tissue replaces the other cells and eventually after years the tubercle becomes calcified, or (b) break down, with *caseation* (Latin: *caseus* – cheese), a soft mixture of dead cells, degenerating cells and tubercle bacilli. Tubercles and caseated areas fuse together, with the development of further degeneration and abscesses; tuberculous abscesses are called cold abscesses, because the inflammation being slow there is little sensation of heat. In the typical chronic tuberculous lesion there is a mixture of reaction — new tubercles being formed, older areas caseating, abscesses forming, and fibrous tissue invading or encircling the whole in an attempt to heal it.

The tubercle bacilli spread from their original focus to local lymph-nodes, in which the same inflammatory processes take place. Bacilli, getting from any infected area into the blood-stream, can be spread throughout the body, causing *miliary tuberculosis* or can invade particular tissues, especially other lymph-nodes, the meninges, the brain, kidneys, peritoneum, joints, epididymis and uterine tubes.

Pulmonary tuberculosis
Primary tuberculosis

A *Ghon focus,* the primary infection of a lung, is a small tuberculous lesion in any part of the lung. A *primary complex* is the combination of Ghon's focus with the associated infected lymph-nodes, both conditions being visible on X-ray. This infection often takes place without causing any general signs of infection; most people do not know they have been infected; and eventually the lesion heals and slowly calcifies. With infection the person's Mantoux reaction changes from negative to positive. However, if the person's resistance is low or he has been massively infected, the lesion may not heal and becomes larger and caseated. Then various complications can develop:
1. Abscess formation.
2. Pleurisy and pleural effusion.
3. A *hilar flare,* due to compression of a bronchus by an enlarged lymph-node and with the collapse of a segment of a lung the production of a *middle lobe syndrome* and bronchiectasis; it is found on X-ray examination.
4. Tuberculous bronchopneumonia.
5. Miliary tuberculosis.

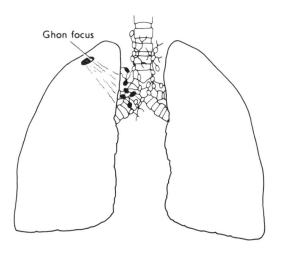

Ghon focus

Fig. 8. Primary complex in tuberculosis of lung, showing a Ghon focus and involvement of lymph nodes.

Infections

Clinical features	Symptoms and signs are often at first slight; general signs of illness usually precede those of signs attributable to the lungs.
General symptoms and signs	Slight recurrent febrile attacks Malaise, fatigue, listlessness, nervousness Loss of appetite, indigestion, loss of weight. Sweating. Anaemia. Amenorrhoea.
Symptoms and signs of chest disease	Cough, expectoration Haemoptysis: varies from slight streaking of the sputum to a massive and sometimes fatal haemorrhage. Pain in chest (due to pleurisy) Hoarseness (due to congestion or tuberculous ulceration of the larynx).

On examination of the chest in the early days nothing abnormal is usually found. With extension of the disease, the affected lung is seen not to expand so well; areas of consolidation are found on percussion and auscultation, and abnormal sounds accompany the breath-sounds. The signs vary with the extent of the disease, the degree of consolidation, the presence of cavities, of fibrosis, or pleurisy and pleural effusion.

Post-primary tuberculosis

This is any re-infection following a primary infection. Tuberculosis is likely to spread in the lungs by direct spread, by lymphatic invasion or by aspiration via the bronchi into other parts of the lung or into the other lung. The same pathological processes take place — the formation of tubercles, their merging, caseation, cavity and abscess formation, and fibrous reaction. So a chronic pulmonary tuberculosis develops. The symptoms will be an intermittent fever, usually higher at night than in the morning, malaise, toxaemia, loss of appetite, cough, expectoration, loss of weight. Toxaemia will be worst with caseating lesions. An extensive fibrosis throws great strain on the right side of the heart, which may show evidence of failure. Tubercle bacilli are present in the sputum either intermittently or all the time. Patients are likely to be in a state of chronic ill-health, with symptoms varying with the degree of deterioration or of improvement. If the infection is unchecked by treatment, death is likely. Most deaths occur in older age-groups.

Complications

Pleurisy, pleural effusion, empyema, haemoptysis, pneumothorax.
Tuberculosis of trachea, larynx; tuberculous ulcers on tongue.
Gastritis, ileitis, fistula-in-ano (from swallowed sputum).

Tuberculous pneumonia

Tuberculous broncho-pneumonia is more common than tuberculous lobar pneumonia. The patient runs a high temperature, coughs and expectorates; patchy broncho-pneumonic consolidation occurs in both lungs and cavities can form. The outlook is poor. Sometimes the consolidation is limited to the lobe of one lung. The clinical picture is very much the same — with pyrexia, cough, haemoptysis sometimes, drenching sweats and severe weight loss; if not adequately treated the patient is likely to die within three months. The consolidation in the lungs in both conditions is visible on X-ray examination and tubercle bacilli are likely to be found in the sputum.

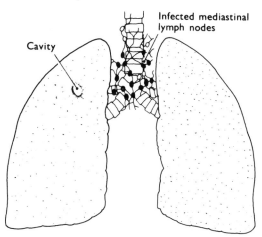

Fig. 9. Miliary tuberculosis (with snow-storm effect on X-ray) following infection of right lung and lymph-nodes in the mediastinum.

Disseminated (miliary) tuberculosis

This is the result of the spread throughout the body of tubercle bacilli via the blood-stream. Tubercles form in many organs and tissues, particularly the lungs and the meninges. The patient is seriously ill with high fever, toxaemia, loss of weight, malaise, profuse sweating and loss of energy. Tuberculous meningitis is common. X-ray of the lungs shows a mottling throughout due to the presence of hundreds of tubercles. Tubercles can be seen in the retina with an ophthalmoscope. The liver and spleen are enlarged. Cyanosis is an indication of greatly impaired respiratory function.

Primary abdominal tuberculosis

This is the result of drinking infected milk. Tubercles are formed in the intestinal tract, peritoneum and abdominal lymph-nodes. Ulceration of the intestine can occur. The infected lymph-nodes matt together and can suppurate, or they heal and calcify. Tuberculous peritonitis can occur. The patient is usually a child. He develops a vague illness, feels unwell, has slight fever, abdominal discomfort or pain, and may waste. The enlarged nodes may be palpable as masses within the abdomen.

Tubercular cervical adenitis

This is caused by bovine tuberculosis. Infection spreads from the pharynx via the lymphatics. The lymph-nodes enlarge and can become attached to the skin (which becomes inflamed and can break down) or they heal, fibrose and calcify. From the infected nodes tubercle bacilli can spread to other parts of the body.

Other causes of enlarged lymph-nodes in the neck are:
tonsillitis
infective mononucleosis, syphilis
Hodgkin's disease and other malignant disease.

Special tests

Sputum: in an 'open' case, tubercle bacilli are present in the sputum, but not in every specimen and one negative result does not indicate abscence of the disease. The bacilli are visible with special staining methods; sometimes it is necessary to inoculate a guinea-pig and examine it later for evidence of tuberculosis.

X-ray of lungs: reveals early lesions long before they can be discovered by ordinary clinical examination; shows presence of consolidation, cavities and fibrosis.

Blood:

(a) sedimentation rate (ESR) is raised; repeated ESRs are useful guide to progress, a fall indicating improvement.

(b) blood count: increased number of lymphocytes.

Tuberculin test: this is a test of the patient's sensitivity to tuberculin, a substance obtained from fluid in which tubercle bacilli have been grown (it does not contain the organisms). In the *Heaf Test* an automatic punch is used to puncture the skin through a film of tuberculin spread on it: a positive reaction is the appearance of an indurated patch in the skin at the site of puncture in 3-7 days. In the *Mantoux Test* an intradermal injection of tuberculin is given: a positive reaction is an indurated area in the skin surrounded by a patch of erythema in 3-4 days. A positive reaction to either of these tests is taken as an indication that the person has at some time had an attack of tuberculosis and developed immunity to it.

Prevention of tuberculosis

1. Better nutrition, better standards of living, better housing.

2. The provision of safe milk by the eradication of tuberculosis from cows and by the pasteurization of milk.

3. The early diagnosis of infection, especially of pulmonary tuberculosis by Mass Radiography.

4. Better ventilation in those industries in which chest diseases such as the pneumoconioses can occur.

5. The adequate treatment of all cases.

6. The tuberculin testing of children, nurses, doctors, other hospital staff, immigrants, and other people especially likely to develop tuberculosis such as sailors.

7. The immunization of people who do not show a positive reaction to a tuberculin test. This can be done by an injection of the Bacillus Calmette-Guérin vaccine (BCG). This is a strain of the tubercle bacillus whose virulence has been weakened by cultivation in adverse conditions. The dose is 0.1 ml given intradermally. A small wheal should be produced and a papule should then form and may ulcerate. Most tuberculin-negative people thus immunized become tuberculin-positive in about 6 weeks and this is taken to mean that resistance to tuberculosis has developed.

8. The use of drugs to prevent disease in positive tuberculin reactors or to prevent the activation of an apparently inactive tuberculosis. Isoniazid (in doses of up to 300 mg daily for 1 year for adults) is the drug usually used because it is effective, acceptable and cheap, and has few side-effects.

Treatment of pulmonary tuberculosis

1. The patient is put to bed and should stay there until his temperature remains normal. With treatment by modern drugs he should cease to be infectious within a few weeks; when this has been confirmed by micro-biological examination of his sputum, precautions against his spreading infection can be relaxed. Admission to hospital is advisable at first for it is essential that he takes rest and especially that he takes all the doses of prescribed drugs; outside hospital patients are very likely to default in taking them.

2. *Drug treatment* is started immediately. The usual method is a combination of:

(a) *streptomycin:* 500 mg-1 g daily by intramuscular injection. Toxic effects are nausea, fever and giddiness (which can become permanent) as a result of damage to the 8th cranial (acoustic-vestibular) nerve.

(b)   *isoniazid:* 300-600 mg daily. Toxic effects are rare with these doses.

(c)   *para-aminosalicyclic acid* (PAS): 10-15 g daily. Toxic effects are usually vomiting and diarrhoea.

(d)   *ethambutol:* 25 mg/kg daily for 2 months, followed by 15 mg/kg; given to patients unable to take PAS.

(e)   *thiacetazone:* 150 mg with 300 mg of isoniazid daily.

(f)   *rifampicin:* 10-20 mg/kg, up to a maximum of 600 mg daily.

None of these drugs is given alone, for the organism may be resistant to it or is likely, if it were given alone, to develop resistance. Intensive treatment is given for 3-6 months and less intensive treatment subsequently for 18-24 months.

Difficulties can arise. An ambulant patient may not turn up for his daily injection of streptomycin and he may give up taking drugs by mouth, particularly PAS which is bulky and unpalatable.

To get over these difficulties (which are particularly great in under-developed countries) other methods of treatment have been devised or other drugs used. These include:

(a)   A combination of streptomycin 1 g daily intramuscularly with isoniazid 300 mg and thiacetazone 150 mg for one month and then the latter two drugs without streptomycin. Toxic effects of thiacetazone are nausea, vomiting, jaundice, exfoliative dermatitis; in some parts of the world the organisms are resistant to it.

(b)   A combination of streptomycin twice-weekly with a high dose of isoniazid (14 mg/kg body weight) twice weekly.

3. *Corticosteroids* may be given for very severe infections, in tubercular meningitis and when there is also tuberculosis of other organs, when there are pleural, pericardial or peritoneal effusions, when the patient is hyper-sensitive to the antituberculous drugs, and in some cases of primary pulmonary tuberculosis. It is essential that the patient is at the same time having a course of the other drugs, because without them there would be a danger of a massive spread of the infection due to a failure of normal defence-mechanisms produced by the corticosteroids.

4. The patient's general health is built up by rest at first and then by gradually increasing exercise, by an adequate food intake, especially of protein, vitamins and iron, and by encouragement. A change of occupation may be required.

5. Surgical removal of any localized lesion in the lung that refuses to heal may be necessary.

SARCOIDOSIS   This is a disease of unknown origin with a world-wide distribution. At various times is has been thought to be an infection of some kind (there are resemblances to the reactions produced by tuberculosis and leprosy), an allergic phenomenon, an auto-immune reaction, or to be due to poisoning by beryllium and other chemicals. It can affect many tissues – especially the lymph-nodes, lungs, bones, heart, liver, spleen, eyes, skin and parotid glands. The clinical features vary with the tissues or organ involved. When the lungs are affected, the patient is likely to be breathless and have a cough; x-ray may show enlarged mediastinal lymph-nodes or a condition resembling miliary tuberculosis. Lymph-nodes in other parts of the body can be enlarged. The parotid glands are sometimes enlarged. Disfiguring skin lesions occur. Involvement of the myocardium can cause irregularity of the heart and heart-block.

The disease can run an acute course, clearing up with or without treatment; or it can begin insidiously, be gradually progressive and not respond to treatment.

Treatment is by corticosteroids, but there is no specific treatment.

TYPHOID FEVER [4]

Other name: enteric fever (also applied to paratyphoid fever)

This is an acute infectious disease caused by *Salmonella typhi.* The organisms are excreted in the faeces during convalescence. Some patients become permanent faecal carriers, excreting the organism for years while themselves suffering no ill effects; urinary carriers are rare.

Infection is the result of ingesting something that has become faecally contaminated. It can occur by taking uncooked food, such as raw milk or salads; by infected meat-carving machines in shops; by shell-fish and watercress from contaminated water; by sewage contamination of water; by direct contact with a patient; laboratory workers have been contaminated by their cultures.

The organisms gain entry to the body via the wall of the small intestine, and having passed along the lymphatic vessels and gained admission into the bloodstream are dispersed throughout the body. They have a liking for lymphatic tissue, packing into and inflaming lymph-nodes, lymphatic tissue in the spleen and elsewhere, and Peyer's patches in the small intestine, which can become acutely inflamed and ulcerate and perforate into the peritoneal cavity. The organisms proliferate too in the bile, infecting the biliary tubes and gall-bladder.

One attack usually — not always — confers immunity. Incubation period: 10-12 days.

Clinical features

Typhoid fever is very variable: it can be a mild illness lasting 1-2 weeks; it can kill a patient within 10 days. Commonly it is — if untreated — a severe illness lasting for 4-6 weeks. Chloramphenicol, an antibiotic, is so successful in treating the disease that it does not often run its full course, although fatal complications can still occur. The description that follows is that of an untreated case.

Onset: usually gradual over several days; intermittent fever, going up and down but tending to be a little higher every day; headache; malaise; loss of appetite, sometimes nausea and vomiting; epistaxis often; slight cough; abdominal discomfort, distension and tenderness; constipation during first fortnight. The patient usually takes to his bed on the 2nd or 3rd day, but can be ambulant until a major complication develops.

Course: over the next 3-4 weeks the temperature swings, rising as high as 41°C (106°F) with sudden falls that chill the patient. Constipation is usually replaced during the 3rd week by diarrhoea, the frequent passing of watery green or grey stools. The abdominal distension and discomfort are worse. The enlarged spleen may be felt. The pulse-rate is often much slower than would be expected in so acute an illness.

[4] *typhoid:* from Greek: *tuphos* – stupor

The rash occurs during 2nd-3rd week. It usually consists of a few small crops of rose-pink spots on the trunk, sometimes on the back and shoulders, less commonly on the limbs; the spots vanish on pressure and fade and are gone within a few days.

The patient may pass into the 'typhoid state' of stupor or delirium with picking at the bedclothes. If he has not been taking adequate amounts of fluid, he is likely now to become dehydrated and wasted, with parotitis[5], sores on his lips and a dry filthy brown furred tongue. Bronchitis may occur. Albuminuria occurs and the organisms are to be found in the urine.

When the patient has been in this state for 3-4 weeks he starts to recover; his temperature falls slowly; abdominal discomfort declines; a clear consciousness returns. A *relapse* is a common phenomenon at this stage, with a slightly raised temperature, sometimes a rash, malaise; it subsides quickly. Convalescence is slow, and it may be several weeks before the patient has regained his normal vitality.

Complications	*Haemorrhage* from bleeding Peyer's patches: can be slight, severe, sometimes fatal; patient becomes pale, has increased pulse-rate, fall in blood-pressure, shortness of breath, fall in temperature; stools become bright red with a big haemorrhage, black and tarry with smaller haemorrhages from high up the intestine.

Perforation of Peyer's patch: very serious, frequently fatal; patient develops acute abdominal pain, rapid abdominal distension, localized abdominal tenderness; shock with rapid pulse and respiration; grey anxious facies.

Special tests	*Blood:* culture of organisms positive in 1st week. Widal reaction (serum from patient clumps the organisms) becomes positive during 2nd week; a negative reaction does not exclude the disease.

    Reduction in the number of white cells, with relative increase of lymphocytes.
Faeces: organisms found in faeces from the second week onwards.
Urine: organisms found in urine from 3rd week onwards.

Prevention	(a) *Public health measures:* provision of safe water supply; safe disposal of human excreta; education of public in hand-washing after defaecation and before preparing and eating food; detection of carriers and prevention of their having anything to do with the preparation and cooking of food; pasteurization of milk; sterilization of meat knives and machines in shops; extermination of flies.

(b)   *Immunization:* there is uncertainty about the best method to use. One method preferred is:

    (i) two injections of 0.5 ml typhoid vaccine subcutaneously, with an interval of over 4 weeks between injections (one dose alone however provides much immunity);
    (ii) a booster dose every 3 years to those exposed to infection.
Vaccines against paratyphoid fever are not very effective; and the TAB combination (typhoid, paratyphoid A and B) causes an unpleasant reaction.

Treatment	1. The patient is isolated.

2. Chloramphenicol(Alficetyn, Chloromycetin) is given at once. The dose for an

[5] *parotitis:* inflammation of the parotid gland

adult is 2-3 g daily by mouth in divided doses until the temperature has fallen to normal (usually on the 3rd day of treatment) and then in doses of 1-1.5 g daily in divided doses for 3-4 weeks. It is more effective if given with cortico-steroids for a few days, e.g. cortisone 200 mg daily for 4-5 days. If a relapse occurs a further course of chloramphenicol is given.

3. The patient requires full nursing care. He should be nursed at first on a ripple-bed and careful attention must be paid to pressure points. Dehydration is prevented by giving fluid in adequate amounts and if necessary by intravenous injection. He is given a diet of milk (2-3 pints daily), sieved broths, eggs, chocolate and other easily digested foods. Vitamin C is given in tablet or fruit juice. Constipation is treated with an enema. Pyrexia is controlled by tepid sponging.

4. Nurses must have been immunized against typhoid and paratyphoid fever. They should wear a gown when attending the patient and be careful to wash their hands after touching him or anything he has touched. His eating utensils are boiled. His excreta can be disposed of untreated into an ordinary sewage-disposal system, but if there is not one they must be disinfected with a suitable disinfectant, e.g. lysol 1:10. Bedclothes should be soaked in a disinfectant before being laundered.

5. Haemorrhage and perforation can occur in spite of treatment by chloramphenicol. Careful observation is maintained for at least 3 weeks. Haemorrhage is treated by morphine sulphate 10.0 mg and blood transfusion. Perforation is treated by operation.

6. Convalescence is long. The diet is gradually increased. At least 3 stools are examined for organisms before the patient is declared free from infection.

7. Treatment of carriers is unsatisfactory. Penicillin in doses of 1 million units daily is given for 10 days. If it fails the patient should have his gall-bladder removed, for the organisms can persist in it. Chloramphenicol has no effect on carriers. A carrier must not engage in any trade in which food is handled nor handle food in his own home, and must be scrupulously careful in personal hygiene. Members of his family should be immunized against typhoid.

PARATYPHOID FEVER

Paratyphoid fever is caused by the paratyphoid A and B bacilli, very similar organisms. The fever they cause is very like typhoid fever, but is usually very much milder and free from serious complications. The treatment is the same as that of typhoid fever.

BRUCELLOSIS

Other names: undulant fever, Malta fever

This is an acute fever due to infection by one of the *brucella* bacteria, of which there are several kinds. *Brucella melitensis,* one of them, is present in goat's milk and used to cause Malta fever; *brucella abortus,* another, causes cattle to abort.

It is common in Mediterranean countries, but can occur in Britain, America and elsewhere. The disease is characterized by prolonged irregular fever, sweating and an enlarged spleen. The body is infected via the alimentary tract, either through drinking infected milk or by handling infected hides, etc. It is an occupational risk of veterinary surgeons, slaughtermen and butchers.

Incubation period: 3-21 days, usually about 14.

Clinical features	*Onset:* headache, loss of appetite, sweating, constipation, sometimes vomiting.
	Course: fever becomes intermittent, with rises and falls of 2-3°C in a day and can be prolonged for months. Sweating is profuse, especially at night. Bronchitis and epistaxis can occur. Intense pain in the chest, back or limbs is common. The spleen becomes enlarged. Death can occur from exhaustion.
Complications	Arthritis Emaciation Anaemia Tachycardia. Depression
Special tests	Blood culture: becomes positive soon. Blood agglutination tests: positive from 2nd week.
Treatment	1. Bed and full nursing care. 2. Tetracycline is doses of 500 mg 6-hourly for 6 weeks; or streptomycin 1 g daily for 21 days. 3. Physiological saline is given subcutaneously when there is dehydration. 4. Cortisone or hydrocortisone is given intravenously when there are signs of adrenal failure. 5. At least one month's full convalescence is required. 6. Carriers are treated with sulphadimidine or sulphadiazine.

WHOOPING COUGH

Other name: pertussis

This infectious disease is due to the *Haemophilus pertussis* and characterized by respiratory catarrh and a paroxysmal cough and whoop. The high mortality in infants, the distress caused by the cough and whoop, and the number and severity of its complications make it one of the nastiest of infectious diseases. It is usually endemic, with epidemics occurring about every 2 years. It usually occurs in the spring and autumn. It is most common in children under 5. One attack usually confers immunity. Incubation period: 7-14 days. Adenoviruses can cause a condition clinically indistinguishable from whooping cough.

Clinical features

Onset: may be slow or sudden; slight fever; upper respiratory catarrh; cough; slight bronchitis.

    Course: the temperature remains raised for about 14 days. The cough gradually becomes paroxysmal, especially at night. Coughing then ends with a whoop; the whoop is due to breathing in air through a glottis in spasm. Bouts of coughing produce congestion and cyanosis of the face, and can cause great distress. Thick sputum may be brought up. Vomiting may occur at the end of the whoop. Sometimes there is no whoop, especially when the disease occurs in an adult. The coughing-whooping stage lasts for 2-6 weeks and then declines.

    Most children recover. The death-rate is high in infants under 6 months.

Complications

Bronchitis, bronchopneumonia, absorption collapse of lung, bronchiectasis.
Lighting up of a focus of pulmonary tuberculosis.
Acute emphysema. Epistaxis; subconjunctival haemorrhages.

Hernia, prolapse of rectum. Ulceration of the frenulum of the tongue.

Asphyxia due to prolonged spasms can produce anoxic, haemorrhagic and degenerative changes in the brain with the production of convulsions, mental retardation, behaviour disturbances, epilepsy, paralysis, and degeneration of sight and hearing.

Special tests

1. *Blood:* shows a lymphocytosis.
2. *Bacterial examination:* the organisms can be grown on suitable medium in a Petri dish on to which the child has coughed.
3. *X-ray of chest:* taken to exclude collapse of lobe or presence of a focus of pulmonary tuberculosis.

Prevention

The incidence of whooping cough has been reduced by injections of pertussis vaccine, usually given with diphtheria and tetanus vaccination. Because of the danger to the child under 1 year, vaccination should begin at 3 months.

Treatment

The patient is isolated in bed. He requires fresh air, food and hot drinks. A young child should be under constant care day and night. During a spasm he should be held head down and have his back patted to prevent the inhalation of secretion and vomit. There is no specific treatment. Steam inhalations are helpful. Sedation by chloral hydrate or phenobarbitone may be required. Preparations of belladonna and ephedrine or tincture opii camphorata are given to relieve cough. Convalescence by the seaside works wonders.

BACILLARY
DYSENTERY

There are two kinds of dysentery — bacillary and amoebic.
Bacillary dysentery is caused by bacteria of the Shigella type, of which there are several kinds. The *Shiga* [6] kind (which is most common in the tropics) causes a very severe dysentery, the *Flexner* [7] kind a moderately severe dysentery and the *Sonne* [8] kind a mild dysentery. The disease is spread by infected faeces from patients or from infected carriers, by faecally infected food and drink, by infected clothing, and by flies. It occurs endemically and epidemically in the tropics, and sporadically and epidemically in Britain, where *Sonne* is the usual organism. It is a disease of poor sanitation and personal care, and epidemics of it are likely to break out in camps, armies, children's homes and mental hospitals. The organism causes an acute inflammation of the colon and rectum, which in the severer cases goes on to ulceration and haemorrhages and severe toxaemia.
Incubation period: 1-7 days.

Clinical features

(a)   *Mild cases:* sudden onset, with slight pyrexia, malaise, abdominal colic, and diarrhoea with a little blood and mucus in the faeces. The illness clears up in a few days.
(b)   *Severe cases:* sudden onset; diarrhoea which becomes very severe; much blood and mucus and sometimes sloughs in the faeces; severe abdominal pain; collapse;

[6] *K. Shiga:* Japanese bacteriologist.
[7] *S. Flexner:* American bacteriologist
[8] *C. Sonne:* Danish bacteriologist

42

Chapter 2

temperature 38.5-39.5°C (101°-103°F); dehydration, thirst, rapid feeble pulse, fall in blood-pressure. The patient may recover, die of toxaemia and exhaustion or pass into a state of chronic dysentery with slight diarrhoea and abdominal pain persisting indefinitely.

Complications (usually *Shiga* infection)

Haemorrhages   Anaemia   Peritonitis   Gangrene of bowel
Stricture of bowel   Polyposis[9]
Arthritis, pericarditis, pleurisy

Special test

The organism can be grown from the faeces or a rectal swab.

Treatment

1. Bed and isolation. The nurse must be careful to wear a gown and to wash her hands thoroughly after attending to the patient. In a children's ward, or home, the nurse who toilets the patients must have nothing to do with the preparation of food or feeding the patients.
2. *Drugs.* A broad-spectrum antibiotic (such as tetracycline, ampicillin or chloramphenicol) is given for 5-7 days.
3. Dehydration is prevented or relieved by fluids by mouth or if necessary intravenously. Electrolyte balance is maintained.
4. Hot applications to the abdomen relieve the pain.

TETANUS [1]

Other name: lockjaw
This is an acute infection due to a bacillus, the *Clostridium tetani,* an organism found in (a) the gastro-intestinal tract of humans (especially farm-workers) and some animals, (b) in soil, especially when it has been manured, (c) occasionally in house-dust, plaster of Paris and the dust on the floors of operating-theatres. The organism can change itself into a *spore,* in which form it is very resistant and can survive for long periods, in soil and in scars. Tetanus is relatively uncommon. Entrance to the body is made through some injury to the skin — through a serious injury such as a wound received in battle, a road-injury, an accidental injury in a garden or on a farm, or a trifling injury such as a scratch or the prick of a needle. The organism produces a toxin which damages nervous tissue. Incubation period: 3-28 days or longer; the shorter the incubation period the worse the disease.

Clinical features

Onset: fever, chill, headache, restlessness, increase in muscle-tone, stiffness of muscles, difficulty in breathing, difficulty in swallowing.
   Course: may be slight or severe. Muscular spasm occurs in jaw (trismus) and spreads to the neck, back, abdomen and limbs. The muscular spasm may be violent: the limbs are extended, the teeth clenched, the mouth is contorted into a grin, the neck and back are arched, the abdomen is held taut. Spasms occur spontaneously or are precipitated by moving the bed, putting on the light, a sudden sound. Fever rises to 39.5°C (103°F). The mind remains clear. About half the infected patients

[9] *polyposis:* multiple polypi in bowel
[1] *tetanus:* from Greek *tetanos* – from *teinein* – to stretch

die of exhaustion, anoxia and heart failure. When he is recovering the patient has fewer and less violent spasms until they cease altogether.

Complications Persistent irritability, sleep disturbance, fits, postural hypotension, pneumonia and EEG abnormalities can occur.

Prevention (a) *Active immunization:* People at risk – children, farm and garden workers, soldiers – should be immunized with tetanus toxoid in two injections of 1 ml each at an interval of 6 weeks; subsequently injections of 1 ml are given every 2 years.
(b) *Passive immunization:* given to non-immunized people who have been injured. After a preliminary test for allergy to the antitoxin, an intramuscular injection of tetanus antitoxin 3,000 units is given.

Treatment 1. Adequate toilet of any wound is carried out.
2. As soon as the diagnosis is made, tetanus antitoxin is given in doses, such as: 200,000 units intravenously or intramuscularly, followed by 10,000-40,000 units, daily, according to degree of severity.
3. Control of spasms is best performed by an anaesthetist carrying out muscle-relaxant treatment under anaesthesia. Severe tetanus should be treated at special centres.
4. Tube-feeding, intravenous drip, tracheostomy and suction are sometimes needed.

ANTHRAX Anthrax is a disease of cattle, sheep, horses and other animals, which become infected by grazing on infected pastures. The *bacillus anthracis* can form a spore (a short, thick-walled form), which is very resistant and can survive for years. In man anthrax is mainly an industrial disease, contracted by workers who handle hides, especially those from the East. Others have been infected by infected shaving brushes and artificial fertilisers containing bone-meal.
    In man the organism gains admission through the skin or through the respiratory tract. It causes an acute inflammation, with blood-stained fluid exudates, haemorrhages, and a severe toxaemia. It is an extremely serious disease and if untreated is often fatal. Incubation period: from a few hours to 3 days.

Prevention Hides are disinfected on arrival. Warning notices are posted in factories where it is likely to occur. Gloves should be worn by gardeners handling bone-meal.

Clinical features (a) *Malignant pustule* follows infection through the skin. A red spot forms, becomes larger, becomes a vesicle, more skin becomes inflamed, and more vesicles are formed. Lymph vessels and nodes become inflamed. Septicaemia is produced with fever, nausea, vomiting, headache and prostration. Meningitis can occur.
    Occasionally there is a generalized infection of the skin without a malignant pustule.
(b) *Respiratory tract infection* (Wool-sorter's disease; 'wool' means hide in the trade). The trachea or a bronchus are infected; mediastinal lymph-nodes become swollen. Common features are: fever, chill, headache, nausea, vomiting, diarrhoea, collapse, septicaemia, broncho-pneumonia, meningitis.

Treatment Treatment begins at once, even if the diagnosis is in doubt, for delay is fatal. It is by benzyl-penicillin 500,000 units 4-hourly for 5-7 days. Tetracycline is sometimes given. An injection of anti-anthrax serum can be given in addition if oedema of the neck occurs.

DIPHTHERIA This is caused by the diphtheria bacillus (*Corynebacterium diphtheriae*). In about 5 per cent of infected people the bacillus is non-virulent; when it is found, its virulence has to be tested on guinea-pigs. Three types are known: the *gravis* (severe), which is more common in epidemics, the *intermedius* (intermediate) and *mitis* (mild).

The disease usually occurs at 1-10 years. Epidemics occur. The organism is usually transmitted by droplet infection directly from one person to another, occasionally by handkerchiefs, rarely by milk or dust. From countries in which the majority of children have been actively immunized, the disease has almost disappeared.

The organism lodges in the upper respiratory tract, producing an exudate of fluid, polymorphs and dead cells, the exudate forms a tough, dirty white or yellowish membrane, which looks like wash-leather. Membrane in the larynx can cause respiratory obstruction and death from suffocation. From any of these sites the bacillus produces a toxin, which enters the blood and affects the heart, kidneys, liver, adrenal glands, cranial and spinal nerves, and can cause death.

Incubation period: 1-4 days.

Clinical features

These vary with (a) the site of infection and (b) the severity of the infection and the degree of the patient's resistance.

Local signs

(a)   If the *fauces* are involved, the pharynx is inflamed; membrane forms on one tonsil and can spread to involve the whole of the soft palate and the other tonsil. Pulling the membrane away leaves a raw bleeding surface. The cervical lymph-nodes are slightly enlarged.

(b)   If the *nasopharynx* is involved, the membrane forms in the nose, sometimes so far forwards as the anterior nares, sometimes spreading up the tympanic tube into the middle ear. The cervical lymph-nodes enlarge, producing a thick 'bull neck'.

(c) If the *larynx* is involved, oedema and membrane produce first hoarseness and cough, then dyspnoea, and finally – if not relieved – cyanosis and suffocation.

Other parts that are occasionally involved are (a) the conjunctiva and (b) wounds and abrasions.

General signs

These vary from very mild to most severe.

Onset: usually malaise, slight fever, a slight sore throat. Little more may develop in mild cases.

Severe cases: severe toxaemia; pallor or cyanosis; high fever; weak rapid pulse; oliguria, albuminuria; death.

Complications

1. *Myocarditis:* Weak rapid pulse; cardiac enlargement, a fall in blood-pressure, circulatory failure.

2. *Neuritis:* (a) paralysis of the soft palate, usually about the 3rd-5th week, with a nasal twang to the voice and regurgitation of food through the nose on swallowing, (b) oculomotor paralysis, producing a squint, (c) facial or laryngeal paralysis, (d) paralysis of the legs, arms, neck or trunk.

Prevention

The Shick Test is performed by injecting into one forearm diluted diphtheria toxin 0.1 ml intradermally. A positive reaction, an area of erythema at the site of the injection within 72-120 hours, shows that the patient is susceptible. A similar amount of inactive toxin is injected into the other forearm to act as a control. A baby born to an immune mother is Shick-negative for the first six months of life, owing to transplacental transfer of antibodies.

Diphtheria is a preventable disease. It can be prevented by:

(a) FT (Formol Toxoid) given in 2 doses of 1.0 ml intramuscularly with 4-8 weeks between injections, preferably done at the age of 8-9 months, with booster doses of 1.0 ml at 5 years, 0.5 ml at 10 years and 0.25 ml at 15 years.

(b) TAF (Toxoid-Antitoxin Floccules) in 3 doses of 1.0 ml, 1.0 ml, and 1.5 ml with 3-4 weeks between injections; usually for adults as it is less likely to produce unpleasant reactions in them.

For schedule of immunization see p. 12.

Treatment	1. The patient must be isolated and given complete bed rest.
	2. Diphtheria antitoxin must be started immediately in doses of 10,000-100,000 units according to the severity of infection.

As diphtheria antitoxin is a foreign protein (horse serum), anaphylaxis can occur. Before it is given:

(a)   the personal and family history of anaphylaxis should be obtained.

(b)   test with 1:10 dilution of antitoxin in saline by either dropping 1 drop in the conjunctival sac or injecting 0.1 ml intradermally and noting if there is any local reaction. If local erythema develops within 30 minutes, the patient is sensitive and must be desensitized by repeated injections of small doses of diluted antitoxin, at first subcutaneously and then intramuscularly.

3. Dehydration is treated by parenteral injections of saline containing dextrose.

4. Intubation or tracheostomy is done if respiratory obstruction develops.

5. The patient is kept in bed for as long as there are signs of cardiac weakness. He is isolated until 2 bacteriological investigations for virulent organisms have been negative on 2 successive days.

6. If paralysis of the diaphragm develops, he is placed in an artificial respirator.

Carriers

If the organism is non-virulent, no treatment is necessary. If the organism is virulent, insufflation of sulphonamide powder should be carried out daily for 8 days. If it fails, penicillin is given. Unhealthy tonsils are removed. The patient is encouraged to get out into the fresh air as much as possible.

LEPROSY

This is a chronic contagious disease due to infection with the leprosy bacillus, *Mycobacterium leprae.* It is common in the tropics and subtropics, but it can occur elsewhere, including Southern and Eastern Europe and Mediterranean islands. It is estimated that there are between 11 and 15 million people infected by it in the world. Infants and young children are very susceptible. It has a very long incubation period: 1-5 years or longer. It is spread, probably through the skin, by close personal contact for long periods and is associated with poor housing, over-crowding, sharing the same pipes, eating from the same dishes. It is associated with much fear and superstition.

Chronic granulomatous changes occur in many tissues which swarm with the organism. Those most affected are the skin, peripheral nerves, reticulo-endothelial system, mucous membrane of the mouth and upper respiratory tract, bones, eyes and testes.

Clinical features

The onset is insidious and progress slow. The skin becomes infiltrated and macules, papules and nodes appear. Infiltration of the face with deepening of the wrinkles produces the so-called 'leonine[2] facies'. Pigmentary changes occur. Involvement of the peripheral nerves produces burning, tingling and then anaesthesia; muscle wasting leads to deformities; the thickened nerves can be felt. Degenerative changes take place in soft tissues and bones of fingers and toes. Joints become fibrosed and ankylosed. Mucous membranes can be swollen and ulcerated. Lymph-nodes enlarge painlessly and feel 'rubbery'. The testes can atrophy. The disease is sometimes slight, at other times runs a prolonged and gradually disabling course. The commonest causes of death are pulmonary tuberculosis and renal failure.

Special test

Skin: scrapings from infected lesions are examined for the organism.

Prevention

Control is difficult. Prolonged contact with infected patients has to be avoided. In countries where the disease is common, patients may have to be segregated in special areas.

Treatment

Treatment is mainly by dapsone in a daily dose of 5 mg increasing to 25 mg. Treatment has to be continued for several years and sometimes for life. Thiambutosine, clofazimine, and other drugs are sometimes given.

[2] *leonine:* like a lion

CHOLERA	This acute infection due to *vibrio cholerae*, a short, curved micro-organism, and is spread by food and water infected with the faeces of patients during an attack or while convalescent. It is predominantly a disease of India and the Far East. It has spread to Africa, Italy, Spain and Portugal. Epidemics occur. Infections vary in severity from mild to fatal. Incubation period: 2-6 days.
Clinical features	The illness usually begins with sudden diarrhoea, vomitting and collapse, but ten per cent of cases have only slight diarrhoea. Profuse watery stools are passed, called 'rice-water' because they are uncoloured by faeces. The fluid-loss is great. Muscular cramps, oliguria and total suppression of urine can occur. Severe attacks can be fatal within a few days, mild ones clear up in 3-4 days with treatment.
Special tests	*Stools:* for culture of the *vibrio cholerae*.
Prevention	Cholera vaccine is given in 2 doses of 0.5 ml and 1.0 ml with an interval of 7-28 days. The degree of protection is poor and lasts for 6 months. Booster doses of 1.0 ml are given at 6-monthly intervals to people at risk. It does not prevent people from becoming carriers.
Treatment	1. Life-saving treatment is fluid by intravenous infusion; normal glucose saline is followed by alkaline hypotonic saline. Fluid replacement then continues by mouth. Hypertonic saline is given if the patient has cramp and fairly good renal function. 2. Tetracyline or chloramphenicol are given.

LEPTOSPIROSIS	*Other name:* Weil's disease This is due to infection by a spirochaete, *Leptospira ictero-haemorrhagiica*. This organism is excreted in the urine of rats and farm animals, and humans become infected either by taking contaminated food or drink or through an abrasion or wound when working or swimming in contaminated water. The disease is an occupational hazard of farmers. Incubation period: 7-14 days.
Clinical features	The onset is sudden with fever, pains in the back and calves, injection of the conjunctivae and sometimes vomiting and diarrhoea. Hepatitis develops in about 65 per cent, producing jaundice and an enlarged painful liver. Nephritis can occur with albuminuria and haematuria. Other signs are purpura, bleeding from the gums, melaena[3], haemoptysis, mild meningeal inflammation. Anuria[4] and uraemia cause the death of a few patients, probably under 5 per cent. Relapses can occur after apparent recovery.
Treatment	Barrier nursing is not necessary. Penicillin is given in doses of 2-3 million units in 24 hours for 7 days. Oxytetracycline 1.5 g 6-hourly can be given.

SYPHILIS [5]	Syphilis is a sexually transmitted disease. It is occasionally transmitted by kissing, rarely in other ways. It can occur in a congenital form.
	   It is due to the *treponema pallidum* (*spirochaeta pallida*), a spirally-shaped, motile and delicate organism. It cannot live for long outside the human body and transmission except by direct contact is unusual.
	   The infection and spread of the disease in the body take place thus:
	   The organisms enter through a tiny abrasion in the skin or directly through a mucous membrane. Then they enter lymphatic vessels, pass along them, and getting

[3] *melaena:* blood in the faeces
[4] *anuria:* failure of urine production
[5] *syphilis:* named after Syphilis, an infected shepherd in an Italian poem of 1530

Fig. 10. Map showing spread of cholera from its original region, India and China.

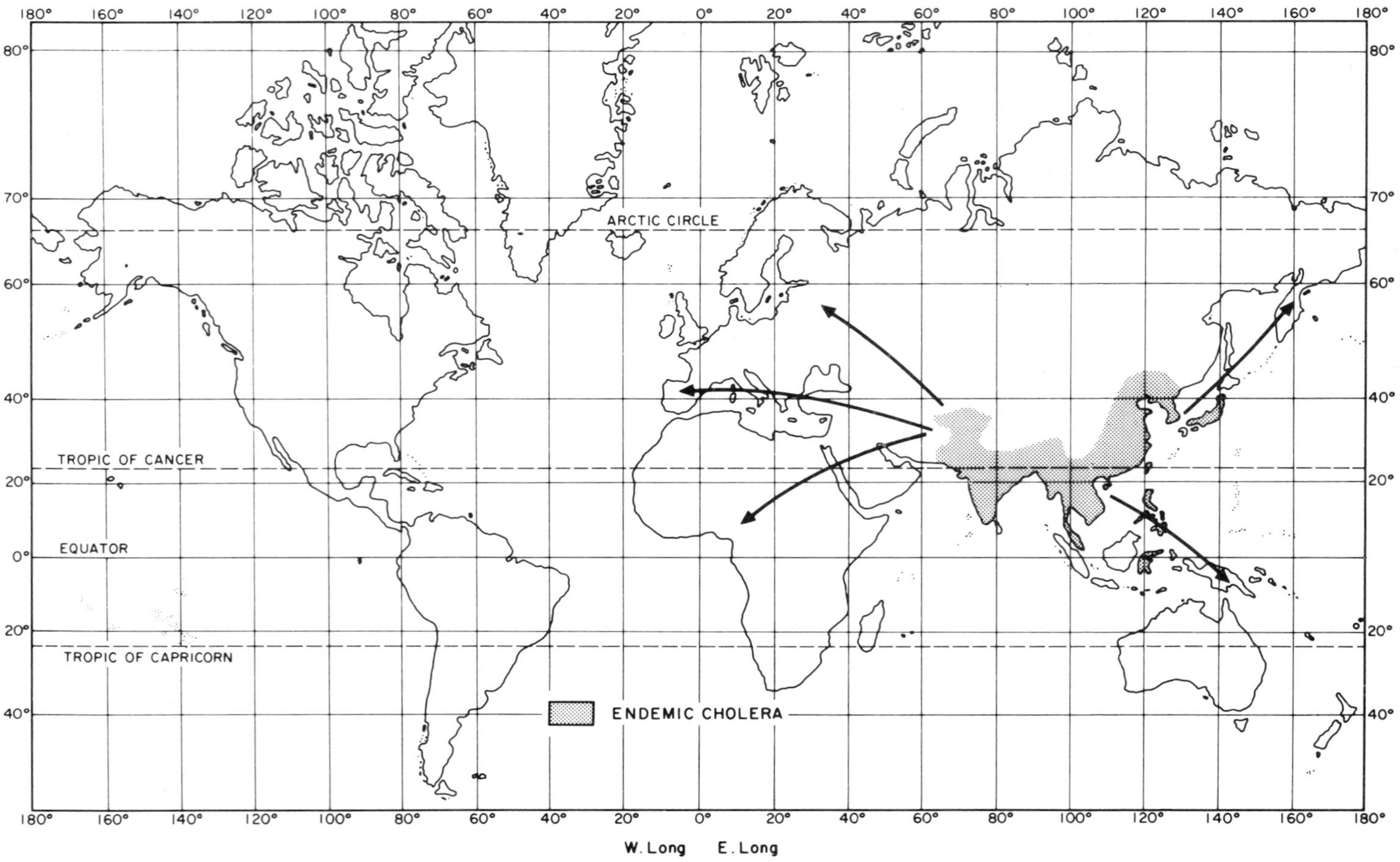
180° 160° 140° 120° 100° 80° 60° 40° 20° 0° 20° 40° 60° 80° 100° 120° 140° 160° 180°
80°
70°
60°
40°
20°
0°
20°
40°
ARCTIC CIRCLE
TROPIC OF CANCER
EQUATOR
TROPIC OF CAPRICORN
ENDEMIC CHOLERA
W. Long
E. Long

into the blood-stream are dispersed, within 24 hours of the infection, throughout the whole body.

The disease is described as taking place in 3 stages:

1. *The primary stage:* The *chancre,* the primary lesion. appears 2-4 weeks after infection at the original site of infection, usually on a genital organ. Lymph-nodes draining the part become enlarged.

2. *The secondary stage:* occurs 6-10 weeks after infection. It is a manifestation of the spread of the disease throughout the body, and the patient usually feels ill, has a slight fever, a rash and other signs of infection. This stage can last for several years and can overlap with the 3rd stage.

3. *The third stage:* occurs 5-25 years after the original infection and usually takes the form of (a) a *gumma,* a chronic syphilitic lesion, (b) aortitis, (c) syphilis of the nervous system, (d) syphilis of the eye.

Both the 1st and the 2nd stage can be absent or minimal, and not every patient is bound to show evidence of tertiary syphilis. Between the 2nd and 3rd stage there is usually a long latent period during which the patient does not show any clinical signs of the disease; special tests on the blood and cerebrospinal fluid will reveal evidence of syphilitic infection. It is not known why the spirochaete can lie dormant for this period, nor what is the stimulus that provokes it into activity.

A patient is infectious during the 1st and 2nd stages, but not during the latent period or 3rd stage. Congenital syphilis is not infectious.

Primary stage

A chancre is a hard nodule. It occurs usually on the genital organs, sometimes in the mouth, on the lips, around the anus or elsewhere. Its surface may become ulcerated with a highly infectious discharge. There is usually a painless and moderate enlargement of the lymph-nodes draining the area; the nodes remain firm, do not ulcerate or matt together and are usually not tender. The chancre usually heals in 2-6 weeks; it may leave a scar. The lymph glands may not return to normal size for several months. Occasionally no chancre appears.

Secondary stage

With a general flare up of syphilis all over the body the patient may feel ill, run a temperature, lose his appetite, have a sore throat, and complain of various aches and pains.

A *rash* appears. It may appear in one of many forms and resemble the rash of some other infection. Macules, papules, pustules and scales may be present at the same time. The papules may be 'coppery' or have the colour of raw ham. Ulcers may appear.

Inside the mouth and on the tonsils and pharynx *mucous patches* may appear; they are silvery-grey and slightly raised.

Condylomata are indurated, slightly raised, moist lesions which appear on the vulva, scrotum, anal region and groins.

A *'split papule'* is sometimes the only sign of secondary syphilis; it is a tiny moist papule at the angle of the mouth.

The discharge from these lesions is very infectious.

Other signs of secondary syphilis are:

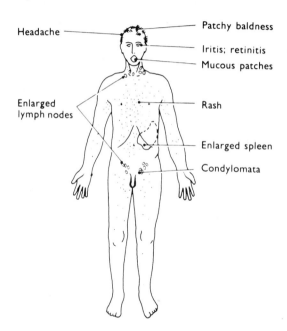

Fig. 11. Common signs of secondary syphilis.

Headache

Patchy baldness

Iritis; retinitis

Mucous patches

Enlarged lymph nodes

Rash

Enlarged spleen

Condylomata

Anaemia,   Pain in bones,   Periostitis,
Headache,   Iritis,   Retinitis.
Enlargement of spleen and lymph-nodes
Alopecia[6], of an irregular 'moth-eaten' type.
    These signs of syphilis may take months or years to clear up.

Third stage (Tertiary syphilis)

(a)   *Gumma:* a hard nodule or granulomatous tissue. More than one can occur. It can appear in almost any tissue, common sites being the skin, the periosteum, bone, testicle, meninges, blood-vessels of the nervous system. It develops slowly and in time one on the skin may ulcerate, forming the typical 'punched out' appearance of a syphilitic ulcer. It can destroy the tissue in which it is growing and cause symptoms by pressing on other organs; one in the brain resembles a slowly growing cerebral tumour. A gumma can gradually disappear and be replaced by fibrous tissue.

(b)   *Aortitis.*

(c)   *Meningo-vascular syphilis; General paralysis of the insane; Tabes dorsalis.*

Treatment

Syphilis is treated by:

(a)   procaine penicillin 600 mg (600,000 units) daily by intramuscular injection for 10 days;

(b)   benzathine penicillin 2.4 g (2.4 mega units) by intramuscular injection once only; this method is used for patients who will not or cannot attend for daily injections; it is possible that this single injection will maintain an adequate level of

[6] *alopecia:* baldness

penicillin in the blood for 14 days, but as there can be a variation in the level, daily injections of procaine penicillin are preferable.

A *Herxheimer reaction* is an acute reaction which can occur on starting treatment. It is not serious in primary and secondary syphilis and quickly subsides; but in tertiary syphilis it can be dangerous and to avoid it only small doses of penicillin are given at first.

If the patient is sensitive to penicillin, he is given tetracycline 750 mg by mouth 6-hourly for 10-15 days.

The patient should come for re-examination once a fortnight or month for 6 months and then every 6 months for 4-5 years. The WR and Kahn tests are repeated on each occasion. During the second year the CSF should be examined for evidence of involvement of the nervous system.

Further courses of penicillin are given for any sign of recurrence.

CONGENITAL SYPHILIS

An infected woman can transmit syphilis to her children for an undetermined number of years after she has been infected. She is most likely to infect a child when her own infection has been recent. The *treponema pallidum* is transmitted via the placenta about the 5th month of pregnancy. The fetus may die and be aborted; later children may be still-born, and eventually a live but infected child is born.

Clinical features
Infancy

The child is usually feeble and fails to thrive or may die. Pemphigus (bullae) appear on soles, palms and buttocks. A copper-coloured rash appears about 3rd month.
Mucous patches appear on mouth, nose and around the anus.
Liver and spleen are enlarged.
The baby has 'snuffles', a nasal discharge.

Childhood

Rhagades, scars from lesions around the corners of the mouth. Hutchinson's teeth, incisor teeth of second dentition are peg-shaped, notched and wide apart.
Periostitis; 'sabre' tibiae. Gummata.
Depression of the bridge of the nose.
Deafness. Interstitial keratitis.

Adolescence

Congenital general paralysis of the insane and congenital tabes dorsalis (both rare).

GONORRHOEA[7]

This is an acute infectious disease produced by the *gonococcus*, a small kidney-shaped organism, which cannot live for long outside the body. It is usually spread by sexual intercourse; the eyes of newly-born babies can become infected during birth producing *ophthalmia neonatorum*. Incubation period: 2-10 days.

Symptoms and signs
In Men

The urethra becomes infected first; there is smarting on micturition and then a purulent discharge. The infection can spread into the prostate gland, producing acute prostatitis and urinary obstruction, and into the epididymis, producing acute epididymitis, which is very painful; the testicle can become swollen and sterility produced. A stricture of the urethra can occur.

In Women

The urethra and the cervix of the uterus become infected first, producing a purulent vaginal discharge. But many women show no signs of infection. Abscesses can occur

[7] *gonorrhoea:* from Greek: *gone* – seed; *rhoia* – flow

in Skene's glands (small glands opening into the urethra) and Bartholin's glands (small glands opening into the vulva near the labia minora). Infections can then spread into the uterine tubes causing acute salpingitis[8], pelvic pain, pelvic peritonitis and abscesses and, if untreated, progressive destruction of the pelvic organs.

Complications

The *gonococcus* gains admission into the blood-stream and is dispersed throughout the body, causing inflammatory changes in various organs.

1. *Gonococcal arthritis* (gonococcal rheumatism) occurs 1-4 weeks after the primary infection, usually in several joints (especially the knees, wrists, ankles), sometimes in one joint only. Teno-synovitis[9] and bursitis can occur. Painful walking may be due to inflammation of the plantar fascia or calcaneal periosteum.

2. *Endocarditis:* (rare), usually affecting aortic valves; can be very severe.

3. *Iritis.*   4. *Meningitis* (rare).

5. *Septic dermatitis:* fever, arthritis, and a rash of papules and pustules.

6. *Metastatic gonorrhoea* (rare): pyrexia, polyarthritis, rashes, due to invasion of blood-stream by gonococcus.

7. *Perihepatitis* (rare): occurs in women with a gonococcal pelvic infection, producing fever, pain in the region of the liver, and signs suggesting peritonitis in the right upper quadrant of the abdomen.

8. *Pharyngeal infection:* usually in male homosexuals.

Special test

Gonococci can be found in the urethral or vaginal discharge, or grown on culture.

Treatment

Early cases: Single dose treatment by (a) ampicillin 2 g with probenecid 1 g, or (b) procaine penicillin 1.2-2.4 megaunits with probenecid 2 g. Probenecid helps to maintain a high blood-level of the antibiotic by delaying its excretion. Most patients are cured by these methods.

Complicated cases: Procaine penicillin by injection 600,000 units 2-3 times a day for 1-2 weeks. Larger doses are given if resistance has developed. Ampicillin may be given in doses of 1 g.

Patients sensitive to penicillin are given kanamycin 2 g intra-muscularly as either a single dose or twice at 24-hour interval; no strain of gonococcus is resistant to it, and it does not affect syphilis (this is important for if signs of syphilis did not appear it might be missed and not treated). Sexual contacts of a patient with gonorrhoea should be traced and persuaded to be examined and if necessary treated.

Ophthalmia neonatorum is an acute infection, usually by gonococci, sometimes by other organisms, of the eyes of a newly-born baby, whose eyes have become infected from the mother's genital passages during birth. The eyes become inflamed, a purulent abscess forms, the eyelids tend to stick together with pus forming behind them, corneal ulcers develop, and the baby can become blind. *Prevention* is by adequate treatment of an infected mother. *Treatment* is by penicillin, sulpha-cetimide or chloramphenical drops. An infected baby must be isolated from other babies.

[8] *salpingitis:* inflammation of the uterine (fallopian) tubes
[9] *teno-synovitis:* inflammation of a tendon and its sheath

LYMPHOGRANULOMA INGUINALE	*Other name:* lymphogranuloma venereum

This is a sexually transmitted disease due to a virus. It is rare in Britain. Incubation period: 3-21 days.

Symptoms and signs

A vesicle or ulcer forms at the site of infection on the genitalia. The inguinal lymph-nodes on one or both sides become greatly enlarged, the surrounding tissues become swollen and hard, the whole area suppurates with the formation of several sinuses through which yellow pus exudes. The patient has a high temperature and may develop arthritis and iritis.

Complications

Scarring and elephantiasis[1] of the male genitalia; proctitis[2], rectal stricture, chronic ano-rectal infection in women.

Treatment

This is by a course of sulphonamide alone or combined with a tetracycline for 3-6 weeks or longer. Aspiration or incision of the abscesses may be necessary.

SOFT SORE

Other name: chancroid.

Soft sore is a rare sexually transmitted disease, caused by the *haemophilus ducreui* (Ducrey's bacillus). Incubation period: 2-5 days.

Symptoms and signs

One or more red spots appear on or around the genitalia and ulcerate. The inguinal lymph-nodes enlarge and may suppurate. The disease differs from syphilis in that: it is caused by a different organism, which can be identified; the incubation period is shorter; and there is no induration of the tissues.

Treatment

The disease is quickly cured by a course of sulphadimidine or other sulphonamide.

REITER'S SYNDROME

This is characterized by urethritis, polyarthritis, conjunctivitis, and other features. Its cause is unknown. In Europe, Asia and North Africa it seems to follow dysentery or non-specific diarrhoea; in Great Britain and North America it seems to follow a sexually-transmitted urethritis. It is predominantly a disease of young men.

The urethritis, the first sign, can cause a purulent discharge and be mistaken for gonorrhoea. The arthritis is multiple, often affecting the fingers, knees, ankles and spine. It may clear up completely or produce painful, crippling deformities. The conjunctivitis is purulent; keratitis, iritis[3] and uveitis[4] can occur. Pericarditis, myocarditis, pleurisy, polyneuritis, thrombophlebitis and amyloid disease have occurred in some cases.

The disease can persist in an acute state for 1-18 months, the majority of attacks lasting for 3 months. A few patients make a permanent and complete recovery; others suffer a prolonged debilitating disease with recurrent iritis, painful deformities of the feet and spondylitis. There is no specific treatment; salicylates are used to relieve the arthritis.

[1] *elephantiasis:* chronic enlargement of skin and subcutaneous tissue
[2] *proctitis:* inflammation of the rectum
[3] *iritis:* inflammation of the iris of the eye
[4] *uveitis:* inflammation of the uvea – the pigmented, vascular layer of the eye, including iris, ciliary body, choroid coat

Infections

3 Diseases of the Cardio-Vascular System

The heart is a pump, and the blood-vessels are the tubes through which the blood passes to get to the tissues and back to the heart. Any disease of the heart is likely to interfere with its pumping action. Disease of the arteries and in particular a rise in blood-pressure increases the work the heart has to do and puts a strain upon it. All the tissues of which the heart is composed — the endocardium which lines the chambers and valves, the myocardium which provides the pumping power, and the pericardium which encloses the rest — are likely to be involved, to some degree or another, in any heart disease. Such a disease can be a congenital deformity, an infection, an interference with its blood-supply through the two coronary arteries, or a degeneration; tumours of the heart are rare.

If the heart is called upon to pump harder — by being compelled to cope with the mechanical difficulties of a stiff or incompetent valve, or of an increase in blood-pressure — it can become larger, its muscle-fibres becoming longer; this is called hypertrophy of the heart.

There is a maximum to which a heart can hypertrophy; and if, when it has reached this maximum, additional strain is put upon it, the muscle stretches and becomes inefficient; this is called dilatation of the heart.

Diseases of the heart are likely in their early stages to produce:
shortness of breath on exertion
increased pulse-rate
palpitations
discomfort in the precordial region (in front of the heart)

fatigue	loss of appetite
giddiness	fainting

More extensive disease of the heart is likely to add to the above some of the following:
shortness of breath even at rest
irregularity of heart action
pain in the precordial region, radiating into the neck, left arm or abdomen

cyanosis[5]	enlargement of the liver and spleen
oedema[6] of the tissues	clubbing of the fingers

[5] *cyanosis:* blueness of skin and mucous membranes due to lack of oxygen in the blood.
[6] *oedema:* excess of fluid in the extra-cellular spaces.

| DISTURBANCES OF CARDIAC RHYTHM | The heart normally beats regularly. *Sinus arrhythmia* is a gradual increase and decrease of heart-rate usually in time with the breathing, increasing during inspiration and decreasing during expiration because of the increased blood-flow into the heart during inspiration, and as such is a normal phenomenon in the young. Occasionally it occurs independently of respiration.
There are several kinds of irregular beat. |
|---|---|
| **Extra systole** | *Other names:* premature contraction, premature systole, ectopic beat
This is a cardiac impulse that starts in some place other than the sinu-atrial node, the place in the heart where the normal beat starts. An extra-systole can start in an atrium, in the atrio-ventricular node, or in a ventricle. The heart beats in response to it; but the next normal beat does not occur because it is stopped by the 'refractory period' (during which no beat can start) and so there is a long pause before another beat occurs. Sometimes extra systoles occur with every heart beat, causing 'coupled beats' (pulsus bigeminus).
An extra systole can occur in healthy people and in heart disease. A person does not notice the extra systole himself; what he notices is the bigger beat that follows it, or sometimes the long pause of a 'dropped beat'. Some people do not notice extra-systoles at all.
Extra systoles are likely to appear when a person is worried or tired; coffee, tea, alcohol and tobacco may make them more frequent. |
| *Treatment* | In the absence of heart disease an extra-systole is of no importance. Reassurance, relief of anxiety, and a diminished intake of coffee, tea, alcohol and tobacco is indicated.
If however extra-systoles are occurring frequently and worrying the patient, lignocaine can be given.
Appropriate treatment is given to the patient with heart disease. |
| **Paroxysmal tachycardia** | *Other name:* atrial or ventricular tachycardia
This is due to a rapid, regular cardiac impulse, which arises in a part of the heart other than the sinu-atrial node and beating at a rate of over 100 times a minute takes over the function of the normal cardiac pace-maker. If the new origin of the heart-beat is in the atrium, both atria and ventricles beat rapidly; if it is in the ventricle, the atria beat at the normal rate and the ventricles at the abnormally rapid rate.
It can occur (a) in health, (b) in heart disease, especially mitral stenosis, myocardial infarction and hyper-thyroidism. Its cause is unknown; alcohol, coffee, tea and tobacco are said to be factors that produce it. Stress and sudden movement may apparently precipitate an attack. |
| *Clinical features* | Attacks are noticed by the patient and cause anxiety. They begin and end suddenly. An attack can last any time from a few minutes to several hours; intervals between them can be anything from a few hours to many years. Associated features are |

Diseases of the Cardio-Vascular System

fainting, giddiness, abdominal disturbances, vomiting, frequency of micturition, migraine and congestive heart failure.

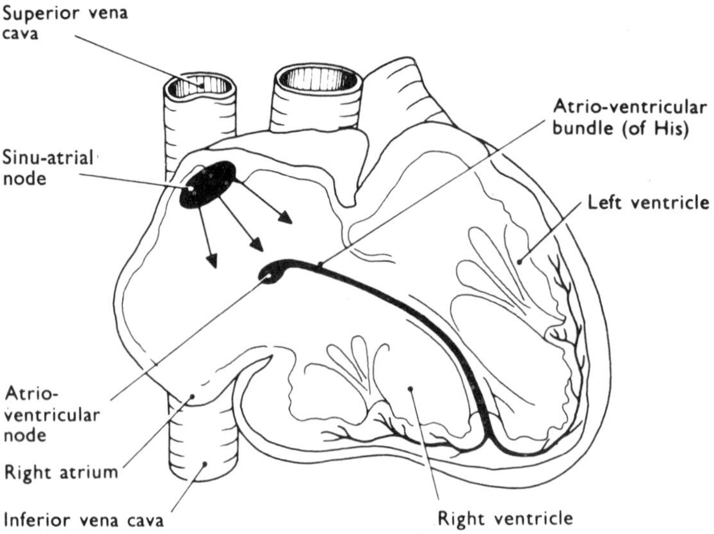

Fig. 12. The cardiac impulse starts in the sino-atrial node and passes through the wall of the right atrium. The atrio-ventricular node is stimulated and the impulse passes down the atrio-ventricular bundle (of His) to reach the bottom of the ventricles. Any interference with the nodes or the bundle can interfere with the cardiac action.

Treatment

1. The patient should be made to lie down and reassured that he is not going to die.
2. The patient may develop a trick of stopping an attack — holding his breath, etc.
3. Direct current counter shock is used.
4. Propranolol 40-80 mg is given 3-4 times daily or practolol (Eraldin) 100 mg 3-4 times daily.
5. Digoxin 1 mg can be given intravenously.

Atrial fibrillation

In this condition the small bundles of muscle-fibres in the atria contract independently at a very rapid rate, sometimes as frequently as 500 times a minute. There is no proper contraction of the atria; and the ventricles, receiving irregular stimuli, themselves contract irregularly and often rapidly.

Atrial fibrillation occurs in (a) heart disease, due to coronary artery disease, mitral stenosis, thyrotoxicosis and constrictive pericarditis; (b) after thoracotomy; (c) occasionally after excessive consumption of alcohol or tobacco. It can occur without known cause.

Clinical features

Attacks can last for short or long periods or become permanent. The patient usually notices that his heart is beating irregularly and may complain of palpitations. If an attack starts suddenly he may collapse. The pulse is 'irregularly irregular' in rhythm and strength, with an irregularity that usually distinguishes it from other forms of cardiac irregularity. Other evidence of heart disease is usually found. Acute cardiac failure can be a complication.

Treatment

1. The cause (e.g. thyrotoxicosis) is treated.
2. Digoxin is given in the following doses:

(a) 1st day: 0.5 mg three times a day,

(b) 2nd-3rd day: 0.5 mg three times a day,

(c) subsequently: 0.25 mg twice a day.

   Such a course should produce 'digitalization' of the heart with slowing and strengthening of the beat. Smaller doses may be effective.

3. Quinidine can be given in an attempt to return the atria to a normal rhythm. After a test dose of 120 mg to reveal any unfavourable reactions, the following doses are given:

(a) 1st day: 300 mg every four hours

(b) 2nd-3rd day: 300 mg every two hours.

A return to normal rhythm should occur on the 3rd day. Treatment is stopped if the patient develops vomiting, diarrhoea, low BP or syncope. Contra-indications are serious organic heart disease, heart failure and pregnancy (quinidine is an abortifacient).

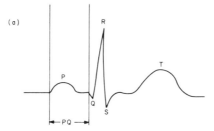

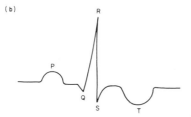

Fig. 13. (a) A normal electrocardiogram (ECG). The ECG is a record of electrical activity in the heart. The P wave is produced during contraction of the atria; the other waves are produced by contraction of the ventricles. The width of P-Q shows the time taken for a contraction-wave to pass down the atrio-ventricular bundle. (b) An abnormal ECG showing an inverted T wave (which can occur after cardiac infarction).

4. *Direct shock.* A DC (direct current) shock is given to the heart through the chest wall to synchronize with the top of the R wave on the ECG (electrocardiogram) and produce a normal sinus rhythm.

Atrial flutter

In this condition there is thought to be a place in the atria from which discharges arise at a rapid rate (up to 300 a minute). The ventricles are stimulated rapidly, but cannot contract at this rate and contract at a lower rate. The condition can occur in any form of heart disease, usually rheumatic heart disease, coronary artery disease or hypertension.

Clinical features

Sometimes little in the way of clinical features is added to the features of heart disease already present. The patient may complain of palpitations. The pulse may be regular; occasionally the heart-rate is suddenly doubled or halved.

Treatment	Digitalis given in the full doses as for atrial fibrillation (see above) sometimes converts the atrial flutter to fibrillation, and if the patient does not then show signs of heart failure, it may be safe to stop the fibrillation by using quinidine (see above). Direct shock is effective.
Treatment by a cardiac pacemaker	A cardiac pacemaker is an instrument that by giving tiny electric shocks to the heart takes over the function of the sinu-atrial node and so stimulates the heart to beat regularly. The following methods are used: 1. A pacemaker is placed on the front of the chest and a shock of 70-150 volts is given to the heart 70 times a minute through the chest-wall. The patient has to be anaesthetized as the method is painful; and as burning of the skin can occur as well, the method can be used only for short periods. 2. A venous pacemaking catheter is passed through the external jugular vein and into the heart until the tip is in the right ventricle. The other end of the catheter is attached to a pacemaker, which is either buried under the skin of the axilla or is attached to the skin. Impulses of 2-5 volts are given. Technical troubles can develop, and the treatment cannot usually be given for more than 9 months. 3. An electrode is sewn into the heart and attached to a pacemaker buried under the sheath of a rectus abdominis muscle. Technical troubles can develop.
External direct current counter shock	This method is used to stop some kinds of cardiac arrhythmias by passing a large electric current once through the heart. The patient is anaesthetized; the electrodes are placed either (a) at the apex of and base of the heart or (b) on the front and back of the chest. The shock should stop the heart, which then usually restarts in a normal rhythm.
HEART BLOCK	In this condition the cardiac impulse is not transmitted from the atria down the bundle of His to the ventricles. The ventricles are not stimulated by the normal impulse and beat independently at a slow rate.
Complete heart block	This can be: (a) congenital (b) due to coronary artery disease, myocarditis, calcification of the aortic valve, diphtheria, syphilis, or (c) due to an overdose of digitalis. The ventricular beat is usually 30-40 times a minute. Fainting is likely if the beat is very slow. Treatment is that of the original condition. No treatment is likely to affect the heart block itself.
Stokes-Adam syndrome	This is an extreme variety of heart block in which the ventricles beat extremely slowly, about 10-20 times a minute. The patient suffers cerebral anoxia, having attacks of unconsciousness without warning; he goes pale, falls unconscious, then develops sterterous or Cheyne-Stokes breathing, becomes cyanosed and may have fits. He can stay in this condition for a minute or more, recovering consciousness without confusion and with a sudden flushing of the face. If the attack lasts for more than 2 minutes, he is likely to die or on recovery have permanent mental deterioration due to damage to brain cells from lack of oxygen.

Complications	Renal failure	Respiratory failure
	Cerebral degeneration	

Treatment This is an acute cardiac emergency for which treatment has to be given promptly and so far as possible on the spot.

1. The patient is laid flat on a hard surface and external cardiac massage is performed by compression of the lower half of the sternum at about 60 times a minute.

2. The air-way is kept clear. Mouth-to-mouth respiration may be necessary or other methods of artificial respiration performed.

3. The following are injected into the heart or jugular vein or given by intravenous infusion:

(a)   either calcium chloride 10 ml of 10 per cent solution or adrenaline 10 ml of 1/10,000 solution: to improve the tone of the cardiac muscle;

(b)   sodium bicarbonate 50 ml of 8.4 per cent solution: to reduce acidosis.

4. To stop ventricular fibrillation an electric shock is given to the heart from a D.C. fibrillator; one electrode is placed on the front of the chest over the apex of the heart and the other on the back just below the angle of the left scapula.

5. After care:

(a)   The pulse and BP are monitored.

(b)   The ECG is observed continuously on an oscilloscope.

(c)   Oxygen is given through a face-mask.

(d)   To prevent the inhalation of vomit, a naso-gastric tube is inserted and the stomach kept dry.

(e)   A catheter is inserted into the bladder in order that any cessation of renal function is detected promptly.

(f)   To prevent attacks the following can be given: (a) ephedrine 30 mg three times a day; (b) slow-release isoprenaline (Saventrine) 30 mg three times a day.

CONGENITAL   Congenital heart disease is the result of failure of the normal development of the
HEART DISEASE   heart and adjoining great blood vessels. The development of the heart in the embryo is a complicated process, for the atria, ventricles, valves, aorta, pulmonary artery and pulmonary veins develop from a simple tube, with a number of intricate manoeuvres having to take place with precise timing. The greater part of this development takes place during the first 2 months of embryonic life, especially from 5th to 8th week. If anything interferes with development at this time, the normal changes may not take place and serious defects can be produced. Likely causes are (a) the mother developing German measles (b) possibly, the mother developing some other virus infection, and (c) metabolic disturbances occurring in the mother. Another set of changes has to take place after birth with the beginning of pulmonary respiration – the closing of the foramen ovale (between right and left atria) and the closing of the ductus arteriosus (between aorta and pulmonary artery).

About 3 babies in every 1,000 are born with congenital heart disease. The death-rate in infancy is high, and any severe abnormality is likely to be crippling if it cannot be treated. Subacute bacterial endocarditis is a serious complication of any congenital heart disease; and before dental extraction, tonsillectomy and any operation likely to set up septicaemia an appropriate antibiotic cover has to be given for the patient, e.g. by procaine benzyl penicillin.

There are many kinds of congenital defect of the heart. Many of them are rare; only the more common are described here.

Fallot's tetralogy [7] In this condition there are four abnormalities:
(a)   stenosis of the pulmonary valve.
(b)   a defect in the wall between the two ventricles,
(c)   over-riding of the aorta, which lies over both ventricles, and
(d)   hypertrophy of the right ventricle.

This is the usual cause of a 'blue baby'. Venous blood can pass into the aorta; the baby is cyanosed from birth or shortly afterwards, and becomes dyspnoeic. He has clubbed fingers and usually fails to develop. Typically the child adopts a squatting position. Without treatment few children with the condition survive into adult life.

Special tests *X-ray of chest:* shows typical heart shadow called 'coeur en sabot' (clog-shaped heart).
ECG: shows hypertrophy of right ventricle.

Treatment Surgery is advisable. Possible operations are:
(a)   total correction of the deformity with relief of the pulmonary stenosis and repair of the defect in the interventricular septum;
(b)   Brock's operation [8]: relief of the pulmonary stenosis;
(c)   Blaloch's operation [9]: an anastomosis between pulmonary artery and a systemic artery.

Coarctation of the aorta [1] This is a congenital narrowing of the aorta, usually just below the origin of the left subclavian artery and at the junction of the arch of the aorta with the descending aorta.

This narrowing produces (a) hypertension in the carotid and subclavian arteries and (b) hypotension in the arteries below the narrowing. There is a big difference between the high BP in the brachial arteries and the low BP in the femoral arteries; the femoral pulse is delayed or absent. The hypertension in the upper part of the body is likely to produce hypertrophy of the left ventricle and retinal artery disease. A collateral circulation is set up between arteries in the upper part of the body and those in the lower, and the pulsation of enlarged arteries in the neck may be visible. Berry aneurysm is an associated condition.

The patient, untreated, is likely to die in middle life of cerebral haemorrhage, heart failure, rupture of the aorta, or subacute bacterial endocarditis.

[7] *tetralogy:* from Greek: *tetra* – four
[8] R. C. Brock: British heart-surgeon
[9] A.Blaloch: American heart-surgeon
[1] *coarctation:* narrowing

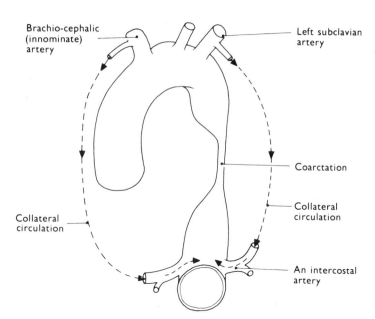

Brachio-cephalic
(innominate)
artery

Left subclavian
artery

Coarctation

Collateral
circulation

Collateral
circulation

An intercostal
artery

Fig. 14. Coarctation of the aorta with the development of a collateral circulation on each side.

| *Treatment* | The results of surgical treatment are good. The best age for operation is 7 - 15 years. The constriction is excised and aortic continuity is then restored by an arterial homocraft[2] or by end-to-end anastomosis[3]. |

Pulmonary stenosis

Congenital stenosis of the pulmonary valve produces an increase of pressure within the right ventricle and atrium and eventual hypertrophy of both. The foramen ovale – connecting the right with the left atrium – may remain open.

Mild pulmonary stenosis causes little or no trouble; severe stenosis causes dyspnoea, attacks of angina and eventually failure of the right ventricle. Subacute bacterial endocarditis is always a likely complication. Untreated, the patient usually dies in early adult life.

Special tests

X-ray of heart: shows hypertrophy of the right ventricle and dilatation of the pulmonary artery beyond the stenosis.
ECG: shows evidence of hypertrophy of the right ventricle.

Treatment

A patient with a mild degree of stenosis that is not operated on should avoid physical exertion. Pulmonary valvotomy is performed for severe stenosis.

Persistent ductus arteriosus

The short tube which before birth allows the passage of blood from pulmonary artery to aorta should close shortly after birth. If it does not close there is a 'shunt' of blood from the aorta into the pulmonary artery and so back into the pulmonary circulation. In order to compensate for the blood thus sent round again, the left ventricle has to hypertrophy.

[2] *homograft:* tissue graft from a donor of the same species (here, from another human body)
[3] *anastomosis:* joining together

Sometimes no symptoms are produced. In severe cases, palpitations and dyspnoea are likely, with cardiac failure developing in middle life and always a risk of subacute bacterial endocarditis. Pulmonary hypertension can be another complication. The

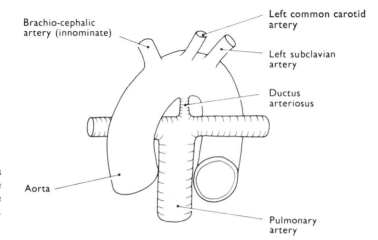

Brachio-cephalic artery (innominate)

Left common carotid artery

Left subclavian artery

Ductus arteriosus

Aorta

Pulmonary artery

Fig. 15. Patent ductus arteriosus connecting the pulmonary artery with the aorta.

diagnosis is made on hearing a typical 'machinery' murmur and discovering the hypertrophy of the left ventricle.

Treatment The duct should be tied or divided, preferably in childhood. The contra-indication to operation is severe pulmonary hypertension.

Atrial septal defect *Other name:* patent foramen ovale
The foramen ovale, the opening between right atrium and left atrium, should close shortly after birth, but, owing to faulty development, sometimes does not do so; and then with every contraction about half the blood in the left atrium is driven back into the right atrium and has to go again, this time uselessly, through the pulmonary circulation.

Clinical features Except for abnormal heart sounds, there may be little evidence of a defect until, in middle life, dyspnoea, heart failure and sometimes pulmonary hypertension develop. Bronchitis can be a complication in later life.

Special tests *X-ray of chest:* shows enlarged and pulsating pulmonary arteries.

Treatment If possible, surgical repair of the hole is performed.

Ventricular septal defect This is a failure of closure of the septum separating the right ventricle from the left. A small hole causes no trouble; a large one will produce abnormal heart sounds and in time cardiac enlargement, pulmonary hypertension and cardiac failure. Subacute bacterial endocarditis is to be dreaded.

Treatment For a large hole, an attempt at surgical repair is advisable.

62

ISCHAEMIC HEART DISEASE [4]

This term describes all conditions in which insufficient blood passes through the coronary arteries to satisfy the demands of the heart for oxygen. Most cases are due to atheroma of the coronary arteries. In some the coronary arteries are normal. Men are more commonly affected than women. In some patients atheroma may start in the twenties. Some atheroma of the coronary arteries is present in almost all people over 40 in Western societies, and in some patients the atheroma is extremely severe. A few very old people may have no atheroma — which is probably the reason why they have reached old age.

The precise causes of this atheroma are unknown. Factors involved are:

(a)   *Heredity:* there is a high incidence of coronary disease, vascular degeneration and hypertension in the close relatives of people with ischaemic heart disease.

(b)   *Abnormal lipid metabolism:* there is evidence that a high consumption of animal fat leads to atheroma; primitive people who eat little animal fat get little or no atheroma; and there is a high incidence of atheroma in those diseases (such as diabetes, myxoedema) in which the serum-cholesterol is high.

The two types of ischaemic heart disease are:

1. angina pectoris
2. cardiac infarction

Angina pectoris

Other name: angina of effort

This is a condition in which attacks of pain are produced by physical effort and relieved by rest. Such attacks are often the first indication of ischaemic cardiac disease, the first indication that the heart is not getting enough blood.

Clinical features

Anginal pain usually begins in the front of the chest, over the heart itself. It may spread to the left side of the chest and less commonly to the right; very commonly

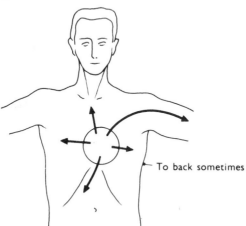

Fig. 16. Distribution of pain in an anginal attack.

it spreads into the arms, usually the left, which may also feel numb and weak. It can spread to the back, into the epigastrium or upwards into the neck and jaw. The chest may feel as if it were being squeezed in a vice. The pain is steady and incapacitating.

[4] *ischaemia:* lack of blood

Diseases of the Cardio-Vascular System

It is usually produced by some physical effort — walking, running for a bus, walking against a wind on a cold day. Emotional stress can bring it on, and it can occur in bed when the patient lies down or has a disturbing dream. Usually the patient has to stop the effort that brought the pain on; some patients claim to be able to 'walk through' it. Usually it lasts for a few minutes and then goes completely. Some patients show anxiety while it is on. With a progressive lesion of the arteries, attacks are brought on by less and less physical effort.

Some patients have an atypical angina which occurs at rest, is not related to emotional stress, can be severe and prolonged, and tends to recur in a regular pattern.

The course of the condition is very variable. With treatment attacks may diminish or vanish and patients may live for many years. Others may become worse; coronary thrombosis is very likely at any time.

Special test   *ECG:* can be normal or show signs of cardiac ischaemia or infarction.
Angiogram of the coronary arteries can be taken.

Treatment   1. An obese patient should be slimmed. This alone may stop attacks.
2. A smoker should stop smoking. This alone may stop attacks.
3. Regular exercise should be taken daily, but not to point of bringing on an attack.
4. Wherever he goes, the patient should take with him a supply of tablets of glyceryl-trinitrate 0.5 mg. He should suck or chew one (the drug is absorbed best from the oral mucous membrane) whenever he has to perform work likely to bring on an attack or whenever an attack comes on. Glyceryl trinitrate dilates the coronary arteries within 2-3 minutes and keeps them dilated for 15-20 minutes. There is no danger of addiction or harming the heart; some patients may feel faint or get giddiness when they first start taking the tablets. The patient should keep tablets by the bedside for use should he have an attack during the night. Penta-erythritol tetranitrate 30 mg is long-acting vaso-dilator which can be taken 3-4 times a day; it is probably less effective than glyceryl trinitrate.
5. Anxiety and stress-provoking situations should be avoided.
6. Rest in bed may be necessary if attacks are frequent.
7. Alcohol is not contra-indicated for it is a mild vaso-dilator and can be taken in moderation.

Cardiac infarction   Cardiac infarction is the damage and death of heart-muscle as a result of a *coronary thrombosis,* the clotting of blood in a coronary artery, blocking the lumen.

The causes of this condition have been described above under the heading of ischaemic heart disease. A coronary thrombosis occurs in a coronary artery already affected by atheroma; but not every atheromatous coronary artery develops a thrombosis. The condition is a common one: it occurs in middle-aged and elderly people of any physical build, mental type and social state; it can occur during sleep or during exercise, at any time of the day, more commonly in the winter than in the other seasons. Hypertension is a factor and so is a high serum-cholesterol, but it can occur in people with a normal BP and an average serum-cholesterol.

Clinical features   *Pain* is the usual symptom. There may be preliminary attacks of slight pain or some malaise, or patients with angina pectoris may experience more frequent or more severe attacks of it. The pain of the infarction can be agonizing; some patients have little pain or — in the 'silent infarction' — none at all. The site and extensions of pain are the same as those of angina pectoris; it is likely to be prolonged for hours or days. Restlessness is common — in contrast with the immobility produced by angina pectoris — and the patient may walk or even run about.

Shock is common — with weakness, fainting, sweating, a clammy skin, a grey anxious face, pale or cyanosed extremities. The BP is low — sometimes so low that no pulse is felt.

Heart failure causes dyspnoea, Cheyne-Stokes breathing, pulmonary oedema. The pulse may be fast or irregular. Congestive heart failure can develop.

Nausea, vomiting and epigastric pain or discomfort are common.

Sudden death can occur in an attack — probably in 1 patient in 4 — at the onset or at any time up to about 10 days. If the patient survives for 3 weeks and does not develop congestive heart failure he is likely to recover. Another attack can occur at any time, but sometimes not for many years.

Complications	Thrombosis of deep veins of leg; pulmonary embolism, pulmonary infarction.

Cerebro-vascular thrombosis or haemorrhage

Pericarditis

Ventricular aneurysm; rupture of heart; haemo-pericardium

'Post-infarction syndrome':- fever, joint-pains, pericarditis, raised ESR.

'Frozen shoulder', 'shoulder-hand syndrome':- shoulder becomes cold, stiff, painful and immobile; hand becomes swollen, stiff and atrophic; spontaneous recovery from both conditions is usual.

Special test   ECG: will show changes confirming the diagnosis and showing the position of the infarction.

Treatment   1. The patient should be given complete bed rest for at least 4 weeks, unless he is old and might develop the complications of immobility.

2. Morphine 15-20 mg or pentazocine 60 mg is given by injection to relieve the pain and anxiety; the dose can be repeated whenever necessary.

3. Passive exercises for the lower limb are started immediately to prevent deep vein thrombosis and joint stiffness.

4. Diet should be light and easily digestible. A small enema is given to relieve constipation and relieve straining at stool.

5. Anti-coagulants may be given in the hope of preventing further thrombosis both in the coronary arteries and elsewhere. Their value is not proved. The patient must be in hospital where laboratory facilities are available for prothrombin time estimation.

6. Further care: after the initial period of rest the patient is gradually promoted to more and more activity and can usually return to work about 3 months later, unless the work is heavy or the infarction has produced extensive heart damage. Obesity must be reduced and smoking stopped.

HEART FAILURE   Heart failure is present when the ventricles become incapable of supplying the body with an adequate amount of blood. A ventricle called on to work harder at

Diseases of the Cardio-Vascular System

first hypertrophies, but if the demand for a greater output persists there comes a time when the hypertrophied ventricle can hypertrophy no more, itself receiving an inadequate amount of blood, and in consequence starts to fail.

Left ventricular failure

This is usually the result of:
(a) hypertension,
(b) disease of the coronary arteries, myocardial infarction.
(c) aortic valvular disease.

Clinical features

These are the result of increased pressure within the left atrium and pulmonary veins:

(a) *Dyspnoea:* increased effort and distress in breathing. At first this is present during severe exertion, but it becomes present on less and less exertion as ventricular failure increases.

(b) *Orthopnoea:* this is the difficulty the patient has on breathing while lying down and is relieved by sitting or standing. Hence his preference for sitting well propped up in bed or an arm-chair.

(c) *Cough and haemoptysis*

(d) *Paroyxsmal nocturnal dyspnoea* (cardiac asthma): occurs when failure is getting worse, or suddenly as a first sign of failure when failure is due to coronary thrombosis. An attack begins when the patient is asleep. He wakes with a feeling of suffocation and with dyspnoea, must sit up in bed or get out of it and rush to a window for air. He has tightness around the chest and coughs up a lot of frothy sputum, sometimes blood-streaked. An attack passes off in about an hour. Death in an attack is rare.

(e) *Pulmonary oedema:* a sign of severe failure. The patient is dyspnoeic and cyanosed and coughs up frothy blood-stained sputum. An attack may be followed by mental confusion and loss of memory.

Examination of the patient is likely to show:
(i) features of the original disease,
(ii) the patient's inability to lie flat,
(iii) fluid in the lungs,
(iv) Cheyne-Stokes breathing in late stages.

Right ventricular failure

Common causes of right ventricular failure are (a) left ventricular failure, (b) mitral valve disease, (c) thyrotoxicosis, (d) following pulmonary embolism.

Clinical features

The patient may already be showing the clinical features of left ventricular failure. He now develops:
(a) fatigue and exhaustion;
(b) dyspnoea;
(c) an enlarged, painful and tender liver; slight jaundice;
(d) oedema in ankles, sacrum, genitalia and abdominal wall;

(e)   ascites[5], pericardial effusion, pleural effusion;

(f)   cyanosis;

(g)   oliguria[6], albuminuria.

Treatment of cardiac failure

1. *Rest.* The amount of work the heart has to do is reduced by rest. The amount necessary depends on the severity of the patient's illness and his response to treatment. Most patients prefer to rest sitting up in an arm-chair; in this position any oedematous fluid tracks down into the legs away from the lungs and there is less risk of thrombosis in the deep leg veins than when the patient is nursed in bed.

2. *Reassurance.* The patient is kept as cheerful as possible. It may be necessary to give morphine 15-20 mg subcutaneously or intramuscularly to relieve distress and over-breathing.

3. *Diet.* Meals should be small and attractive. Food-intake reduction is not usually necessary unless the patient is obese or the cardiac failure severe. A low salt diet is advisable, certainly in the early days of treatment, but it is not always welcomed and persisted in by the patient. Fluid-intake need not be reduced. Alcohol is allowed in moderation.

Smoking should be discouraged.

4. *Drugs*

(a)   *Digitalis* improves failing heart muscles, causes the heart to contract more powerfully, and increases the output of blood with each contraction. The heart becomes smaller; venous congestion is reduced; the output of urine is increased; oedema is reduced.

Preparations of the drug in use are:

(i)   *digoxin:* initial dose 1 mg intramuscularly or intravenously; followed by 0.5 - 0.75 mg until digitalisation has been achieved; total dose not more than 4 mg.

(ii)   *digitoxin:* initial dose 1-1.5 mg in divided doses; maintenance dose: 0.05 - 0.2 mg daily.

The usual technique is to give digitalis in large amounts at first in order to produce a rapid 'digitalization' of the heart and then, when the pulse rate has fallen to 70-80 per minute, to reduce the dose to an amount sufficient to keep the heart under control. Administration by mouth is usually adequate. In emergencies digoxin and digitoxin can be given intravenously, but not to a patient who has had any preparation of digitalis by mouth during the preceding fortnight.

The nurse should be on the look-out for signs of overdosage by digitalis. Loss of appetite is the first sign and is likely to be followed by nausea, vomiting, headache and diarrhoea. Excessive slowing of the heart, coupling of the beats, extra-systoles and paroxysmal tachycardia are indications of a serious depression of the heart's action.

The patient may notice that everything he sees looks yellow (xanthopsia). Toxic signs can persist for several days after the drug has been stopped. They are particularly likely to occur in old people.

[5] *ascites:* fluid in the peritoneal cavity
[6] *oliguria:* reduction in the amount of urine formed

Lantoside C is another drug with actions similar to the preparations of digitalis.

(b)   *Diuretics* are drugs that increase the production of urine. They are indicated when the patient has oedema. Among those used are:

chlorothiazide (Saluric): 200 mg-2 g daily for 4-5 days and then on alternate days.

chlothalidone (Hygroton): 100-200 mg 2 or 3 times a week.

ethacrynic acid (Edecrin): 50 mg, increasing to 200 mg daily by mouth; 50-100 mg by intramuscular injection.

frusemide (Lasix): 25-300 mg daily by mouth; 20-60 mg by intramuscular or intravenous injection.

Excessive secretion of urine can cause a serious loss of potassium, which has to be replaced by potassium chloride or citrate by mouth.

5. *Oxygen* is given by mask or tent when there is a reduction in the usual amount of oxygen in the arterial blood and the patient is cyanosed.

6. *Venesection* reduces venous pressure and relieves congestion; 350-750 ml of blood are withdrawn at a time from the antecubital vein in the arm.

7. If these measures do not reduce the oedema and relieve congestion, it may be necessary to tap the pleural and peritoneal cavities to remove the fluid in them. Occasionally the oedematous fluid in the legs has to be allowed to drain away through multiple incisions in the skin.

SHOCK
This is a condition in which there is a sudden severe fall in cardiac output. It is likely to be produced by:

(a)   severe injury, haemorrhage, burning, crushing;

(b)   cardiac infarction;

(c)   other severe sudden illness, such as perforation of the stomach or intestine, pancreatitis, peritonitis, pulmonary embolism, or massive septicaemia.

There is depression of all vital functions. Syncope may occur, but usually the patient, although collapsed, does not lose consciousness. He may be restless or lie still. The pulse is rapid and feeble, the skin pale and clammy, the BP is low.

Treatment
Shock is an acute medical emergency — to be prevented if possible, to be treated promptly and efficiently if it occurs. The patient should be put to bed or made comfortable. Pain is relieved by morphine given intramuscularly. Shock due to injury or haemorrhage requires a transfusion of blood, plasma or dextran; if these are not available, saline or glucose saline is given as a temporary measure.

SYNCOPE
Syncope is a sudden short interruption of consciousness due to a sudden circulatory failure, which may be:

(a)   physiological fainting, occuring when the patient is standing up, or

(b)   pathological due to haemorrhage, heart disease or disease of the autonomic nervous system.

Fainting (vaso-vagal syndrome) is a common form of syncope caused by lack of vaso-motor control of the blood-vessels with the blood-vessels in the muscles becoming dilated and the BP in consequence failing. Precipitating causes are prolonged standing, emotional stress, stuffy atmosphere, pregnancy, etc. The patient feels faint, goes pale, sweats, breathes quickly, has a slow pulse; unconsciousness lasts for only a few seconds. Convulsions, shock, and death may occur if there is a serious organic cause of the condition and the syncope is prolonged.

Postural hypotension is a fall in BP when the patient stands up. It is due to a failure of the normal mechanism whereby blood-vessels are constricted and BP is maintained. It can occur in some chronic diseases of the nervous system and when the sympathetic nervous system (which maintains tone in the blood-vessels) is interfered with by bilateral sympathetectomy. Pressure on the carotid sinus by a tumour, by throttling or by a sharp movement of the neck can cause a fall in BP and syncope. It is a common side-effect of anti-hypertensive drugs.

Syncope due to cardiac disease can occur when there is a disturbance of normal heart rhythm, in heart-block, in cardiac infarction and other severe cardiac disease.

Treatment	The patient should lie flat. Fainting usually stops spontaneously within a few seconds. Drugs such as ephedrine or amphetamine are used in chronic syncope to prevent attacks by their action in constricting blood-vessels.

ACUTE PULMONARY EMBOLISM

In this condition the pulmonary artery or one of its branches is suddenly blocked by a clot of blood that has become detached either from the right side of the heart or from a large vein in the leg, pelvis or abdomen. A clot of blood can form in the heart as a result of a cardiac infarct, severe anaemia or a chronic wasting disease such as cancer. A clot can form in a vein of the leg, pelvis or abdomen as a result of prolonged immobility, fever, operation, injury, or childbirth; a clot that becomes detached from any of these sites will pass up the inferior vena cava, through the right atrium and ventricle into the pulmonary artery and there stick. It will block, according to its size, the pulmonary artery or one of its branches. Multiple small emboli can eventually build up a large obstruction.

Clinical features

The patient collapses on the spot with severe post-sternal pain, which may suggest he is having a coronary thrombosis. He can die on the spot. If he survives the onset, he is likely to have air-hunger, signs of right ventricular dilatation and failure, pleurisy, cough, haemoptysis, enlarged pulsating veins in the neck, and an enlarged tender liver.

Death is common: about 80 per cent of patients with this condition die on the spot or within a few hours or days.

Prevention

It is of the utmost importance to prevent this condition. Any patient immobilized in bed should have frequent changes of posture and have both passive and active leg movements whenever his condition allows it. During operation tissues must be handled gently. If in spite of all care thrombosis in the veins does develop, it must be checked by anti-coagulants. In severe or recurrent cases, the femoral or iliac vein or the inferior vena cava may have to be tied.

69   *Diseases of the Cardio-Vascular System*

Treatment	1. The patient is nursed flat in order to maintain his cerebral circulation while his BP is low.
	2. Oxygen is given with a mask or tent.
	3. Morphine 15-20 mg is given to relieve pain.
	4. If a thoracic team is on the spot, the clot can be removed by operation, but this heroic measure is rarely possible and has a high death-rate.

COR PULMONALE

Other name: pulmonary heart disease
This can be caused by:
chronic bronchitis, emphysema, asthma;
any condition causing fibrosis of lung (e.g. a pneumoconiosis);
severe chest deformities   obesity
primary sclerosis of the pulmonary arterioles.

Patients are very often those pulmonary characters — heavy smokers living in a dirty atmosphere unaffected by smokeless-zone regulations. Increasing failure of pulmonary function leads to an increase in pressure in the pulmonary arteries, hypertrophy and then dilatation of the right ventricle, failure of the tricuspid valve, hypertrophy and then dilatation of the right atrium, and finally right-sided heart failure. An acute pulmonary infection is likely to produce a disaster.

Clinical features

The patient will already have the clinical features of chronic lung disease. These will now become worse; he will show more and more respiratory embarassment — shortness of breath, cyanosis, cough, haemoptysis, and then enlargement of the heart, congestive heart failure, enlarged veins in the neck, an enlarged tender liver, clubbing of the fingers. An infection makes everything worse. Death within a year is likely, but treatment may prolong life and relieve symptoms.

Treatment

1. Rest in bed is necessary during an acute phase.
2. An appropriate antibiotic is given for any infection of the lung.
3. Oxygen in tent or by mask is necessary in any cyanotic emergency.
4. Appropriate treatment is given for heart failure.
5. In emergencies, such as an acute infection, tracheostomy and artificial respiration are necessary.
6. The patient should stop smoking. If possible, he should move into a smokeless zone. Obesity should be reduced by slimming.

PULMONARY
HYPERTENSION

Normally the BP in the pulmonary arteries is not higher than: systolic 30 mm, diastolic 15 mm, of mercury. Hypertension in them can be due to:
(a)   mitral valve stenosis, with increased pressure in the left atrium and the pulmonary veins,
(b)   any congenital lesion of the heart in which there is a shunt of blood from the left to the right side — atrial septal defect, ventricular septal defect, ductus arteriosus,
(c)   blocking of small branches of the pulmonary artery by multiple emboli which

have become detached from a venous thrombus in pelvis, abdomen or leg, usually during the puerperium[7],

(d)   a narrowing of the pulmonary arterioles (cause uncertain, possibly a collagen disease).

Clinical features   The patient is likely to have a cough, dyspnoea, syncope and angina pectoris, especially on exertion. Signs of hypertrophy and eventually of failure of the right ventricle appear.

Treatment   The treatment is that of the primary condition. Anti-coagulants are given for pulmonary emboli.

DISEASES OF THE HEART VALVES   The types of heart valve disease are:

mitral stenosis
aortic stenosis
tricuspid valve disease.

mitral regurgitation
aortic regurgitation
pulmonary stenosis or incompetence

Mitral stenosis   This is the most common of the diseases of the heart valves. It is almost always due to a previous attack of acute rheumatism (rheumatic fever, chorea); rarely is it

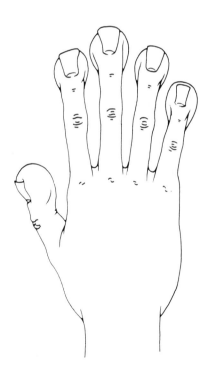

Fig. 17. Clubbing of the fingers.

[7] *puerperium*; period of time after childbirth until uterus and other tissues have returned to normal

congenital. The valve is fibrosed, thickened and hardened and presents an obstruction, of varying degree, to the normal flow of blood through the valve from left atrium to left ventricle. There is an increase of pressure in the pulmonary circulation and eventually, if the condition is progressive, in the right ventricle with the production of congestive heart failure.

The patient usually has a typical 'malar flush' — a patch of congestion in the cheek over each malar bone. He is likely to be short of breath, have a cough, develop bronchitis and bring up blood-streaked sputum. On auscultation of the heart a number of abnormal murmurs are heard.

In some patients the stenosis is slight and does not progress. A patient with a severe, untreated stenosis is not likely to live beyond 50. There is always a risk of subacute bacterial endocarditis.

Special tests

ECG: to show atrial fibrillation, right ventricular hypertrophy.
X-ray of heart: likely to show dilated pulmonary arteries, ventricular hypertrophy.

Complications

atrial fibrillation

congestive heart failure

pulmonary oedema

subacute bacterial endocarditis

thrombi in left atrium (liable to break off and form emboli in the systemic circulation)

thrombi in deep leg veins (liable to break off and form emboli in the pulmonary circulation)

Treatment

1. A mild case requires no treatment, the patient himself reducing exertion to what is tolerable.

2. All other cases must be considered for surgery -- for mitral valvotomy (division of the valve) or its replacement by a synthetic valve. Contra-indications to surgery are age under 20 (rheumatic changes likely to be continuing) or over 65, active rheumatic disease, subacute bacterial endocarditis, uncontrolled atrial fibrillation, heart failure.

3. Appropriate treatment is given for atrial fibrillation and congestive heart failure.

4. Benzyl procaine penicillin 600,000 units are given twice daily for 5 days while a patient is undergoing dental extraction, tonsillectomy or other operations in which there is a risk of causing subacute bacterial endocarditis.

Mitral regurgitation

In this condition the mitral valve is enlarged and incompetent, blood passing backwards, with each cardiac contraction, from left ventricle into left atrium. Regurgitation is often associated with stenosis. Incompetence of the valve can be due to dilatation of the right atrium as a result of acute rheumatism, or to dilatation of the left ventricle as a result of hypertension or aortic valve disease.

Disability is usually slight. An abnormal murmur is likely to be heard during systole. No special treatment is indicated.

Aortic stenosis

This can be congenital or due to rheumatism or atheroma of the valve. The fibrosed, narrow, puckered valve can in time become calcified.

As a result of the extra work it has to do in driving blood through a narrowed stiff opening, the left ventricle hypertrophies; later, when the work becomes too much, it dilates and left sided heart failure sets in.

Clinical features The patient may not show any symptoms before the start of dilatation and failure. He may be short of breath on exertion and have paroxysmal dyspnoea at night. The reduction of blood-supply to the heart is likely to cause attacks of angina pectoris and fainting. A 'thrill' can be felt when the hand is placed over the pre-cordium[8] and a murmur can be heard.

Special tests *ECG:* will show evidence of left ventricular hypertrophy.
X-ray of heart: is likely to show ventricular hypertrophy and sometimes calcification in the aortic valve.

Treatment Surgical division of the stenosis and valve-replacement have been attempted. Treatment is otherwise by moderation in physical activity, rest periods, the treatment of angina pectoris and heart failure, and appropriate penicillin cover when an operation is pending (see mitral stenosis).

Aortic regurgitation In aortic regurgitation an incompetent aortic valve allows blood to pass in the wrong direction during systole. The amount of blood that can return in this way may amount to half the stroke-output (i.e. the output from the ventricle with each contraction). The left ventricle has to hypertrophy to make this return good and can in time fail.

The common causes are:
acute rheumatism (in Britain)
syphilis of the aorta.

Less common causes are hypertension, rupture of an atheromatous valve-cusp, subacute bacterial endocarditis, a congenital lesion of the valve.

Clinical features A slight degree of aortic regurgitation causes few or no symptoms. With greater degrees and the onset of ventricular failure, the patient is likely to develop dyspnoea on exertion, attacks of dyspnoea at night, and angina pectoris. The pulse is a tap, collapsing rapidly as some of the blood falls back into the left ventricle and the rest rushes on into the dilated arterioles. The heart shows left ventricular hypertrophy and a distinctive murmur is audible during diastole, due to the rush of the blood back through the valve.

A patient can live for years with a mild degree of this disability, but if heart failure develops the expectation of life is not more than 3 years.

Complications Heart failure
Subacute bacterial endocarditis.

Treatment The only effective treatment is a replacement of the defective valve by an efficient plastic one.

[8] *precordium:* part of the chest-wall in front of the heart

Diseases of the Cardio-Vascular System

The patient should live within his cardiac limits. Heart-failure is treated appropriately. If the condition is due to syphilis, anti-syphilitic treatment is given but will not cure the leak. To prevent subacute bacterial endocarditis, penicillin cover is given when teeth are taken out or ENT operations performed.

Tricuspid valve disease

The tricuspid valve (between right atrium and right ventricle) can be stenosed or incompetent. Both these states can be a result of acute rheumatism. Incompetence can be caused by stretching of the periphery of the valve in a general dilatation of the right side of the heart. Stenosis is sometimes congenital.

The clinical features are those of a progressive congestive heart failure, for which the usual treatment is given.

INFECTIVE ENDOCARDITIS

This is an infection of the endocardium by certain organisms — most commonly the *streptococcus viridans* (a normal inhabitant of mouth and throat), sometimes other kinds of streptococci, staphylococci, other micro-organisms, fungi. The infection occurs in a heart that has a congenital lesion or a valve damaged by an attack of rheumatic fever; rarely does it affect a healthy heart. The infection follows a bacteriaemia — a transient occurrence of micro-organisms in the blood, as after dental extraction or surgical operation. The organisms invade the heart valves, setting up an inflammation; vegetations (outgrowths of inflammatory tissue) appear on the edge of the infected valve-cusps; being soft, the vegetations easily break off and bits of them can be swept along in the blood-stream to form emboli in the systemic or pulmonary circulations. Most cases occur over the age of 50. The infection can occur as a terminal infection in a dying patient.

Clinical features

The patient feels vaguely ill, is listless, and loses his appetite. He runs a slight temperature. He is anaemic and develops a 'café-au-lait' complexion. The spleen may be enlarged. Later clubbed fingers and heart failure can develop.

The emboli produce typical features of the disease:
(a)   in the skin: tiny, tender, red spots;
(b)   under the nails: thin 'splinter' haemorrhages (they can occur in normal people and in uncomplicated rheumatic endocarditis);
(c)   in the kidneys: haematuria, renal failure;
(d)   in the retinae: tiny haemorrhages, papilloedema;
(e)   in the lungs: fever, patchy consolidation, recurrent pulmonary infarction, pleurisy;
(f)   in the brain: hemiplegia, mental changes.

The death-rate is about 30 per cent. Death is usually due to perforation of a valve, embolism, rupture of an aneurysm or renal failure.

Special tests

Blood-culture: for diagnosis and sensitivity-tests of organisms.
ESR: raised.   *RBC and HB:* low.
White cell count: leucocytosis.

Prevention

Patients at risk, (those with a congenital or rheumatic lesion of the heart) should be given 'penicillin umbrella' protection if they have to have a dental or surgical operation. Procaine benzyl penicillin 600,000 units or some other form of penicillin is given twice daily for 1 day before operation and 3 days afterwards. People at risk should practise good oral hygiene.

Treatment	The patient is given full bed-rest. A course of antibiotic treatment is given for at least 6 weeks or until the patient becomes afebrile, the ESR has fallen to normal, and blood-cultures are persistently negative. Penicillin is the usual antibiotic used. Streptomycin may have to be given as well or the antibiotic to which the organism is sensitive. Treatment for heart-failure may be required. As relapse can occur the patient should be followed up for several months.

ACUTE MYOCARDITIS	Acute myocarditis can be due to: (a) virus infection — especially influenza virus, Coxsackie virus, echoviruses; (b) infective mononucleosis; (c) any of the acute infectious diseases of childhood.
Clinical features	Myocarditis produces a rapid and irregular action of the heart, and muscular pain. Pericarditis can occur with or without a pericardial effusion. Complete recovery is usual, but sudden death can occur.
Special tests	ECG shows various abnormalities.
Treatment	There is no specific treatment. Sodium salicylate is given if the patient has pericarditis. Prolonged inactivity is probably bad for convalescent patients, for whom a course of graded exercises is advisable.

PERICARDITIS	Pericarditis is an inflammation of the pericardium. It may be (a) dry — without an effusion (b) with effusion (fluid in the pericardial cavity) (c) constrictive — with fibrosis and calcification. Common causes of pericarditis are:

rheumatic fever   tuberculosis
septicaemia and other infections   collagen disease
cardiac infarction   cancer of bronchus
uraemia

The term benign or idiopathic pericarditis is given to a pericarditis of unknown origin, occurring at any age, usually mild, clearing up spontaneously, sometimes recurring.

In *dry pericarditis* the inflamed, roughened, shaggy surfaces of the pericardial layers, rub together with each cardiac movement. In addition to the features of the original disease, the patient is now likely to develop pain in the precordial region or in the neck or shoulder. The inflamed surfaces may be heard or felt to rub together.

In *pericarditis with effusion* fluid is poured out into the pericardial cavity. With a large effusion, cardiac function is embarrassed — the increased pressure within the cavity compresses the venae cavae and prevents the return of blood to the heart; cardiac output is reduced. The patient is likely to complain of precordial discomfort; the apex-beat is displaced and the area of cardiac dullness to percussion is increased. The pericardial rub may persist or disappear when there is an effusion.

Rheumatic pericarditis occurs in about 10 per cent of patients with rheumatic fever. Pyogenic pericarditis can be the result of septicaemia, pneumonia or a staphylococcal infection. Tuberculous pericarditis can produce a blood-stained fluid. A cardiac infarction, involving pericardium as well as myocardium, can produce a small dry pericarditis. Pericarditis can occur in the terminal stages of uraemia or follow invasion of the pericardium by a cancer of the bronchus.

Constrictive pericarditis is usually the result of tuberculosis, never of rheumatic fever. The pericardium becomes fibrosed and then calcified. This greatly embarrasses the heart, limits cardiac movements, and produces clinical features similar to those of congestive heart failure — venous congestion, dyspnoea, ascites, hepatic congestion and eventually cirrhosis.

Special test
X-ray of heart: in pericardial effusion the heart-shadow is typically pear-shaped and enlarged; in constrictive pericarditis patches of calcification (when the disease has progressed so far) become visible.

Treatment
1. Treatment for the original condition is necessary.
2. A very large effusion may have to be tapped if it is interfering with cardiac function.
3. In constrictive pericarditis, surgical removal of the tissue is performed. Chemotherapeutic cover for tuberculosis is advisable.

HYPERTENSION
Other name: high blood-pressure
The level of the BP depends normally on (a) the output of the heart and (b) the resistance of the arterioles. The normal BP of a young person at rest is about 120/80; by the age of 60 it may have risen to about 150/90. A BP that is persistently raised above the normal is usually the result of:
essential hypertension,
renal disease.

Rare causes of hypertension are coarctation of the aorta, Cushing' syndrome, phaeochromocytoma, and obstruction of a renal artery.

Essential hypertension
The cause is unknown. Heredity would appear to be a factor. Possibly it is not a disease but the absolutely top limit of the normal BP. The tone of the arterioles increases; this reduces their size and increases the resistance of the arterioles to the flow of blood. The arterioles eventually degenerate.

Clinical features
A moderate degree of hypertension may not cause any symptoms and the subject can live a life of average length. In some young people the pressure can fall to normal without treatment. Severe degrees are likely to affect the cardio-vascular system.

(a)   *Heart:* the left ventricle hypertrophies in order to overcome the peripheral resistance and in time can fail. Hypertension is the commonest cause of heart disease and of death from it.

(b)   *Cerebral arteries* are involved in the increased tone and the degeneration. The patient is likely to have headaches and may die of cerebral haemorrhage. A *hypertensive encephalopathy* is an acute condition brought on by a sudden increase in an already high BP: the patient is likely to have confusion, disturbed speech, transient paralysis, fits and unconsciousness.

(c)   *Retinal arteries* (visible with an ophthalmoscope): likely to become narrow and tortuous, and to press on the veins; haemorrhages and papilloedema can occur.

(d)   *Kidneys:* the renal arteries are involved; albumin may be excreted; renal failure is unusual.

Malignant hypertension

An extreme form of hypertension, with the diastolic pressure over 140 mm of mercury, occurs mostly in young and middle-aged men. Renal failure is common and death probable within 3 years of onset.

Complications

Left-sided heart failure   Renal failure
Hypertensive encephalopathy   Cerebral haemorrhage.

Treatment

Hypertension is treated (a) to relieve symptoms and (b) to prevent deterioration and cardiovascular disease.

Several drugs which reduce blood-pressure are available.

Mild degrees of hypertension are usually treated with guanethidine sulphate by mouth in doses of 10 mg daily, increased by 10 mg daily every 5-7 days until a satisfactory fall of BP is achieved, up to a maximum of 300 mg daily in divided doses. Side-effects of the drug are diarrhoea and postural hypotension.

Malignant hypertension, hypertensive encephalopathy and left ventricular failure due to hypertension are treated with intravenous or intramuscular injections of guanethidine sulphate, and when pressure has fallen to a safer level by the same drug given by mouth. Methyldopa, diazoxide or clonidine may be given by injection, with or without diuretics, instead of guanethidine.

Tolerance to drugs can occur. Patients have to be convinced of the need to take the drugs by mouth as they tend to default when symptoms are relieved.

ATHEROMA

Atheroma is the commonest form of arterial degeneration. Beginning in early adult life, it gradually involves more and more arteries. The aorta and its branches, the arteries of the limbs, the arteries of the heart, brain and kidneys are all likely to be involved, especially where arteries divide.

Atheroma begins as small patches of degeneration in the intima, the inner lining of an artery, usually first in the places most exposed to stress — the aorta and its large branches and the place where an artery divides. The degenerating areas form a rough, raised yellowish-grey patch, which may ulcerate and gradually spread and thicken, obstructing the flow of blood and eventually stopping it altogether.

Thrombi are likely to form on the rough surface of the patch; bits of these thrombi can become detached and pass on to block a smaller vessel or a big thrombus can block the artery in which it has formed.

Atheroma is thus a cause of gangrene, of cerebral vascular disease, of ischaemic heart disease (angina pectoris, cardiac infarction), and other diseases. It is a complication of diabetes mellitus and nephrosis.

The cause of atheroma is obscure. An accumulation of lipids has suggested that the disease is in part due to an over-consumption of lipids (lipoids), particularly cholesterol. Atheroma is most common in countries where large amounts of animal fats are eaten and least common in countries where vegetable fats rather than meat fats are eaten. At present this high-cholesterol theory is unproved. Atheroma is more likely to be present in smokers than non-smokers.

Treatment It is occasionally possible to remove surgically part of a large atheromatous artery and replace it with a graft. There is otherwise no specific treatment for atheroma. A fat patient should be slimmed; a smoker should stop smoking. It would be advisable to reduce the consumption of fat meat.

ACUTE ARTERIAL BLOCKING

Other name: acute arterial occlusion

A main artery can become suddenly blocked by:

(a)   a clot of blood that has become detached from the left atrium in a heart affected by mitral stenosis or atrial fibrillation,

(b)   a detached vegetation in subacute bacterial endocarditis,

(c)   a detached thrombus after a cardiac infarction,

(d)   the clotting of blood on an atheromatous patch.

The embolus cuts off the blood-supply. If there is a good collateral supply, the affected part will recover, but when there is not a good collateral supply, the tissues are likely to die.

Clinical features The patient is smitten suddenly with severe pain in the affected part, which becomes pale and cold; sensation and function are impaired. The arterial pulse cannot be felt beyond the block.

Treatment 1. The affected part is kept cool (to reduce its demands for oxygen) while the rest of the body is warmed (e.g. by an electric blanket) to promote reflex dilatation of vessels.

2. Anti-coagulants are given.

3. Embolectomy is performed if these measures do not restore the circulation within 4 hours.

DISSECTING ANEURYSM OF THE AORTA

In this condition, following a degeneration of the middle layer of the aorta, a split forms in the wall of the aorta and blood is forced down inside it. The tear usually starts in the thoracic aorta and can go down to the bifurcation of the aorta or upwards towards the heart. The

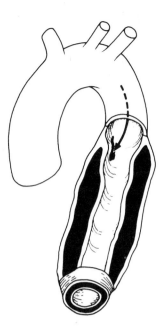

Fig. 18. Dissecting aneurysm of the aorta, blood forcing its way within the wall of the aorta.

patient, usually an old man, may have hypertension and atheroma, but the atheroma is not the cause of the tear. There is a high incidence of the condition in Marfan's syndrome[9].

Clinical features

The patient is seized with an agonizing pain in the chest, spreading to the back. He is likely to have shock and die quickly. He may improve for a short time only to die later of rupture into the pericardium. Only a few patients survive.

Treatment

Morphine or pentazocine is given for the relief of pain.

SYPHILIS OF THE AORTA

Syphilis affects the aorta in the tertiary (third) stage of the infection, usually 5-30 years after the primary infection. The disease is most common in men of 30-60 years. The small vasa vasorum (the tiny arteries that supply the wall of an artery with blood) become involved in a syphilitic inflammation, which eventually obliterates them. The effects of this are: (a) elastic tissue is replaced by fibrous tissue; (b) the weakened aorta stretches; (c) stretching of the aortic ring to which the cusps of the valve are attached causes aortic regurgitation; and (d) in some patients the weakened wall stretches so much that an aneurysm is formed. The cusps of the aortic valve can become involved and thickened. The intima, the internal lining of the aorta, shows inflammatory and degenerative changes, and as this is very likely to occur in the lower part of the ascending aorta, just above the aortic valve, the openings of the coronary artery become blocked and the patient develops ischaemic heart disease.

Congenital syphilis does not usually cause aortitis.

[9] *Marfan's syndrome:* a congenital anomaly; patient has long thin bones, spider-like fingers and toes, hypotonic muscles, little body fat; may also have congenital lesions of heart

The disease has probably been present for months or years before the first symptoms appear. The patient is then likely to complain of a dull ache behind the sternum and then to have attacks of angina pectoris. Aortic incompetence leads to left-sided heart failure. Signs of tertiary syphilis may be found in other parts of the body.

Syphilitic aneurysm of the aorta

In this extreme form of syphilitic aortitis, the weakened fibrosed wall of the aorta bulges out in a thin-walled sac. This happens usually to the ascending aorta and the arch, but it can happen in the descending aorta and any of the major branches of the aorta. It is predominantly a disease of men engaged in heavy manual work.

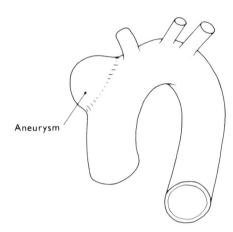

Aneurysm

Fig. 19. An aneurysm of the arch of the aorta.

The sac bulging forwards causes pain in the front of the chest, and eroding the chest-wall can present as a pulsating swelling under the skin. It can press backwards and eroding the vertebral column cause severe pain in the back. It can press on the trachea and bronchi, producing a 'brassy' cough and collapse of a lung; it can press on the oesophagus and cause difficulty in swallowing; it can press on the left recurrent laryngeal nerve (which hooks round under the arch of the aorta) and produce hoarseness; it can press on the great veins and cause venous obstruction in the neck. Eventually it can rupture through the skin or into an internal organ or tissue and so kill the patient.

Special tests

Blood: WR and Kahn test positive in most cases.
X-ray of chest: shows aortic dilatation and aneurysm if present; may also show syphilitic calcification of the aorta.

The outlook for life for patients with syphilitic aortitis is very variable. With early treatment the outlook is good, but if gross structural changes have occurred nothing can be done to put them right. The patient may die suddenly from complete blocking of a coronary artery. A syphilitic aneurysm may progress rapidly and burst, but in another patient the aneurysm may appear to be stationary for several years.

Treatment

Antisyphilitic treatment is given.

First potassium iodide 500 mg is given three times a day for three weeks. This should cause inflammatory changes to subside and prevent the occurrence of a

Herxheimer reaction[1] when penicillin is given. If such a reaction did take place, the coronary arteries might be suddenly blocked and the patient killed. A course of penicillin is then given — usually 1 million units daily for 14 days. If the WR and Kahn test have not become normal in 3 months a second course of treatment is given.

GIANT CELL
ARTERITIS

Other name: temporal arteritis.
This is a chronic degeneration of arteries of unknown origin, mostly commonly affecting branches of the external carotid artery. It gets its name from the large multi-nucleated cells found in the degenerating tissue. It occurs over the age of 60.

Clinical features

Headache in the distribution of a temporal or occipital artery is almost always present. The arteries are tender and sometimes nodular, and the skin over them may be red. Pain in the face, jaw and mouth is due to involvement of the facial, maxillary or lingual arteries. The patient may have fever, sweating, malaise, loss of weight, and muscular pains and weakness.

Complication

Impairment of vision or blindness, due to involvement of the arteries to the optic nerve and disc.

Special tests

ESR: raised, usually above 100 mm per hour.
Biopsy: 1 cm of the superficial temporal artery is excised and examined microscopically.

Treatment

Corticosteroids are given quickly and in high doses, e.g. prednisone 60 mg daily for 3 days, followed by 20 mg daily for 6-12 months, according to patient's response and ESR. Smaller maintenance doses may be required indefinitely.

RAYNAUD'S
SYNDROME [2]

This is a condition in which the arteries to the fingers (and less commonly to the toes, cheeks, ears and nose) go into spasm. It occurs in:
(a)   collagen disease;
(b)   young women who are hypersensitive to cold;
(c)   some blood diseases;
(d)   syringomyelia;
(e)   cervical rib;
(f)   butchers, fishmongers and people using vibrating tools, as an occupational disease.
　　　Women are affected ten times more often than men. In severe cases the arteries degenerate.

[1] *Herxheimer reaction:* an acute reaction that can take place when syphilis is first treated
　　　　　　　　with penicillin etc.
[2] *M. Raynaud* (1834-81): French physician

Attacks of spasm occur. They cause the fingers and hands to go cold, white and pulseless; sensation is impaired and fine movements cannot be performed accurately. In time the spasm passes off and then the affected parts become blue and then red and tingle and throb. In severe cases with degeneration of the artery the tips of the fingers can develop gangrene.

Treatment

1. The patient should keep warm, wear loose gloves in cool and cold weather, and not put hands in cold water. Immersion in warm water often ends an attack.
2. Rauwolfia in small doses dilates the blood-vessels.
3. Sympathectomy can be performed. It will relieve spasm; but arterial degeneration will not be improved. Surgical amputation of the tips of the fingers may be necessary.
4. Smoking is prohibited.

THROMBO-ANGIITIS OBLITERANS [3]

Other name: Buerger's disease[4]

In this disease the arteries and veins to the legs (and less commonly those to the arms) become thickened and eventually obliterated. Once it occurred almost entirely in men, but now more women are being affected. This may be because the affected person is practically always a smoker. It begins at 25-45 years.

The patient develops intermittent claudication[5] and attacks of pain in the legs at night. With complete blocking of the blood-supply affected parts eventually become gangrenous. Deep vein thrombosis can occur. Cardiac infarction can cause sudden death. The course of the disease is usually progressive, but sometimes it stops spontaneously.

Treatment

is by stopping smoking, by the use of vaso-dilator drugs such as tolazoline 25 mg three times a day, by scrupulous care of the feet, and by sympathectomy.

VENOUS THROMBOSIS

Thrombosis is the clotting of blood within a blood-vessel.

Deep vein thrombosis (phlebo-thrombosis) is thrombosis of deep veins of the calf. It can occur:

(a)   in the course of any severe prolonged illness,
(b)   after operation or childbirth,
(c)   in heart failure,
(d)   in some cases of cancer,
(e)   in thrombo-angitis obliterans.

It is particularly liable to occur in dehydrated, seriously ill or elderly patients who do not move about in bed.

Clinical features

These may at first be slight; sometimes the first indication is a pulmonary embolism. The patient has a slight rise of temperature. He may complain of pain in the calf, which becomes swollen and tender. Dorsi-flexion of the foot is very likely to cause pain.

Complication

Pulmonary embolism from a detached part of the thrombus.

[3] *thrombus:* a clot of blood; *angiitis:* inflammation of blood-vessel
[4] *L.Buerger* (1879-1943), American physician.
[5] *intermittent claudication:* attacks of pain in calves and limping, produced by exercise, relieved by rest.

Prevention Seriously ill and elderly patients should be encouraged to move their legs as much as possible. If they cannot, passive movements should be performed. Dehydration is prevented.

Treatment If thrombosis has occurred, the affected part is kept still for fear of producing a pulmonary thrombosis; but passive movements should be performed.

A course of anti-coagulants is given (if the patient is in hospital with facilities for estimating the pro-thrombin time) until a week after the patient is free from symptoms.

Superficial vein thrombosis is less serious as pulmonary embolism hardly ever occurs, but it is occasionally an indication of a cancer somewhere in the body. The affected vein is painful and tender and can be felt as a rounded cord.

The affected part should be bandaged and rested. Anti-coagulants are not required.

Diseases of the Cardio-Vascular System

4 Diseases of the Respiratory System

Diseases of the respiratory system are conveniently divided into: (a) diseases of the upper respiratory tract — the nose, pharynx, larynx, trachea and associated structures, and (b) diseases of the lower respiratory tract — the bronchi, lungs and pleura. The division is not absolute, for disease of one can spread into and involve the other.

The most common diseases of the upper respiratory tract are relatively mild infections — such as a cold, pharyngitis, tonsillitis and laryngitis. Some of these infections can, however, have serious complications — such as a sinusitis (an infection of one of the nasal sinuses within the maxillae, frontal, ethmoid and sphenoid bones); and serious disease — such as cancer of the larynx — can occur. Common symptoms and signs of disease in the upper respiratory tract are:

cough	pyrexia
discharge from the nose	bleeding from the nose
sore throat	
hoarseness	loss of voice

Diseases of the lower respiratory tract are usually serious, for they are likely to be extensive and to impair the normal function of the lung, in the place where oxygen is absorbed into the body and carbon dioxide excreted from it. Common diseases here are infections, both acute and chronic, asthma and new growths. Symptoms and signs of disease of the lower respiratory tract are likely to be:

pyrexia		rapid respiration
cough	sputum	haemoptysis[6]
pain on breathing		cyanosis[7]

Severe chronic disease of the lungs is likely to cause a serious impairment of respiratory function and to have a damaging effect on the heart, with which the lungs are functionally closely connected.

EPISTAXIS   *Other name:* Nose-bleeding

Epistaxis is most commonly due to a punch on the nose, picking the nose, the onset of any acute infection, and — in late adult life — hypertension. Other causes are rare — new growths in the nose, leukaemia, any bleeding disease.

The bleeding usually comes from a small area near the front of the nasal septum.

[6] *haemoptysis:* coughing up blood
[7] *cyanosis:* blueness of skin and mucous membranes due to lack of oxygen in the blood

Treatment	In young people epistaxis usually stops spontaneously. If it is due to hypertension, a little blood-letting does no harm. It can usually be stopped by squeezing the nose firmly between finger and thumb for 5 minutes, the patient sitting forwards and breathing through his mouth. If this does not stop it the nose may have to be packed with ribbon-gauze. Only rarely are more heroic measures — such as post-nasal packing or a blood transfusion — required. Any nasal packing should be removed within 2 days as there is a risk of infection. If repeated bleeding is found to come from a clump of dilated vessels on the septum, the offending vessels can be sealed by electric cauterisation.

ALLERGIC RHINITIS	This is an allergic condition, the patient being sensitive to some 'allergen' in the air; the same patient may suffer from hay fever and asthma. In this particular sensitivity, the nasal mucous membrane becomes oedematous and pours out secretion. The condition is often inherited. If it begins in infancy, it may diminish in adult life, but it can begin at any later age and persist.
Clinical features	The patient complains of attacks of nasal obstruction, sneezing and a discharge from the nose, sometimes associated with conjunctival irritation and an excess of tears.
Special tests	*Transillumination and X-ray of sinuses:* may be opaque owing to thickened mucous membrane and fluid. *Nasal smears:* show excess of eosinophils (acid-staining white blood-cells).
Treatment	1. Antihistamine drugs usually control the rhinitis. 2. Any nasal polypi are removed; infected sinuses are drained; diathermy of the inferior turbinate bone relieves oedema. 3. If a specific allergen is found, desensitisation against it can be attempted.

SINUSITIS	Sinusitis is an inflammation of any of the nasal sinuses (maxillary, frontal, sphenoid or ethmoid). More than one may be affected.
	    In *acute sinusitis* the mucous membrane becomes inflamed and oedematous; the cilia, which by their movements keep the sinuses free from dust and bacteria, are immobilized; and if the outlet of the sinus into the nose becomes blocked, pus forms in the sinus. The infection can be due to a common cold, an allergic rhinitis, or to infected water being forced into a sinus when the person dives.
	    A *chronic sinusitis* follows an acute sinusitis, when the acute condition is not completely cleared up, possibly because the patient has a physical defect in his nose — a deviation of the septum markedly to one side, an enlarged inferior turbinate bone, a polyp (a small benign growth, several of which may be present); any of these can stop drainage from an infected sinus. A chronic sinusitis of the maxillary sinus (antrum) can be caused by a dental abscess from one of the teeth just below it in the upper jaw.

Clinical features   In *acute sinusitis* the patient has stuffiness of the nose, a nasal discharge, and a headache made worse by stooping. He gets pain over the affected sinus if its exit into the nose is blocked. A maxillary sinusitis can cause toothache in adjoining teeth. A frontal or ethmoid sinusitis causes headache, pain in and around the eyes, and oedema of the eyelids.

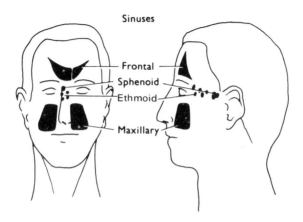

Sinuses

Frontal
Sphenoid
Ethmoid
Maxillary

Fig. 20. The position of the nasal air-sinuses.

In *chronic sinusitis* there may be persistent headache and some nasal catarrh, and there often is an associated tonsillitis, laryngitis or bronchitis.

Complications of frontal and ethmoidal sinusitis
Infections of the orbit, osteomyelitis
Meningitis, cerebral abscess, cavernous sinus thrombosis.

Special tests   *Transillumination and X-ray of sinus:* shows opacity due to thickened mucous membrane, fluid or pus.

Treatment   In *acute sinusitis* the patient should go to bed. He is given nasal decongestant sprays followed by nasal inhalations every 4 hours. Pain is relieved by acetyl-salicylic acid (aspirin) or other analgesic. Antibiotics are given for severe or potentially dangerous infections. In *chronic sinusitis* it is important that an affected sinus should be free to discharge into the nose, if necessary a new hole is made for drainage, a deviated septum is straightened, polyps and enlarged turbinates are removed.

TONSILLITIS   This common infection of children and young adults is usually due to a haemolytic streptococcus and spread by droplets; milk, when not pasteurized can be the means of spread.

Clinical features   The child complains of sore throat, difficulty in swallowing, and feverishness. The temperature can be raised to 39.5°C. (103°F.). Lymph-nodes in the neck are likely to be enlarged and inflamed. Earache is usually 'referred' from the tonsils, but the ear-drum is inspected, for the pain can be due to acute otitis media.

The tonsils are swollen, reddened and perhaps exuding pus, and adjacent parts of the fauces are likely to be inflamed and coated with mucus.

It is important to distinguish acute tonsillitis from diphtheria, which is rare in countries where immunization programmes have been carried out. In diphtheria there is a characteristic smell in the breath, the membrane — the congealed exudate — spreads from the tonsils on to the fauces, cannot be removed easily and when removed leaves a raw bleeding surface behind it.

Complications	Chronic tonsillitis	Adenoids, enlargement of
	Quinsy	Acute otitis media
	Acute rheumatism	Acute nephritis

Treatment   The patient should go to bed until he is better. Acetyl-salicylic acid relieves pain and inflammation. Only in severe cases, when glands are very enlarged or complications develop, is it necessary to use an antibiotic.

CHRONIC
TONSILLITIS   Recurrent attacks of tonsillitis can occur, with the tonsils and cervical lymph-nodes becoming chronically enlarged and the adenoids causing obstruction.

Treatment   If the tonsils are grossly enlarged, acute attacks recur, adenoids are troublesome, and particularly if attacks of acute otitis media occur, the tonsils are removed.

ADENOIDS   The adenoids are the naso-pharyngeal tonsil, a pad of lymph tissue on the roof and posterior wall of the naso-pharynx. Healthy ones atrophy and vanish in early adult

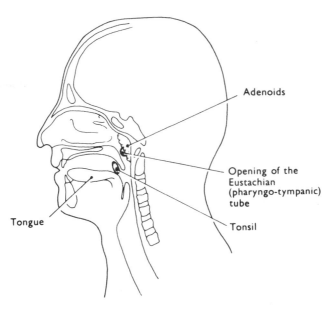

Fig. 21. Section of the head showing how the opening of the Eustachian (pharyngo-tympanic) tube can become obstructed by overgrowth of the adenoids.

Adenoids

Opening of the Eustachian (pharyngo-tympanic) tube

Tongue

Tonsil

Diseases of the Respiratory System

life, but chronic infection and hypertrophy can occur in childhood and diseased ones persist.

Clinical features   The child has nasal obstruction and becomes a mouth-breather. He is likely to have a nasal whine in his voice, to snore and to cough at night. Blocking of the opening into the naso-pharynx of the lower end of the auditory (eustachian) tube (the other end opens into the middle ear) is likely to cause earache and acute otitis media. The nasal sinuses can become infected and attacks of bronchitis occur; the child's general health is likely to suffer.

Treatment   This is by surgical removal at the same time as tonsillectomy is performed.

EPIGLOTTITIS   This acute infection of the epiglottis occurs in children and adults.

Clinical features   Sore throat, cough, voice changes, difficulty in swallowing and pyrexia can be followed in a few hours by laryngeal obstruction, toxaemia and death.

Treatment   Antibiotics, and a tracheotomy if symptoms of laryngeal obstruction appear.

LARYNGITIS   Laryngitis can be acute or chronic. Acute laryngitis occurs as a complication of the common cold, of measles and other acute infectious diseases, and as a non-tuberculous complication of pulmonary tuberculosis. It is an occupational risk of costermongers, auctioneers, schoolmasters, lecturers, clergymen, public speakers and singers, particularly if they have not been trained in voice-production. Chronic laryngitis follows attacks of acute laryngitis; factors in its persistence are smoking, drinking, working in stuffy, dusty, ill-ventilated rooms, and having chronic nasal infection and obstruction.

Clinical features   In acute laryngitis the patient loses his voice to a variable degree, is hoarse and has a cough and slight temperature. In chronic laryngitis there is a persistent hoarseness, aching in the throat, and loss of voice.

If laryngitis becomes chronic the throat should be examined by a laryngologist, who will look in particular for 'singer's nodes' (tiny swellings, the result of haemorrhages) and for cancer of the larynx.

Treatment   In acute laryngitis, the patient is confined to bed in a warm room with the air kept slightly moist by a steam-kettle. To rest his larynx adequately, the patient should not speak at all and be made to communicate all his needs by writing or signs. Smoking is forbidden. Steam inhalations are given 3-4 times a day; cough is relieved by codeine linctus.

Chronic laryngitis is treated by resting the voice, treating nasal or dental infection, forbidding smoking, and using saline sprays for the throat.

CANCER OF THE LARYNX   This usually occurs in middle-aged or elderly men, less commonly in women, and rarely before 30 years of age. Factors in its causation are smoking, the inhalation of dust and fumes, the consumption of alcoholic drinks especially spirits, and chronic laryngitis. The usual site of the cancer is on the anterior half of a vocal cord.

Clinical features   Hoarseness is the first and most persistent symptom, and any person who has hoarseness for more than a few weeks should be seen by a laryngologist. Later features are pain referred to the ear, difficulty in swallowing, respiratory obstruction and enlarged cervical lymph-nodes.

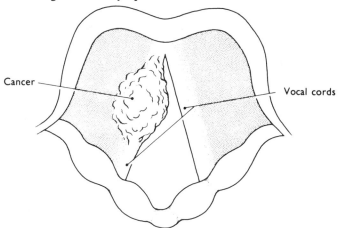

Fig. 22. A cancer of the larynx growing on a vocal cord.

Treatment   This is by radiotherapy for early cases; about 80 per cent of cases so treated are curable by radiotherapy, with full return of function to the voice. If the case is too advanced for radiotherapy, it is necessary to carry out partial laryngectomy or complete laryngectomy with block dissection of the cervical lymph-nodes. Antimetabolites and alkylating agents (fluorouracil, cyclophosphamide) are given for inoperable neck metastases. Rehabilitation by a speech-therapist is necessary after operation, and a speech-aid may be required.

FUNCTIONAL APHONIA   This is a loss of voice likely to occur in nervous women. There is usually no associated disease, but it can develop if the patient has a cold or other respiratory tract infection. The cause is usually thought to be psychological. The voice may be lost entirely or the patient may be able to speak in a faint whisper. Treatment is by reassurance that the voice will return and by alleviating if possible any psychological difficulty. Relapse is very likely.

TRACHEITIS   Tracheitis can be acute or chronic; it is usually associated with upper respiratory tract infection and bronchitis. It can be due to:
(a)   infection: by any organism that causes upper respiratory tract infection — viruses, streptococci, etc; and as a complication of influenza, measles, whooping cough, diphtheria, typhoid fever;
(b)   exposure to a foggy, cold and damp climate or working conditions;
(c)   inhalation of steam or poisonous fumes;
(d)   a foreign body in the trachea.

Clinical features   In acute tracheitis the patient runs a temperature, feels ill and has a headache. Then he develops a cough and post-sternal irritation and rawness. He has hoarseness and loss of voice if the larynx is involved. He coughs up pellets of mucus, likely to be blood-streaked. The acute symptoms subside in a few days, but the patient may be left with a persistent cough. Repeated attacks lead to a chronic tracheitis with persistent hoarseness, cough and post-sternal irritation.

Treatment   Treatment is as for laryngitis.

HAEMOPTYSIS   This is coughing up of blood: it is not a disease but a sign of disease. The amount brought up may vary from a streak in the sputum to a large amount. Death from haemoptysis is rare. Common causes are:

cancer of the lung   pulmonary tuberculosis
bronchitis   bronchiectasis   lung abscess
mitral stenosis   infarction of the lung
acute left ventricular failure.

    Haemoptysis has to be distinguished from haematemesis, the vomiting of blood. The differences are:

Haemoptysis	*Haematemesis*
1. The patient may have a history of lung or heart disease.	1. The patient may have a history of abdominal disease.
2. The patient knows he coughed.	2. The patient knows he vomited.
3. The blood is bright red and mixed with sputum.	3. The blood may be dark red and mixed with food.

Special tests   *X-ray of lung:* for evidence of pulmonary disease.
Sputum: examined for cancer cells and tuberculosis bacilli.
Bronchoscopy: if cancer of the lung is suspected.

Treatment   If the haemorrhage is severe:
1. The patient is put to bed with absolute rest, usually in the semi-propped up position.
2. If he is anxious he is reassured and can be given morphine 10-15 mg which also relieves cough.
3. For severe haemoptysis a blood transfusion is given.
4. Diet should be liquid for 24 hours and then gradually increased.

ASTHMA [8]   Asthma is characterized by attacks of wheezing and difficult breathing, due to spasm of the bronchi and the accumulation of secretion within them. It is a common condition, occurring in about 2 per cent of the British population.
    1. *Extrinsic asthma[9]* is an allergic state. Attacks begin in childhood (usually before 5 years) or adolescence. In about 70 per cent of asthmatic children attacks stop at adolescence. Before puberty, boys are, for reasons unknown, affected twice

[8] *asthma:* from Greek: *asthma* — difficult breathing
[9] *extrinsic:* arising from factors outside the body

as often as girls. There is usually a family history of allergic disease and the patient himself may have had eczema or urticaria. Sensitivity to the hair of hamsters can be a cause.

2. *Intrinsic asthma[1]* begins later in life, sometimes not before 60 or 70 years. Some attacks are precipitated by a respiratory tract infection; allergy does not seem to be an important factor. The house dust-mite (a tiny insect) is the likely cause of asthma produced by house-dust; they are present in house-dust in large numbers, especially in damp houses. In some women, especially just before the menopause, attacks precede menstruation. It can be associated with polyarteritis nodosa.

Psychological factors are important in the precipitation of attacks at any age. In children attacks seem to be precipitated by emotional stresses – such as over-protection by parents, the rejection of the child by a parent, anxiety in parents who strive for perfection in their children. In older life attacks can be precipated in stress and anxiety – by threats to security, bereavement, sex and marriage problems, financial difficulties, assaults, frights, etc. Fear of an attack of asthma is an added and justified complication.

In many patients many factors are inter-related – allergy, emotional problems, infection, exposure to cold and wet.

In an attack there is a spasm of the muscle of the bronchi. The bronchi become narrow; their mucous membrane swells; plugs of thick mucus form in them.

Clinical features Asthma occurs in paroxysms. An attack begins suddenly, often during the night, and lasts for 1-2 hours. The patient has difficulty in breathing and tightness of his chest: he wheezes, is distressed, uses all his accessory muscles of respiration to aid him, and with difficulty coughs up plugs of mucus. Exhausted after an attack he is likely to fall asleep. Between attacks he can be well; or he may have over several days a chronic wheeze with sharper bouts now and again. If attacks are frequent and severe he is likely to finish up with emphysema and chronic bronchitis. *Status asthmaticus* is a continuous asthma going on for a long time, such as for more than 24 hours, terminating in exhaustion or sometimes death.

Complications Emphysema   Chronic bronchitis
Collapse of the segment of a lung (due to obstruction of a bronchus by a plug of mucus)
Spontaneous pneumothorax   Failure of respiratory function

Special tests *Inhalation test:* to see if inhalation of a suspected allergen brings on asthma.
Skin test: a spot of a solution of a suspected allergen is put on the skin and a scratch made through it; a positive reaction is the appearance of a weal within 15 minutes.
Blood: if due to allergy, there is likely to be an increase of eosinophil granular white cells.

Prevention Attacks are likely to recur whatever is done to prevent them. Attempts at prevention are by:
(a)   taking ephedrine 30-60 mg (15 mg for young children) 2-3 times a day;
(b)   taking courses of respiratory exercises from a physiotherapist;

[1] *intrinsic:* arising from factors within the body

(c)   trying to identify an allergen and taking measures to avoid it: e.g. not giving a child milk in any form if he is sensitive to it; a housewife whose attacks are caused by house-dust has to give up house-cleaning or wear a mask when she does it; a family pet may have to be given away.

(d)   trying to desensitize a patient whose attacks are due to an identified allergen by giving him subcutaneous injections of at first very small, and then progressively larger doses of the allergen weekly until large doses produce no reaction; desensitization against pollen must not be attempted when the pollens are actually in the air; adrenaline must be available for injection during and after treatment should the patient develop any reaction.

(e)   solving emotional stresses and improving parental attitudes;

(f)   hypnosis and auto-hypnosis;

(g)   avoiding the wind and the rain;

(h)   having adequate treatment for any respiratory infection.

Treatment   (a)   Broncho-dilator drugs such as salbutamol and orciprenaline are self-administered during an attack. Patients using aerosols have to be trained in the technique, and must appreciate that overdosage is dangerous and can cause death. Oral preparations of the drugs are used for some cases.

(b)   Prednisone and prednisolone are taken by mouth in short courses when attacks do not respond to bronchodilators. Continuous corticosteroid treatment may be necessary for severe asthmatics, but it can suppress adrenal function and is a potential danger to life.

(c)   Infections known to precipitate attacks of asthma are treated with a broad-spectrum antibiotic, such as tetracycline, ampicillin and co-trimoxazole.

The treatment of status asthmaticus is by:

(a)   admission to a hospital with facilities for intensive respiratory care

(b)   corticosteroids

(c)   continuous oxygen

(d)   oro-tracheal intubation and intermittent positive-pressure ventilation, if the patient does not improve with the above treatment.

BRONCHITIS   This can be acute or chronic. The causes are the same as those of tracheitis, with which bronchitis is often associated, although when the smaller bronchi are involved the trachea may escape completely or almost completely. Attacks of bronchitis are common in infants and old people, and are particularly likely to be precipitated by cold, damp weather or 'smog'. The sufferer from chronic bronchitis is likely to belong to the lower socio-economic groups, to be a chronic cigarette smoker, and to live in urban, dirty atmospheric conditions. The death-rate from chronic bronchitis is about 20 times higher in those who smoke more than 25 cigarettes a day than it is in non-smokers.

Clinical features   Acute bronchitis begins with malaise, a sore chest, aching limbs, and a temperature which can rise to 39.5°C (103°F). The patient has a cough, dry at first and later moist. Sputum may be blood-streaked. He has a flushed face and his respiratory-rate is likely to be raised. After a few days of acute illness he starts to improve, but he is likely to be left with a persistent cough.

Chronic bronchitis may follow attacks of acute bronchitis or be a gradual development where a person is exposed to smoke and dust and fog. At first the patient develops a cough after a cold; then the cough occurs in the winter, then in winter and summer but worse in the winter, and finally is bad all the year round. He brings up sputum. With the development of emphysema and fibrosis of the lung he develops a shortness of breath that becomes progressively worse. He is likely to finish up with cor pulmonale and heart-failure.

Complications of bronchitis		
Bronchopneumonia	Lobar pneumonia	Aspiration pneumonia
Pulmonary tuberculosis	Bronchiectasis	Emphysema
Fibrosis of lung	Heart disease	

Treatment
Acute bronchitis
The patient should go to bed in a warm room. Inhalations of steam from a kettle are given every 4-6 hours. The cough is relieved by codeine linctus. Antibiotics are not usually necessary.

Chronic bronchitis
If possible the patient should live in a warm, dust-free climate, but for many this is impossible. He should give up smoking. Acute exacerbations are treated with antibiotics. Postural drainage helps to get rid of bronchial secretions.

BRONCHIECTASIS
This is a condition in which one or more of the bronchi are dilated. *Bronchiolectasis* is a dilation of the bronchioles, the branches of the bronchi.

Bronchiectasis is caused by:

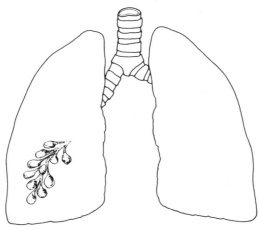

Fig. 23. Bronchiestasis as revealed by a bronchogram (the injection of a radio-opaque fluid into the respiratory tubes).

(a)   any infection of the lung (e.g. pneumonia of any kind, pulmonary tuberculosis) by causing weakness and degeneration of the wall of the bronchi;
(b)   the strain of asthma, chronic bronchitis, emphysema;
(c)   obstruction by a foreign body, a plug of mucus during an anaesthetic, a cancer, pressure on the bronchus by an enlarged lymph-node;

Diseases of the Respiratory System

(d)   chronic pleurisy, pleural adhesions;

(e)   a congenital malformation or a failure of lung-expansion after birth.

Both lungs are usually involved. The dilated bronchi usually fill up with pus, adjacent parts of the lung degenerate and abscesses form.

Clinical features   Usually the patient has had a pulmonary disease. A sudden unexplained onset would suggest that he has inhaled a foreign body.

Cough and expectoration are early symptoms. The sputum increases in amount and becomes foul-smelling. The amount brought up varies with the position of the patient. Haemoptysis can occur.

The general health can remain good until the disease becomes extensive and abscess-formation produces malaise, fever, loss of appetite and wasting. On examination affected parts of the lungs are dull to percussion, air-entry is diminished and abnormal sounds are heard. The patient is likely to have clubbed fingers.

Without treatment the condition becomes progressively worse.

Complications

Pleurisy	Empyema	Bronchopneumonia
Abscess of lung	Septicaemia	Pyaemia
Abscesses in brain and elsewhere		Septic pericarditis.

Special tests   *X-ray of lungs* is taken before and after the injection of iodized oil which will fill the dilated parts of the bronchi.
Sputum: to exclude pulmonary tuberculosis and to test for sensitivity of organisms.

Treatment   Prevention is by breathing exercises after any pulmonary infection and by the prevention of mucus or infected material getting into the lungs during an operation. Treatment is by: (a) postural drainage 1-2 times a day indefinitely; (b) antibiotic treatment for any infection; (c) surgical removal of a segment or lobe of a lung.

CANCER OF THE
BRONCHUS   *Other name:* cancer of the lung
This is the commonest form of cancer in men in Britain; it is 4 - 5 times more common in men than in women. It begins usually as a cancer of the bronchus within a couple of inches of the bifurcation of the trachea and thence spreads into the lung and elsewhere.

Factors in its cause are:

(a)   cigarette smoking: this is undoubtedly the commonest cause; the more cigarettes a person smokes the more likely is he to develop cancer of the lung;

(b)   cigar and pipe smoking;

(c)   certain industrial diseases of the lung, especially asbestosis;

(d)   possibly air pollution from petrol engines, etc; this is uncertain.

Clinical features   The patient is usually middle-aged with a history of smoking for years. He develops a persistent cough. Later he brings up sputum and is likely to have a haemoptysis. Occasionally mass radiography will reveal a tumour before it is producing symptoms. With the spread of cancer into the lung, the patient develops wheezing, pain in the chest, shortness of breath and wasting. There may be evidence of spread into other parts of the body. In the untreatable case death occurs in about 9 months.

Complications 1. Spread of the cancer into the lung and pleura: collapse of a lung-segment; lung abscess; pleural effusion; empyema, pneumonia.

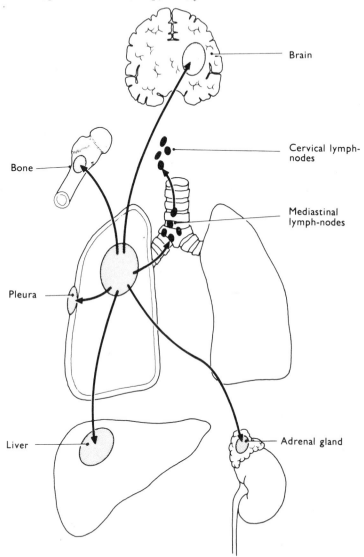

Brain

Cervical lymph-nodes

Mediastinal lymph-nodes

Bone

Pleura

Liver

Adrenal gland

Fig. 24. Diagram of common sites of secondary tumours of cancer of the lung.

2. Spread into the heart interfering with cardiac function, producing pericardial effusion.

3. Pressure on superior vena cava producing thrombosis in it, causing aching and pain, oedema of face and arms.

4. Secondary deposits in brain (a tumour here may be the first sign), liver, lymph-nodes, adrenal glands, skin, etc.

Special tests	*X-ray of lung:* to show presence of tumour, abscess, etc. *Sputum:* cancer cells present in about 60 per cent of cases. *Bronchoscopy:* for inspection of tumour and removal of specimen for biopsy. *Lymph-node:* removal of enlarged node for biopsy.
Prevention	Every pressure should be put on people not to start smoking or to give it up if they have started. Even people who have been smoking heavily for years have less chance of developing cancer if they give it up.
Treatment	Surgical removal of a lung or a lobe of a lung is the only cure, but few patients present themselves early enough. Radiotherapy of the inoperable case may relieve symptoms for a time. Anti-mitotic drugs used in the treatment of some cancers are not effective, except thiotepa for malignant effusions.
EMPHYSEMA	This is the condition of the lungs in which there is a dilatation of the air-spaces beyond the bronchioles. Affected parts of the lungs lose their elasticity and become

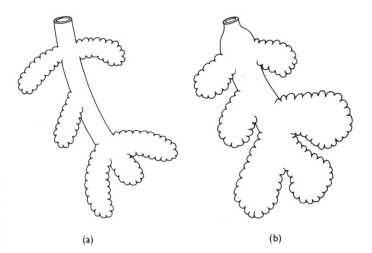

(a) (b)

Fig. 25. Diagram of (a) normal bronchiole and alveoli of a lung and (b) how they become distended in emphysema.

enlarged; larger sacs called bullae appear. The actual mechanisms by which these changes take place are obscure. The conditions can occur:

(a) in chronic bronchitis or asthma,
(b) in pneumoconiosis and other dust diseases,
(c) possibly where there is an inherited weakness of elastic tissue,
(d) in some cases for no known reason.

   Effects on respiration can be serious. The lungs become chronically over-inflated; the 'fixed volume' of gases in them is increased, and this means that inspired air is mixed with a greater volume of gas in the lungs. The transfer of gases – of oxygen and carbon dioxide – between the alveoli and the pulmonary capillaries is impaired; and to compensate for these inadequacies the patient has to breathe harder.

Clinical features	The condition usually occurs in middle life; it is more common in men than women; occasionally it begins in childhood.
	Dyspnoea[2] is the characteristic symptom. At first it occurs only on exertion, but later it can be present at rest. In some patients the rate of development of the condition is slow and they suffer little disability; others can become 'respiratory cripples' within a few years, being unable to make the slightest effort without becoming short of breath.
	The chest becomes enlarged and 'barrel-shaped'. The lungs are hyper-resonant and breath-sounds weak. The patient may become cyanosed and have clubbed fingers.
Complications	Bronchitis Asthma Pulmonary tuberculosis
	Pneumo-thorax (from rupture of a bulla)
	Heart failure from cor pulmonale.
Special test	*X-ray of lung:* will show over-translucency in lungs, particularly where there are bullae.
Treatment	If possible the patient should live in a warm, dry climate. If he cannot do this, he may be able to change his job or live outside an urban, smoke-ridden atmosphere.
	He should be taught to breathe not with the upper half of his chest but with the lower half and the diaphragm. Bronchitis is treated.

THE PNEUMONIAS

Pneumonias are acute infections of the lungs. They can be classified, on the distribution of the infection in the lung, as *lobar,* when one or more lobes is involved, or *bronchopneumonic,* when there is a patchy distribution of infection around the bronchi. Here they will be classified according to the infecting organism:

Pneumonoccal pneumonia   Staphylococcal pneumonia
Virus pneumonia   Influenzal pneumonia
Tubercular pneumonia   Rare infections.

Pneumococcal pneumonia

The infecting organism is the *pneumococcus.*

It can occur at any age. It is common in young children; it may prove the end of life for the old and the weak and the alcoholic; but it can occur in people who have previously enjoyed excellent health. It is more common in the winter than in the other seasons. It usually occurs sporadically, but small epidemics can occur where there is over-crowding, poor housing and inadequate ventilation.

Affected parts of the lungs become engorged with blood and there is an outpouring into the pulmonary tissues of cells and exudate, causing the lung to become 'consolidated'. Pleurisy occurs. The heart may become dilated and its action impaired. Pneumococci are found in the lungs and in severe cases in the blood.

Clinical features

The onset is sudden. The patient feels ill and has a chill, shivering or a rigor. He may vomit. A child may have a fit. The temperature rises sharply, sometimes as high as

[2] *dyspnoea:* difficult breathing

40.5°C. (105°F.). He develops a cough and a sharp pain in the side (due to the associated pleurisy), which makes breathing and coughing very difficult. The pulse-rate is raised and the breathing rapid and shallow. Herpes may appear on the lips. A little 'rusty' sputum is brought up.

As the diagnosis is usually made by this time and appropriate treatment started, the further course of the disease is cut short.

Untreated, the patient would remain ill for several days. Signs of 'consolidation' would appear in the lungs, the patient's temperature would remain high, the respiratory rate be raised, the patient be acutely ill, until either the temperature came down suddenly (by 'crisis') or he died.

With appropriate treatment by antibiotic or sulphonamide, the temperature should fall to normal within 48 hours and the patient improve rapidly. Signs of consolidation should disappear during the next few days.

Complications   These can still occur in spite of apparently adequate treatment.
1. Delayed resolution: the consolidation persists for weeks instead of clearing up in a few days; this suggests that the patient might have a tubercular infection or some other underlying disease of the lung such as a cancer or bronchiectasis.
2. Pleurisy, a pleural effusion, empyema.
3. Involvement of the heart: endocarditis, myocarditis, pericarditis, pericardial effusion, irregular action, heart failure.
4. Uncommon complications: parotitis, arthritis, otitis media, meningitis, pulmonary fibrosis and bronchiectasis.

Special tests   X-ray of lung to show consolidation. Cultured organisms for drug sensitivity.

Treatment   The patient should be put to bed in a warm, well ventilated room.
The following drugs should be given:
(a)   Benzyl-penicillin; 300 mg (500,000 units) 6-hourly for 24 hours; then 8-hourly for another 24 hours; then 12-hourly for 24 hours; followed by procaine penicillin 600 mg (600,000 units) daily for several days; or
(b)   Tetracycline, 500 mg 6-hourly for 5-7 days, if the patient is sensitive to penicillin or the organism resistant, or
(c)   Sulphadimidine (Sulphamezathine): initial dose of 2 g followed by 1 g 6-hourly until the temperature has been normal for 36 hours and then in smaller doses for several days.

The patients should at first have a fluid diet of 5-6 pints of milk, water and fruit-drinks, but as soon as he starts to feel better he can be given food, such as fish, eggs, bread and butter. If pain is severe he is given pethidine or morphine. If he is cyanosed, he is nursed in an oxygen-tent or given oxygen through a nasal catheter or mask.

Breathing exercises to promote full expansion of the lungs should begin when the temperature has fallen to normal and should be continued for several weeks.

Staphylococcal pneumonia   This is due to an infection of the lungs by the *Staphylococcus pyogenes*. It usually affects children and young adults. It can be due to a staphylococcal septicaemia in which the organisms have entered the blood-stream from a boil or carbuncle, to a staphylococcal mastoiditis or to a peri-nephric abscess[3]; but in some cases no such primary infection has occurred.

The onset is usually sudden with malaise, vomiting and sometimes a rigor. A cough and pain in the chest develop. The temperature is usually swinging and sweating profuse. Sputum is purulent and blood-streaked.

Complications	Lung abscess, which may burst into a bronchus. Empyema. Spontaneous pneumothorax.
Treatment	The usual treatment of pneumonia is instituted (see pneumococcal pneumonia). Drug treatment is by (a) cloxacillin (Orbenin) orally in doses of 500 mg, 6-hourly; or (b) methicillin (Celbenin) 1 g, 4-hourly for 6 days; or (c) benzyl-penicillin 1.0 mega unit intra-muscularly 6-hourly.
Virus pneumonia	A broncho-pneumonic virus infection can occur. There is a gradual onset with malaise, loss of appetite, headache, muscular pains and a cough. The temperature rises over several days to 38°-39.5°C. (100°-103°F.). Patchy areas of consolidation develop in the lungs. Pleurisy can occur. The condition usually clears up in about a fortnight, but convalescence can be slow.
Complications	Complications are uncommon. A pleural effusion can occur.
Treatment	The patient should stay in bed until a week after his temperature has fallen to normal. No special treatment is usually required, but tetracycline 500 mg. can be given 6-hourly for several days.
Influenzal pneumonia	An attack of pneumonia can be a serious complication of influenza and a common cause of death. It is most common during epidemics. Toxaemia is due to a mixed influenzal and staphylococcal infection. The patient passes in a few hours into a grave condition, with a rapid respiratory rate, blue-grey cyanosis, and circulatory collapse.
Treatment	The patient should be placed in an oxygen tent. Benzyl-penicillin 1.0 mega unit, cloxacillin 500 mg and ampicillin 500 mg are given intramuscularly every 6 hours in the hope of combatting the dual infection. Circulatory failure is treated by hydro-cortisone hemi-succinate 100 mg intravenously followed by cortisone 200 mg daily for several days.
Tubercular pneumonia	Tuberculosis can occur as a broncho-pneumonic or lobar pneumonic infection. It is not infrequently mistaken for a pneumococcal pneumonia, until a failure to respond to the ordinary treatment suggests that the patient has another kind of infection. Examination of the sputum reveals the tubercle bacillus.

[3] *peri-nephric:* around the kidney

Treatment	This is as for an acute tubercular infection.
Rare infections	Rarely pneumonia is caused by:

psittacosis.   Friedlander's bacillus
typhoid bacillus.   anthrax bacillus.

**Aspiration pneumonia
(pneumonitis)**

This is an infection of the lung due to the aspiration of mucus during a cold or a sinus infection, to blood trickling into a bronchus or to the spilling over of vomit or food into the bronchial passages in a patient who is unconscious or has oeso-phageal obstruction. The inhaled material blocks a bronchus or bronchiole; the part of the lung cut off collapses and an infection of it can follow. The patient develops a cough, malaise and fever and shows signs of involvement of a part of the lung. The area involved can be detected on X-ray examination. Treatment is on the usual lines.

COLLAPSE OF LUNG

A bronchus can become blocked by (a) a plug of mucus from an upper respiratory tract infection, (b) a clot from blood that has trickled down into it, (c) a foreign body that has been inhaled, (d) a cancer of the bronchus, or (e) pressure from an aneurysm or from a lymph-node enlarged by cancer, tuberculosis or Hodgkin's disease. Following this blocking, the part of the lung involved collapses. A lung will also collapse if it is pressed on by a pneumothorax or pleural effusion.

With a large collapse, the mediastinum shifts towards the affected side, the diaphragm rises, and unaffected parts of the lung or the opposite lung become dis-tended as a result of the extra work they have to do. The gases in the alveoli are absorbed into the blood and not replaced. This absorption can be followed by infection and the infection can go on to abscess-formation. If the lung is not ex-panded to its normal size within a month, it is likely to be permanently shrunk.

If collapse follows operation, signs are usually apparent within 2-3 days. The patient has shortness of breath and sometimes pain in the chest, he breathes rapidly and may have cyanosis. On examination the affected part of the lung is found not to move, there is dullness over the area, breath sounds there are diminished, and the mediastinum is found to have shifted.

Prevention

Prevention is by pre-operative care. Before any non-emergency surgery in which a general anaesthetic is going to be used: (a) any sinus or dental infection is treated; (b) the patient is not operated on if he has a cold, (c) he is given instruction in breathing exercises, and (d) smoking is forbidden.

Treatment

Treatment is by (a) postural drainage in the hope that the obstruction will move, (b) encouraging the patient to cough; if this is painful he is given morphine. If these measures are ineffective, bronchoscopy is performed and the mucus or blood aspirated. Oxygen is given for cyanosis and antibiotics if infection threatens.

LUNG ABSCESS

A lung abscess can be due to:
(a)   the inhalation of septic material during a dental operation, tonsillectomy or

other operation on the throat or nose, or by the inhalation of vomit during un-consciousness.

(b)   infection around a cancer of the lung, a foreign body in a bronchus, a stenosis of a bronchus or bronchiectasis.

(c)   blood-borne infection during a staphylococcal septicaemia, a pyaemia, septic thrombo-phlebitis, a right-sided bacterial endocarditis.

(d)   a perforating wound or a bullet in the lung;

(e)   degeneration in a lung during any pneumonia.

(f)   the rupture of a hydatid cyst or amoebic abscess through the diaphragm, or of a mediastinal abscess, into a lung. For some abscesses no cause can be found.

Clinical features   Symptoms develop quickly. The patient complains of malaise, loss of appetite, shivering and sweating. He has a raised temperature, a cough and sputum. Haemo-ptysis can occur. A foul smell in the breath precedes the coughing up of pus from an abscess that has burst into a bronchus.

With a chronic abscess, the patient continues to have a swinging temperature, rigors and sweating, to cough up purulent sputum.

Complications

Pleurisy	Empyema	Pyo-pneumothorax
Mediastinitis		Pericarditis
Fibrosis of the lung		Bronchiectasis
Abscess in other parts (especially the brain)		Meningitis

Special tests   *X-ray of lung:* will show position and extent of the abscess.
Blood: polymorphonuclear leucocytosis will be present.
Sputum: if available, should be tested for sensitivity of organism.

Treatment   An appropriate antibiotic should be given in maximum doses. If the sensitivity of the organism cannot be detected, benzyl-penicillin should be given in doses of 600 mg (1 million units) 12-hourly with streptomycin 500 mg 6-hourly.

Postural drainage is carried out several times a day, the precise position depending on the position of the abscess as determined by X-ray examination.

If the abscess is not healed by these methods, surgical removal of the infected lobe will be required.

CYSTS OF THE LUNG   Cysts of the lung are congenital (as a result of the failure of development of part of the lung bud from which the lung develops) or acquired, being secondary to emphysema or to some infection of the lung that has caused a breakdown of the walls of alveoli.

Congenital cysts with a valve-like opening into a bronchus can cause respiratory distress in infancy if air can get in but not out, the cyst getting bigger with each inspiration. Cysts can become infected and behave then like abscesses.

When possible cysts are removed surgically, but acquired cysts are often multiple and too much lung tissue is involved to make removal possible.

PNEUMOCONIOSES   *Other name:* dust diseases
These are diseases resulting from the inhalation, in various industries, of dusts which damage the lungs:

101   *Diseases of the Respiratory System*

(a)   *silicosis* – due to the inhalation of fine particles of silica; it can occur in some coal-mines, in the pottery industry, in sandstone and granite industries, and where silica-containing substances are used in grinding processes;

(b)   *asbestosis* – due to the inhalation of asbestosis fibres, which contain magnesium silicate;

(c)   *byssinosis*[4] – probably an allergic reaction to proteins in cotton dust.

Any of these will in time produce a cough, shortness of breath and fibrosis of the lung; and a person seriously involved is likely to become a respiratory cripple. Tuberculosis and cancer of the lung are complications.

Prevention is by recognition of the risk, the provision of adequate ventilation, the wearing of masks where it is feasible, and the removal from the occupation of a workman who is showing evidence of involvement.

FAILURE OF RESPIRATORY FUNCTION

This can be a complication of any severe pulmonary disease and of some other conditions. The functions of the lungs are to keep the arterial blood adequately oxygenated and to discharge any excess of carbon dioxide, both functions being carried out through the alveolar walls. Respiratory function has failed when disease of the respiratory tract produces serious abnormalities in the amount of oxygen or of carbon dioxide in the blood. Cigarette-smoking is often a contributory factor.

The causes of failure are:

1. *obstruction in the air-passages*

(a)   excess of mucus and swelling of mucous membrane in chronic bronchitis.

(b)   spasm of the bronchial muscles in asthma.

2. *failure of alveolar function*

(a)   the number of functioning alveoli is reduced by fibrosis of lung, emphysema, pleural effusion, surgical removal, etc.

(b)   there is a failure of gaseous exchanges owing to some alveoli containing air that cannot move in or out.

3. *restriction of respiratory movements*

(a)   lungs cannot expand owing to congestion, fibrosis, pleural thickening, pneumothorax, etc.

(b)   paralysis of the respiratory muscles by acute poliomyelitis, myasthenia gravis, neuritis.

(c)   obstructive physical deformities – kypho-scoliosis, gross obesity.

4. *depression of respiratory centre in brain*

(a)   poisoning by barbiturates, morphine, etc.

(b)   shock.

(c)   intracranial haemorrhage.

(d)   terminal illness.

Clinical features   Lack of oxygen in the blood causes cyanosis and confusion. Excess of carbon dioxide causes tachycardia, twitchings and confusion.

[4] *byssinosis* – from Greek: *byssos* – flax

Special tests:	1. *Match test:* a person with healthy lungs should be able to blow out with his mouth open a match 20 cm from his lips. The lips must not be pursed.
	2. *Expiration test:* a person with healthy lungs should after taking a deep breath be able to expire 75 per cent of his vital capacity[5] in 1 second.
	3. *Analyses* of gases in blood and lungs.

Treatment
Acute failure

1. The original disease is treated.
2. Postural drainage at frequent intervals for removal of mucus.
3. Oxygen shortage is relieved by giving oxygen 30 per cent with air through a mask. Greater concentration of oxygen produces a dangerous rise of carbon dioxide in the blood.
4. Nikethamide (Coramine) 2-10 ml is given intravenously to stimulate deep breathing.
5. If other measures fail, it may be necessary to perform tracheostomy and carry out intermittent positive pressure respiration.

Chronic failure

1. The patient should give up smoking.
2. He should when necessary give himself broncho-dilator drugs with an aerosol.
3. He should have oxygen available in a portable cylinder.
4. If possible he should move to a smoke-free climate.

PLEURISY

Pleurisy is inflammation of the pleura, the membrane whose inner layer clothes the lungs and whose outer layer lines the inner surface of the chest-wall. Pleurisy can be due to:

(a)   any infection of the lung — pneumonia, pulmonary tuberculosis, lung abscess, etc.
(b)   a pulmonary infarction;
(c)   a cancer of the lung;
(d)   bronchiectasis;
(e)   injury, e.g. a bullet-wound, a stab-wound, a broken rib perforating the lung;
(f)   any generalized infection of the blood — septicaemia, pyaemia, typhoid fever, acute rheumatism;
(g)   spread of infection through the diaphragm from an intra-abdominal infection — peritonitis, subphrenic abscess, hepatitic abscess, etc.;
(h)   chronic nephritis.

A pleurisy begins as a *dry pleurisy,* in which a patch of pleura becomes inflamed and roughened and a little fibrous exudate is produced. Such a condition can clear up completely or leave some permanent pleural thickening behind or go on to develop pleurisy with effusion. *Pleurisy with effusion* is the form of pleurisy in which there is a pouring out of fluid into the pleural cavity, the space between the two layers of the pleura. *Empyema* is the condition in which there is pus in the pleural cavity.

[5] *vital capacity:* maximum amount of air that can be taken into the lungs in one breath

Diseases of the Respiratory System

Dry pleurisy
Clinical features

The patient develops a sharp pain in his side. It is made worse by breathing, coughing and sometimes moving; the patient can cry out if an involuntary cough or deep breath catches him unawares and he may hold his chest-wall to minimize his breathing. Sometimes he lies on the affected side, sometimes on the healthy, sometimes on his back. His temperature rises a little, perhaps as high as 38.5°C (101°F). The rub of the inflamed surface can be heard through a stethoscope as the patient breathes.

Diaphragmatic acute pleurisy is pleurisy of the pleura between lung and diaphragm. It can be due to any of the causes of acute pleurisy and in particular to an infection coming up through the diaphragm. The pain can be 'referred' to the abdomen or to the tip of the shoulder (because the fibres of the phrenic nerve which supplies the diaphragm come from cervical nerve-roots whose main sensory distribution is to the shoulder and neck). The affected side of the diaphragm is held motionless; there may be 'guarding' of the upper abdominal muscles. Hiccough can be a nuisance.

Complications

Pleurisy with effusion   Empyema
Chronic pleural thickening

Treatment

The patient is put to bed. Strapping is applied to the affected side. A kaolin poultice helps to relieve pain. Morphine 10-15 mg or pethidine 100 mg relieve pain. If these measures prove ineffective and pain persists, an artificial pneumothorax can be performed, gas being injected to separate the inflamed layers of pleura.

Pleurisy with effusion

The amount produced can be as much as 3.5 litres (6 pints). The fluid is clear and pale and may coagulate when it has been withdrawn from the chest. As the fluid increases, the lung collapses, the mediastinum is displaced to the healthy side, the diaphragm is pushed downwards.

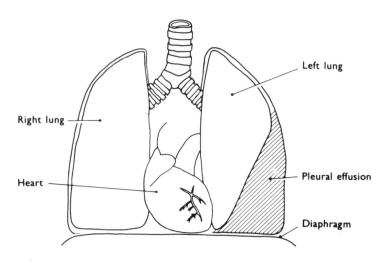

Fig. 26. Pleural effusion with compression of the left lung and the heart displaced to the right.

The patient starts with the pain of acute pleurisy, but as fluid is produced the inflamed surfaces of pleura becomes separated and pain diminishes. But if a lot of fluid is produced quickly, the sudden collapse of the lung is likely to cause dyspnoea. The affected side moves little; the area is dull to percussion; breath sounds are absent or diminished and voice-sounds are not transmitted. The liver and spleen can be felt if they are pushed down below the costal margin.

With an effusion of moderate size, the temperature falls to normal in about 10 days and the fluid is completely absorbed within a month. Larger effusions take longer. Sometimes absorption of the fluid appears to be stimulated by the removal of a small amount for examination.

Complications	Empyema	Acute oedema of lung	Cardiac failure

Special tests *Fluid:* a specimen is aspirated for examination, in particular for evidence of tuberculosis.
X-ray of chest: will show opacity due to fluid, lowering of diaphragm, displacement of mediastinum.

Treatment The patient is confined to bed. Apart from the withdrawal of a small amount of fluid for examination, aspiration is not at first necessary unless there is a large effusion with dyspnoea. Later, if there is evidence that the fluid is not being absorbed, if the patient is seriously ill with high fever, or if there is acute oedema, the fluid is aspirated.

EMPYEMA In empyema the pleural effusion is purulent. Organisms commonly causing infection are pneumococci and streptococci. The fluid may have any degree of purulence from slight turbidity to thick pus; the colour of the fluid varies from grey to green; some fluids smell offensive.

Clinical features These stem from a dry pleurisy or from pleurisy with effusion. The patient's condition becomes much worse. The temperature rises higher – to 40°C. (104°F.) or higher. The patient is likely to sweat profusely, to have dyspnoea; he may have a rigor. The physical signs are those of a pleural effusion; but in addition, there can be bulging of an intercostal space, oedema of the chest wall, and 'pointing' of the abscess through the chest wall.

Some empyemas become localized and separated from the rest of the pleural cavity by adhesions. This can happen as an *apical empyema* at the apex of a lung, as an *interlobar empyema* between two lobes of lung, as a *diaphragmatic empyema* at the base of a lung.

Complications *Perforation* of the empyema through the chest wall, into the lung and a bronchus, into pericardium, into oesophagus.

Formation of a *fistula* between pleural cavity and external surface of chest or an internal organ.

Gangrene of lung

Permanent collapse of a lung or lobe of a lung, with chronic pleural thickening, flattening of chest wall, scoliosis, drooping of shoulder.

Special tests   *Fluid:* aspiration of specimen; bacteriological examination and sensitivity-test of organism.
X-ray of chest: will show opacity due to empyema.

Treatment   The chest is aspirated and as much of the purulent fluid is removed as possible. A specimen is sent for examination of the organism and its sensitivity. Meanwhile the first aspiration is followed by an injection of benzyl-penicillin 600 mg (1 million units) in 10 ml of sterile water into the pleural cavity and a course of penicillin is begun.

Aspiration is repeated on alternate days. Treatment is continued with intrapleural and parenteral antibiotics of the kind the organism is now known to be sensitive to.

If the fluid is too thick to be aspirated, a rib-resection is performed and the empyema drained surgically.

A course of breathing exercises is given by the physiotherapist to ensure that there is full expansion of the lung.

HYDROTHORAX   This is fluid in the pleural cavity due to transudation from the capillaries, not — as in pleurisy with effusion — to inflammation. It occurs as part of a general oedema of the tissues with fluid in the peritoneal cavity (ascites) and in the pericardial cavity.

Common causes are: (a) heart failure, (b) acute or chronic renal disease, (c) famine oedema.

Clinical features   These are those of the original disease with those of the presence of fluid in the pleural cavity — collapse of the lung, displacement of the diaphragm and mediastinum, dyspnoea, cardiac embarrassment, and cyanosis. There is no fever.

Treatment   Treatment is of the primary condition and removal of the fluid by aspiration.

HAEMOTHORAX   This is blood in the pleural cavity. It can be due to a perforating wound, fracture of a rib, a new growth, rupture of an aneurysm, or the blast of an explosion. The blood is largely defibrinated and does not clot. The lung collapses. Intra-pleural adhesions can form on recovery. It can be a cause of sudden death. The clinical features combine those of a haemorrhage with those of fluid in the pleural cavity. Treatment is by aspiration, blood-transfusion, antibiotics to prevent infection, and if bleeding continues a thoracotomy [6] to find and tie bleeding points.

PNEUMOTHORAX   This is air in the pleural cavity. It can be due to:

[6] *thoracotomy:* surgical opening of the chest

(a)   air getting in from the lung or bronchi; this is the cause of 95 per cent of cases; usually air gets in through a ruptured emphysematous bulla;

(b)   a penetrating wound, ulceration into the pleural cavity from an abscess, a mediastinal growth, or perforation of a peptic ulcer through the diaphragm to which it has become attached by adhesions.

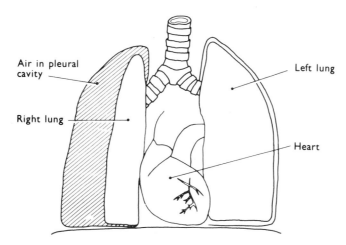

Fig. 27. Diagram of a right-sided pneumothorax, with compression of the lung.

A spontaneous pneumothorax can occur at any age as a complication of a chronic lung disease; but it occurs most commonly in previously healthy young men as a result of a rupture of a symptomless cyst of the lung into the pleural cavity, the apex of a lung being the commonest site.

Clinical features   The onset can be sudden or slow. It is sudden when an emphysematous bulla bursts and slow when there is a slight leak from the lung. With a sudden onset there is an abrupt rise of pressure from the normal negative pressure to atmospheric pressure. The patient has an acute pain in the chest and feels that something has given way. He is likely to collapse, with a fear of sudden death, and to go cold, clammy and blue. His pulse is rapid and feeble, his breathing rapid and shallow. Death can occur. On the affected side there is no movement of the lung, the heart is pushed over to the other side, breath-sounds cannot be heard and the area is hyper-resonant.

Complications   Fatal asphyxia
Pleurisy, effusion, empyema.
Permanent collapse of lung.

Special tests   *X-ray of chest:* will show the air in the pleural cavity; is repeated to check absorption of air.
Puncture of chest: air can be withdrawn.

Treatment   In an emergency a needle is plunged into the pleural cavity through an intercostal space and then connected by a rubber tube to a water-seal, extractor-pump or pneumothorax apparatus. In severe but not dangerous conditions a rubber catheter is introduced into the pleural cavity through an intercostal space; the other end is

Diseases of the Respiratory System

connected to an under-water seal, and the patient is told to cough gently. In mild degrees of pneumothorax the air is spontaneously absorbed.

FARMER'S LUNG

This is an allergic reaction to dust from mouldy hay inhaled by a person who by previous exposure has become allergic to it. It is an occupational disease of farmers, their wives and children, animal and bird-house attendants, and workers in bird-seed factories. *Bird-fancier's disease* and *mushroom worker's lung* are similar conditions due one to the inhalation of dust from birds' feathers and droppings and the other to the inhalation of spores from compost used in growing mushrooms.

Clinical features

A few hours after exposure to the dust the patient develops a chill, headache, nausea, vomiting, muscle pains, retro-sternal pain, difficulty in breathing, and a dry or productive cough, the sputum sometimes being blood-stained. The temperature rises to about 40°C. (104°F.) The patient has a raised heart-rate, rapid shallow breathing, cyanosis, and signs of congestion in the lungs. An acute attack lasts for a few days, but can be followed by long debility; death in it can occur. Repeated attacks cause fibrosis of the lungs, emphysema, a diminution of pulmonary function, cor pulmonale, and death in early adult life.

Special test

X-rays: lungs show a fine diffuse mottling in an acute attack and fibrosis in the chronic state.

Prevention

An affected farmer should give up farming, but this is economically not always possible. Modifications of farming practices can be made to reduce the dust; a mask is not effective because the dust-particles are tiny.

Treatment

1. The patient should be removed from all contact with the dust and go to bed.
2. Cortico-steroids (e.g. prednisone) are given.
3. Oxygen is given to relieve cyanosis.

5 Diseases of the Blood, Lymphatic System and Spleen

Haematology is the study of the blood and its diseases. It should be recalled that:

(a)   Red blood cells (erythrocytes) are formed after birth from cells in the bone-marrow. The cells from which they have developed contained nuclei, and the appearance in the blood-stream of nucleated red cells (normoblasts) or of cells with a fine network in the cytoplasm (reticulocytes) is an indication either of disease of the blood-forming tissues or of a severe anaemia, which has caused immature red cells to be rushed hastily into the circulation. The red cells require for their development certain amino-acids, iron and cobalt (which is obtained from vitamin B_{12}), and shortage of any of these will cause anaemias of various kinds. Diseases in which there is an excess of red blood cells are uncommon. Red cells live for about 120 days, being then broken down in the liver, spleen and bone-marrow. In some diseases there is an excessive breakdown of red cells, which in these conditions can have a short life.

(b)   The white cells are of several kinds: granulocytes, lymphocytes, monocytes. An excessive number of some of these occurs in infections and in the leukaemias.

(c)   Platelets are tiny granules which have important functions in the clotting of blood and the stopping of bleeding. A decrease in their number below the normal can lead to excessive bleeding.

The *plasma* is the fluid part of the blood. It plays an important part in the fluid-balance of the body, and disorders of it are described in Chapter 7.

The *spleen* (which is involved in the destruction of red blood cells, the storage of iron, and the formation of lymphocytes) becomes enlarged in some blood-diseases and in some infections, notably malaria. It has to be enlarged about 3 times before it becomes palpable below the left costal margin. As it enlarges, it pushes downwards towards the umbilicus and right iliac fossa. It presents as a firm mass with a smooth surface and a notched anterior margin.

The *lymph-nodes* can become enlarged in several conditions, particularly infections, malignant new growths, lymphadenoma (Hodgkin's disease) and leukaemia.

TERMS AND TESTS
The following terms and tests are used in haematology:

Red blood cell: the normal red cell count is 4 - 6 million per mm^3.

Reticulocyte: an immature red cell with a fine network in its substance found in blood when there is an urgent demand for new red cells from the bone-marrow, e.g. after a haemorrhage.

Normoblast: an immature red cell with a nucleus, normally in the bone-marrow, found in the blood when there is an urgent demand for red cells.

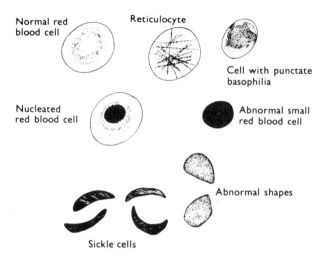

Fig. 28. Normal and abnormal red blood cells.

Haemoglobin: average amount in normal blood is 14.8 g per 100 ml.

Packed-cell volume (Haematocrit value): volume occupied by red cells in 100 ml of centrifuged blood; normally about 45 ml per cent.

MCHC (Mean corpuscular haemoglobin concentration): obtained by dividing Hb in grams per 100 ml by the packed-cell volume and multiplying by 100. Normal: 32-38 g per cent. Value below 32 shows need for treatment by iron.

MCV (Mean corpuscular volume): is average volume of a single red blood cell: normal 80 - 94 cu. micron.

Colour Index: Hb percentage divided by red cell count percentage; indicates haemoglobin content of a single red cell. Normal range 0.9-1.1

White cells (leucocytes)

Total count: Normal range:	4,000 - 11,000 per mm^3.
Granular cells: normal range:	
neutrophil granulocytes:	2,500 - 7,500 per mm^3.
eosinophils:	150 - 400 per mm^3.
basophils:	0 - 100 per mm^3.
Lymphocytes: normal range:	1,500 - 2,700 per mm^3.
Monocytes: normal range:	350 - 500 per mm^3

Leucocytosis: an increase in the number of white cells above the normal range.

Leucopenia: a reduction in the number of white cells below the normal range.

Granulocytosis: increase in number of granular cells (usually seen in acute infections and in myeloid leukaemia)

Lymphocytosis: increase in number of lymphocytes (usually seen in some chronic infections and in lymphatic leukaemia)

Eosinophilia: increase in number of eosinophils (seen in some parasitic infections).

Platelets: Normal count: 250,000-500,000 per mm^3.

ANAEMIA	Anaemia is present when there is insufficient haemoglobin to carry oxygen in adequate amounts to the cells of the body. It is most commonly due to:

1. A deficiency of iron. Iron is an essential part of haemoglobin and lack of it causes iron deficiency anaemia.

2. A deficiency of vitamin B_{12}. Vitamin B_{12} is essential for the formation of haemoglobin and lack of it causes megaloblastic anaemia.

3. A deficiency of folates (folic acid). These are essential for the formation of haemoglobin and lack of them causes an anaemia similar to that of pernicious anaemia.

4. Excessive destruction of red blood cells as occurs in several blood-diseases, e.g. spherocytosis, thalassaemia.

5. Haemorrhage of any kind.

6. Diseases of the bone-marrow that prevent the formation of red blood cells.

Iron deficiency anaemia

Other name: hypochromic[7] microcytic[8] anaemia
This anaemia can be due to (a) a failure of intake of adequate amounts of iron, (b) a failure of the absorption of iron from the intestine, or (c) loss of blood. It is common during pregnancy and in middle-aged women whose iron-store has been depleted by pregnancies, lactation and loss of iron at the menstrual periods and who have not taken adequate amounts of the iron-containing foods (meat, eggs, green vegetables) to compensate for this loss. It is common too among elderly people of both sexes who have taken inadequate amounts of the same foods because of their cost, of difficulties in cooking them, of difficulty in eating them because of lack of teeth or of badly fitting dentures. This anaemia can be caused by partial gastrectomy and similar operations, the partially digested food not having a chance to get into the duodenum or being hurried through it. Any large or persistent haemorrhage can cause this anaemia – menorrhagia[9], ulcer of the stomach, ulcer of the intestine, injury, hook-worm infestation in the tropics.

Clinical features

The patient complains at first of being tired and later of shortness of breath, palpitations, anginal attacks, a sore tongue and difficulty in swallowing. Pallor of the skin and mucous membranes is seen. The tongue is smooth and raw from loss of epithelium from its surface. The ankles can be oedematous and the spleen just palpable. The nails can be spoon-shaped, with typical hollowing of the centre. (koilonychia[1]).

Complications

Myocardial infarction. Cancer of tongue or pharynx, following degeneration of epithelium.
Pernicious anaemia, a shift from hypochromic to hyperchromic anaemia.

Special tests

RBC: normal or reduced in number; small; central pallor of cell. *Hb:* low.

[7] *hypochromic:* lacking colour (here, haemoglobin)
[8] *microcytic:* red cells smaller than normal.
[9] *menorrhagia:* excessive loss at menstrual periods.
[1] *koilonychia:* from Greek: *koilos* – hollow; *onyx* – nail

Gastric juice: achlohydria[2] in 40 per cent of patients.
Faeces: for blood.
X-ray of chest: for cancer or tuberculosis.

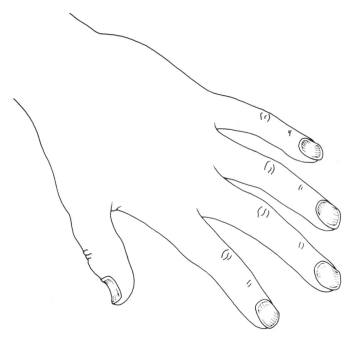

Fig. 29. Spoon shaped fingernails as seen in anaemia

Treatment

1. Ferrous sulphate 200 mg 3 times a day between meals (it is not well absorbed if given with food). If there is no response (as shown by RBC count and Hb estimation) the dose is not increased.
2. Ferrous gluconate 600 mg 3 times daily is given if ferrous sulphate causes gastro-intestinal upset.
3. Iron-dextran complex (Imferon) 50-100 mg is given intra-muscularly if iron by mouth is not tolerated, anaemia is severe or if it is suspected that the patient is not taking the drug.
4. A blood transfusion is given for severe anaemia.
5. The patient should take plenty of meat, eggs and green vegetables.

Pernicious anaemia

This anaemia is due to a deficiency of intrinsic factor. The usual reason is a failure of absorption of vitamin B_{12} because of an inherited deficiency of secretion by the gastric mucosa of the 'intrinsic factor' necessary for the absorption of the vitamin. There is a high incidence of pernicious anaemia, iron deficiency and gastric achlorhydria in near relatives. Pernicious anaemia usually begins between 40 and 70 years, occasionally at a much younger age. It is more common in women than men and in white races than in those of African or Asiatic stock. It can follow prolonged iron-deficiency anaemia and be a complication of diabetes mellitus, thyrotoxicosis and myxoedema.

[2] *achlorhydria:* lack of hydrochloric acid in gastric juice

Much less common causes of vitamin B$_{12}$ deficiency are: (a) strict vegetarianism, (b) following gastrectomy or in cancer of the stomach, (c) malabsorption syndromes, (d) after any operation on the small intestine in which a blind loop is formed — microorganisms in the loop taking up the vitamin.

Clinical features

The onset is slow and the patient may be seriously anaemic by the time he presents for examination. He is likely to complain of tiredness, shortness of breath, palpitations and giddiness; old people may also complain of angina pectoris and intermittent claudication. Gastro-intestinal symptoms are common: sore tongue, loss of appetite, nausea, vomiting, diarrhoea.

Subacute combined degeneration of the spinal cord occurs in about 10 per cent of cases. Patients who are developing it are likely to complain of tingling in the hands and feet and of weakness and difficulty in walking.

The patient is likely to be pale. The tongue is smooth and raw, the spleen palpable. The patient may have a slightly raised temperature. Death can occur from cardiac failure or pulmonary oedema.

Complications

Subacute combined degeneration of the spinal cord.
Haemorrhage into retina.   Cancer of stomach.

Special tests

Blood:
   RBC: cells reduced in number, increased in size; abnormal types present.
   Hb: slightly reduced.
   WBC: decreased to 3,000-4,000 per mm^3.
   Platelets: may be decreased
   Serum vitamin B$_{12}$: usually below 150 μ + 4 g. per ml. (normal: 450 μ + 4 g. per ml).
Bone-marrow puncture: megaloblasts and other abnormal cells present.
Gastric juice: complete achloryhdria; if histamine produces hydrochloric acid the patient has
   not got pernicious anaemia.

Treatment

The diagnosis must be made before treatment is begun because treatment obscures the findings in the blood.

Vitamin B$_{12}$ (cyano-cobalamin) is given by injection in doses of 1,000 mcg twice weekly for 5 injections and then weekly until the blood is normal and then every 4-8 weeks for life. The patient should start to feel better within 2-3 days and a normal blood-picture can be expected within 6-8 weeks.

If the patient also has subacute combined degeneration, a dose of 1,000 mcg has to be continued twice weekly for at least 6 months.

Folate deficiency anaemia

Folic acid is a synthetic substance, but the name is also given to a number of substances called folates with similar activities found in meat, green vegetables, nuts, etc. Deficiency can be due to (a) shortage of it in the diet; (b) an increased demand in pregnancy; (c) decreased absorption following disease or removal of the small intestine; (d) in scurvy; (e) in liver disease; (f) certain drugs, especially phenytoin and primidone. The same changes occur in the blood as in pernicious anaemia.

Treatment

Treatment is by folic acid 5 mg daily by mouth.

113   *Diseases of the Blood, Lymphatic System and Spleen*

HEREDITARY SPHEROCYTOSIS [3]	*Other names:* acholuric family jaundice[4], congenital haemolytic jaundice In this disease the red blood cells are more spherical than normal. The ratio of cell-surface to cell-volume is reduced, and in consequence the cells show increased fragility in hypotonic saline. The cells have an abnormally short life (normal: about 120 days). The disease is an hereditary one, the abnormality being transmitted as a mendelian dominant. Half the children of an involved parent are likely to be affected; the other half are likely to transmit it. It affects mostly people of European stock. Although the condition is present at birth, signs of it may not appear until much later − or may not appear at all, being discovered possibly at some routine examination.
Clinical features	The patient is likely to complain of jaundice, giving a history of having always been slightly jaundiced or having recurrent attacks of jaundice. There is no bile-pigment in the urine − hence the name 'acholuric'. Usually slight anaemia is present and the spleen slightly enlarged. From time to time, for no apparent reason, the production of red cells ceases, cells already in circulation are destroyed, the spleen becomes painful and tender, and there is a sharp increase in jaundice and anaemia. In infancy the disease may be severe and fatal. Occurring in later life, the dangers are less, gall-stones being the most troublesome feature.
Complications	Gall-stones Chronic ulceration of the legs (cause unknown).
Special tests	*RBCs:* rounded, of variable size; usually reduced to 3-4 million per mm³; show increased osmotic fragility. *Reticulocytes:* at least 10 per cent of RBCs. *Van den Bergh test:* a raised indirect reaction occurs in haemolytic anaemia; if a gall-stone blocks the common bile-duct and causes obstructive jaundice, the test gives a positive direct reaction.
Treatment	*Splenectomy* stops the abnormal destruction of blood cells, the blood count returns to normal, jaundice vanishes, leg ulceration clears up. The operation can be dangerous if performed in infancy, because it appears to increase the dangers of any infection that might occur; an operation should, if possible, be postponed until the child is older. Cholecystectomy is performed for gall-stones and may have to be preceded by a blood-transfusion.
THALASSAEMIA [5]	This is a group of genetic diseases in which anaemia is produced as a result of a failure of proper production of one or more of the globin chains of haemoglobin. The RBCs are abnormal and have a short life. The disease occurs mainly in the Mediterranean littoral, Near East, Persia, India, Thailand, China, Phillipines and parts of Central Africa. It has occurred in people of pure British stock.
Clinical features	The disease occurs in two forms: 1. *Thalassaemia minor:* anaemia slight; symptoms mild; patient may live a normal life-span. 2. *Thalassaemia major:* severe anaemia; large spleen and liver; typical facial appearance − bossing of frontal and parietal bones, prominent malar bones, depressed bridge of nose, slanting eyes; retardation of physical and mental development; symptoms begin in infancy and patient usually dies before reaching adolescence.
Special tests	*X-ray of bones:* large medullary cavity, thin cortex; skull shows changes resembling hair standing on end.

[3] *spherocyte:* red cell that is rounded instead of biconcave
[4] *acholuric:* from Greek: *a* − not; *chole* − bile; *ouron* − urine
[5] *thalassaemia:* from Greek − *thalassa* − the sea (i.e. the Mediterranean)

114

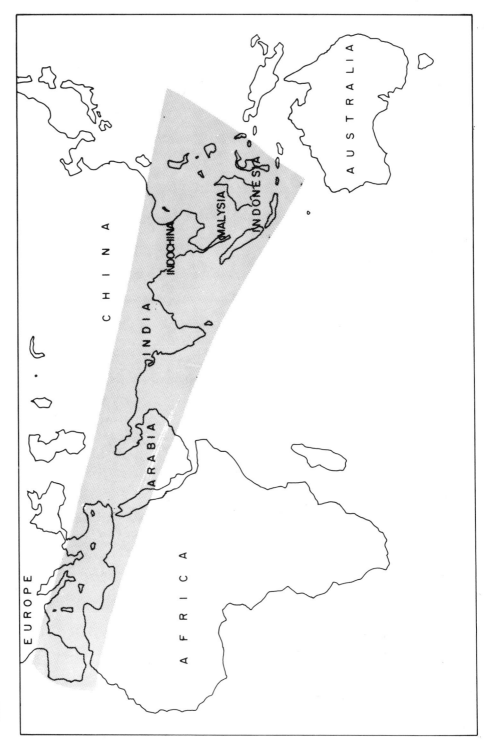

Fig. 32. Map showing thalassaemia areas.

(by courtesy of Wellcome Institute of Medical Science).

Diseases of the Blood, Lymphatic System and Spleen

Blood: hypochromic anaemia with reticulocytes and normoblasts present.

Treatment	Blood transfusions; prevention of infection; splenectomy in some cases; the removal of excess iron by a chelating agent; the maintenance of an adequate level of folic acid.

Sickle-cell anaemia

In this anaemia many of the RBCs are sickle-shaped and readily destroyed. The disease is due to an inherited abnormal haemoglobin called haemoglobin S (Hb S). It occurs in people of the Negro race.

Clinical features

It begins in infancy and the patient usually dies before 30. He has anaemia, slight jaundice and an enlarged spleen; every now and again he has crises of pyrexia, pain in the limbs, and intra-vascular clotting. Between crises he is listless and depressed. Chronic ulceration of the legs is common.

Special tests

RBCs: up to 60 per cent may be sickle-shaped; number is reduced to about 3 million per mm^3 and less during crises.

Treatment

There is no effective treatment. Splenectomy sometimes does good. Transfusions are given for severe anaemia.

Aplastic anaemia

In this condition there is destruction in the bone-marrow of the cells from which red cells, white cells and platelets are formed. *Agranulocytosis* is a destruction of the cells from which granular leuococytes are formed.

The causes of aplastic anaemia are:

(a)   unknown – idiopathic aplastic anaemia (most cases),

(b)   exposure to X-rays or radio-active substances,

(c)   some drugs – chloramphenicol, tridione, sulphonamides, etc.,

(d)   industrial poisons – benzol and its derivatives, etc.

Clinical features

The disease usually develops slowly over months, but a haemorrhage or infection can precipitate a crisis. Anaemia is produced by the destruction of red cells; fever and ulceration of the throat are due to the body's inability to withstand infection as a result of the destruction of white cells; purpura and haemorrhages are the result of the destruction of platelets.

About half the patients die within 3 months of the diagnosis being made; some survive for a little longer; about half recover with treatment.

Treatment

1. The cause is if possible removed.

2. Blood-transfusions are given regularly; in some patients the bone-marrow eventually starts to function normally.

3. Penicillin or other appropriate antibiotic is given for infection.

MULTIPLE MYELOMA

Other name: plasmocytoma

In this disease multiple tumours develop in bone; an abnormal protein is present in the plasma and an abnormal one in the urine. The tumours arise from plasma cells[6] in various bones – especially the skull, spine, ribs and pelvis. As they grow they erode the bone, which gives way under pressure or strain with the production of deformity or spontaneous fracture. Occasionally only a single tumour is present. Tumours of similar cells are sometimes present in liver, spleen, kidneys, testis, ovary or tonsil.

The disease occurs in the later half of adult life. It is always fatal; about half the patients die within a year, a few live for more than 5 years.

[6] *Plasma cell:* a relatively large cell with a single nucleus, normally present in bone-marrow and other tissues

Clinical features	The patient complains of pain in the affected parts, which are tender to percussion. Deformities of spine and leg are likely; the disease is a common cause of spontaneous fracture. The patient becomes anaemic. Pneumonia is a common cause of death.
Complications	Paraplegia[7], due to compression-fracture of a vertebral body. Renal failure, if tumour grows in kidney.
Special tests	*X-ray of bone:* shows characteristic punched-out holes. *Blood:* contains abnormal protein of uncertain origin; serum calcium raised to 16-17 mg per 100 ml. (normal 8-10 mg); *ESR:* raised to 100 mm. or more in 1 hour (normal: 3-7 mm in 1 hour). *Sternal puncture:* shows excess of plasma cells. *Urine:* shows Bence-Jones protein in about half the cases: it is a protein which shows as a cloud when urine is heated to 55°C. disappears on heating to 85°C., reappears on cooling.
Treatment	Treatment may produce temporary remissions. Bone-marrow depressant drugs such as melphalan (Alkeran) or cyclophosphamide (Endoxana) are used. The whole body can be irradiated. Cortico-steroids are sometimes used. Severe anaemia is relieved by blood-transfusion.

PURPURA [8]	Purpura is the occurrence of haemorrhages in the skin or just under it. The sizes of the haemorrhages can vary from tiny spots to large haematomas. Purpuras are divided into: 1. Thrombocytopenic purpuras, in which there is a reduction in the number of platelets in the blood to below about 40,000 per mm^3. 2. Non-thrombocytopenic purpuras, in which the platelet count is in the normal range.

THROMBO- CYTOPENIC PURPURAS [9] **Essential** **thrombocytopenia**	This rare disease of adolescents and young adults occurs in an acute and a chronic form. It appears to be an auto-immune disease in which there is decreased platelet production or in which antibodies destroy blood-platelets. It is characterized by purpura and bleeding from the nose, gums, gastro-intestinal tract, renal tract and uterus. Haemorrhages into brain and eye can cause serious complications. The spleen may be palpable.
Secondary **thrombocytopenic** **purpuras**	These can be due to: 1. bone-marrow damage from excessive irradiation or the action of cytotoxic[1] drugs (used for malignant disease) 2. sensitivity to certain drugs — quinine, quinidine, Sedormid, etc. 3. disease destroying the bone-marrow — leukaemia, lymphadenoma, etc. 4. in enteric fevers, chicken-pox, German measles. 5. excessive destruction of platelets by the spleen.

[7] *paraplegia:* parlaysis of legs
[8] *purpura:* from Greek: *porphura* — purple dye
[9] *thrombocyte:* platelet. - *penia:* few
[1] *cytotoxic:* cell-damaging

NON-THROMBO-CYTOPENIC PURPURAS

Allergic purpura

Other names: Anaphylactoid purpura. Henoch-Schonlein syndrome
This disease of childhood and adolescence is possibly a result of a streptococcal infection, for it can follow a sore throat or other mild infection and may produce an acute nephritis.

Purpura is associated with urticaria, haemorrhages into the tissue around a joint (causing joint-pain), into the gastro-intestinal tract (causing melaena) or in the renal tract (causing haematuria). Most patients recover spontaneously. Those with recurrent attacks of haematuria can finish with renal failure.

Treatment is unsatisfactory; steroids and immuno-suppressive drugs are sometimes given.

Purpura simplex

This occurs in otherwise healthy people, usually women in the 30-45 age group. Such a woman usually has a history of bruising easily and of menorrhagia. The usual site is on the trunk and legs. A psychogenic purpura can occur.

Senile purpura

This occurs on the forearms and backs of the hands of old people as the result of receiving minor injuries on skin that has lost its elastic tissue. Purpura can appear on the legs of old people with varicose veins.

Vitamin C deficiency

Vitamin C is necessary for the health of capillary walls and lack of it can so cause purpura; platelets contain a large amount of vitamin C.

Uraemia

In its late stages this can cause purpura.

Steroid therapy

Used in the treatment of purpura, steroid therapy can itself cause purpura, if its use is prolonged, by causing loss of elastic tissue and atrophy of the skin.

Mechanical purpura

This purpura is produced by fits, bouts of severe coughing, vomiting. The purpura is likely to occur on the heads and necks of infants and young children, sometimes in adults with bronchitis and emphysema.

HAEMOPHILIA [2]

This is an inherited sex-linked recessive condition, transmitted by females, who show no signs of it, to males, who show signs of it (see Chap. 11). There are theoretical grounds for believing that rarely a female could show signs of the disease and in practice about 1 in 200 cases is a female. There is a family history of haemophilia in about 75 per cent of cases. Should a boy develop the condition without any family history, there has probably been a gene-mutation in the chromosomes of his mother, any more children she has being likely to show or transmit the disease according to mendelian principles.

Haemophilia is characterized by a marked increase in the coagulation time and therefore by long, uncontrollable haemorrhages. This increase is due to lack of factor VIII, one of the substances necessary for the clotting of blood. The usual type

[2] *haemophilia:* from Greek: *haima* – blood; *philein* – to love

of haemophilia is called Haemophilia A or classical haemophilia; an uncommon and often mild type called Haemophilia B or Christmas disease[3] is due to lack of factor IX.

Clinical features The abnormal bleeding is usually noticed in early childhood. Tiny scratches bleed for days on end; any trivial knock can cause a big bruise. A dental extraction can cause a massive haemorrhage; some patients cannot use a tooth-brush because the gums bleed so much. Haemorrhages into joints cause pain, swelling and loss of function and can cause permanent crippling ankyloses[4] and contractures. Sub-periosteal haemorrhages can form large haemorrhagic cysts.

With modern treatment patients are now living much longer than they used to, and if they can survive into adult life there seems to be a tendency for the condition then to become milder.

Special test *Coagulation time:* is prolonged (normal: less than 10 minutes)

Prevention Unaffected males are the only members of a haemophilic family who can be guaranteed not to have haemophilic children or to transmit the disease. The other members should be warned accordingly.

The patient should be protected as far as is reasonable from accidental knocks and cuts. Intramuscular injections are not given because intramuscular haemorrhage is likely. Aspirin should not be taken as it can increase bleeding. Any bleeding from the skin should be treated with light pressure and the application of Russell's viper venom and thrombin. No operation should be performed unless absolutely necessary and only where full facilities for stopping haemorrhage are available. See *Treatment*.

Treatment When haemorrhages are occurring and before any operation, the patient's factor VIII level is raised by the injection of lyophilized human AHG (a freeze-dried preparation, rich in factor VIII, obtained from plasma), or of cryoprecipitate (cryoglobulin) (a protein rich in factor VIII obtained from plasma), or of plasma. The blood-level has to be kept raised for 1-4 days.

Similar preparations rich in factor IX are available for Christmas disease.

POLYCYTHAEMIA
VERA [5] This is a disease in which there is a great increase of RBCs and haemoglobin.

Polycythaemia can also occur: (a) as a temporary condition when the blood is concentrated following dehydration; (b) in any chronic cardio-pulmonary disease causing anoxia[6], and (c) as an apparently normal condition in some over-active plethoric people.

Polycythaemia vera occurs during the second half of adult life; there may be a family incidence. There is a marked increase in the amount of the red bone marrow (from which RBCs are formed); the medullary cavities of the long bones, instead of being occupied by fatty tissue, are packed with red marrow.

[3] *Christmas disease:* named after the family in which it was discovered
[4] *ankylosis:* fusion of bones at a joint, producing a stiff joint
[5] *polycythaemia:* from Greek: *poly* – many; *kutus* – container; *haima* – blood. *vera:* true
[6] *anoxia:* lack of oxygen

Clinical features	Common symptoms are headache, loss of weight and strength, shortness of breath, angina pectoris, itching of the skin, and temporary cerebral attacks with confusion, paralysis, aphasia[7] and visual disturbances. The patient is typically deep red or cyanosed, with blood-shot eyes, a large spleen and sometimes a large liver.
	The patient may live for several years if efficiently treated. Death from a vascular accident can occur. Some patients pass into a remission which can be followed by anaemia or leukaemia, but it is possible that these are the result of radio-therapy.
Complications	Cerebral haemorrhage Haemorrhage from nose, lungs, gastro-intestinal tract, etc. Venous thrombosis.
Special tests	*Blood:* RBCs: 7-14 million per mm³. Hb: 18-25 g per 100 ml. Haematocrit reading: over 60.
Treatment	1. *Bleeding* is performed twice weekly at first, 1 pint of blood being removed on each occasion, and then, when blood has become normal, at longer intervals as necessary. 2. *Radio-phosphorus* is given to reduce bone-marrow activity. The usual dose is 3-7 millicuries intravenously as a single dose; half this dose may be given 3-6 months later and again 3 months later. Further courses of treatment may be necessary. 3. Any surgical operation should if possible be postponed until the patient has responded to treatment. Anticoagulants are not given because they can start off a haemorrhage.

LEUKAEMIA

In leukaemia there is an overgrowth of the tissues that form white blood cells and in consequence a large increase of white cells in the blood.

It is generally regarded as a cancer. Hereditary factors may be involved. There is a relatively high incidence of leukaemia in mongolism, possibly because the same chromosome is involved in both conditions. It can be a result of exposure to radiation: it is more common in radiologists than in other doctors; it has occurred in patients with ankylosing spondylitis who have been subjected to irradiation of the spine; there has been a high incidence of it in survivors from atomic bomb explosions; there appears to be a risk of it appearing in infants whose mothers have, during pregnancy, had a diagnostic X-ray. The incidence in Britain and other countries this century suggests that some other factor, so far unidentified, is at work. There is evidence — but so far no proof — that this factor is a virus.

Leukaemia can be classified: (a) according to the particular kind of white cell predominantly involved; and (b) according to whether it is acute or chronic.

Acute leukaemia

Acute leukaemia can be *lymphatic* (when there is an increase in the number of lymphocytes in the blood), or *myeloid* (when there is an increase in the number of myelocytes i.e. granulocytes) or *monocytic* (when there is an increase in the number of monocytes).

More males than females are affected. Acute lymphatic leukaemia is most common in children under 5 years; the other two types of acute leukaemia can occur at any age.

[7] *aphasia:* loss of speech due to brain disease

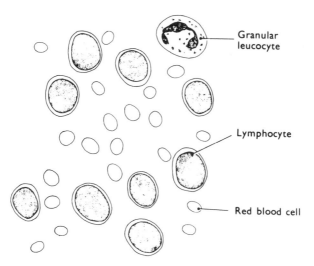

Fig. 31. Film of blood in lymphocytic leukaemia showing an excessive number of lymphocytes.

Granular leucocyte

Lymphocyte

Red blood cell

Clinical features The disease can be:

(a) acute from the onset: with fever, sore throat, purpura, bleeding from the nose and gums, bleeding after dental extractions and minor operations.

(b) insidious at first, with fatigue, pains in the gums, pains in the bone; and then a sudden shift into the acute form.

The patient is very pale. The gums swell and bleed like those of scurvy. The lymph-nodes, particularly those in the neck, are enlarged. The liver and the spleen are enlarged, the tip of the spleen being sometimes as much as 4 fingers' breadth below the costal margin.

The salivary glands (parotid, submandibular, sublingual) and the lacrimal glands are enlarged in acute lymphatic leukaemia.

Effusions into the joints, pericarditis, endocarditis, pleurisy and broncho-pneumonia can occur. Children with the disease can develop leukaemic meningitis — with headache, drowsiness, fits and paralysis of cranial nerves.

A spontaneous remission can occur and last for months or years. It is usually followed by relapse and death. The average length of life from the onset is about 12 months in a child and less than that in an adult, but with modern drugs there is a chance of recovery. The usual causes of death are cerebral haemorrhage, acute gastro-intestinal ulceration, or an acute infection.

Special tests *Blood:* White cells: there may at first be a reduction in the number of white cells or a normal white cell count; this is followed by an increase to 20,000-50,000 per mm³ of which 90 per cent are immature white cells.
RBC and Hb: both reduced.
Bone-marrow puncture: shows over-growth of primitive white cells.
X-ray of chest: to show enlarged lymph-nodes within chest and enlarged thymus.

Treatment 1. Anti-leukaemic drugs are given singly or in combination. These include: vincristine, asparaginase, daunorubicin and cystine arabinoside.

121   *Diseases of the Blood, Lymphatic System and Spleen*

2. Corticosteroids (usually prednisolone) are given with the anti-leukaemic drugs.
3. An appropriate antibiotic is given for any infection.
4. Blood transfusion is given for severe anaemia.

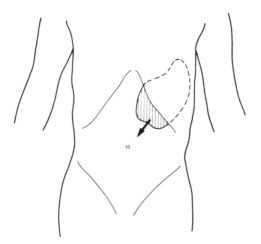

Fig. 32. Enlargement of the spleen.

Myeloid leukaemia

Other name: chronic myelocytic anaemia

This type of leukaemia occurs in both sexes and begins usually in the 30-55 year age group; it is rare before puberty.

Clinical features

The disease begins insidiously and it may be several years before the patient feels ill enough to go to his doctor.

He complains of fatigue, loss of strength, and gastro-intestinal disturbance. In this type of leukaemia the spleen becomes enormously enlarged; the patient may be aware that his abdomen is getting bigger or have a chronic dragging pain in his left side. There may be bouts of slight fever separated by long afebrile periods.

The patient is pale. The most distinctive feature of the disease is the spleen, which may be enlarged as low as the umbilicus and the right iliac fossa. The liver may be palpable. Lymph-nodes enlarge later. With the development of the disease the patient becomes emaciated and has oedema and ascites[8].

About half the patients die within 2½ years; some can live for more than 5 years. Remissions can be produced by drugs in about 50 per cent of the patients.

Complications

Impairment of vision due to haemorrhage into the retina.

Deafness and Ménière's syndrome due to involvement of the inner ear.

Special tests

Blood: White cells increased to 100,000-1,000,000 per mm³, mostly granulocytes.
RBC and Hb: reduced.
Chromosomes: An additional chromosome (No. 21) is found in cells of bone-marrow and in some granulocytes in blood.

[8] *ascites:* fluid in the peritoneal cavity

Chapter 5

Treatment	1. Courses of antileukaemic drugs are given. Drugs used include vincristine (VCR), cytosine arabinoside (ARA-C), thioguanine (TG) and daunorubicin (DAUNO). Combinations of drugs are more effective than any one drug given alone. Courses lasting for 5 days are given with intervals of 2-3 weeks between them, for the drugs are too toxic to be given continuously.

2. Fluid and electrolyte replacement is often necessary. Packed red cell and platelet transfusions may be necessary.

3. Antibiotics are given for any infection.

Lymphatic leukaemia

Other name: chronic lymphocytic leukaemia

In this form of leukaemia there is an overgrowth of lymphatic tissue in the body and an increase in the number of lymphocytes in the blood.

It is a disease of late middle life, the average age of incidence being 60, affecting men twice as often as women. Children are hardly ever affected.

Clinical features

The disease begins very insidiously and the patient may have had slight symptoms for years before he goes to his doctor.

The usual complaints are of fatigue, shortness of breath and loss of weight. There may be bouts of slight fever separated by long afebrile periods.

Lymph-nodes are enlarged in many parts of the body; they are moderately hard and separate, not matting together. The spleen may be moderately enlarged — 2-3 fingers' breath below the costal margin; the liver may be palpable.

Tumours of lymphatic tissue can develop in many parts of the body — in the skin, breast, tonsils and within the chest. The salivary and lacrimal glands are sometimes enlarged.

The course of the illness is prolonged. About half the patients die within 5 years; some are alive 10 years after the onset.

Complications

Auto-immune haemolytic anaemia (5-10 per cent of cases)
Thrombocytopenic purpura (in patients with a large spleen)

Special tests

White blood cells: increased to 10,000-100,000 per mm^3, 95-99 per cent of them are lymphocytes.
RBC and Hb: reduced.

Treatment

This is not very effective. The following are tried:
1. Splenectomy if the spleen is much enlarged; can be followed by a long remission.
2. Radiotherapy with X-rays or radio-active phosphorus.
3. Chlorambucil, a drug that prevents cells from multiplying, in 3-6 week courses.
4. Cortico-steroids for acute haemolytic anaemia.

DISEASES OF THE LYMPH-NODES

Enlarged lymph-nodes are found in:
1. *Local infections:* lymph-nodes draining an infected part become enlarged, painful and tender.

2. *General infections:* tuberculosis, secondary stage of syphilis, infective mono-nucleosis, German measles, toxoplasmosis, cat-scratch fever.
3. *Cancer:* by spread from a primary growth.
4. *Blood diseases:* in lymphatic and myeloid leukaemia.
5. *Disease of the lymphatic system:* in lymphadenoma (Hodgkin's disease).
6. *Drug reaction:* as a reaction to some drugs, phenytoin and its derivatives.

LYMPHADENOMA

Other names: Hodgkin's disease [9], lympho-granulomatosis
This is a disease of unknown origin (thought by some to be a kind of new growth, by others to be an infection, possibly by a virus). Lymph-nodes become enlarged, at first in one of the superficial groups, eventually in all the lymph-nodes and tissues of the body. The lymph-tissues show at first an overgrowth of lymph cells and in some cases a development of large primitive cells, possibly of a sarcomatous nature. The disease, one of adult life, is progressive and fatal unless treated promptly.

Clinical features

The lymph-nodes first affected are usually a group in the neck. They become enlarged and rubbery hard and after a time matt together. In time other lymph-nodes are involved. The spleen and the liver become enlarged and palpable because of the overgrowth of lymph-tissue in them. The patient feels ill and tired, becomes anaemic, runs a temperature (often with long afebrile periods), itches and wastes. A typical phenomenon is that taking alcohol produces pain in bones and other structures.

The length of life after the onset of this disease is very variable. Patients showing the rapidly growing 'sarcomatous' type of cell-change with the large primitive cells, go downhill very quickly and die within a year. In others the disease can be prolonged for 20 years.

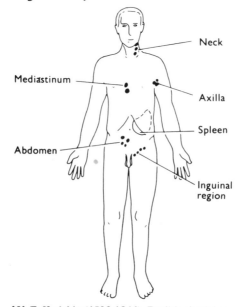

Neck

Mediastinum

Axilla

Spleen

Abdomen

Inguinal region

Fig. 33. In lymphadenoma (Hodgkin's disease), enlarged lymph-nodes in the neck are the first sign in most patients, but occasionally it begins in one of the other sites indicated.

[9] T. Hodgkin (1798-1866), English physician

Complications	Collapse of lung — due to pressure from enlarged nodes at the roots of the lungs. Obstructive jaundice, ascites — due to overgrowth of lymph-tissue in the liver. Collapse of vertebral body — due to growth of lymph-tissue in vertebrae. Intra-cranial and intra-spinal growths, producing pressure symptoms.
Special tests	*Biopsy:* a gland is removed for histological examination. *Blood:* slight anaemia; leucocytosis in about half the cases; raised ESR during acute stages.
Treatment	Treatment can produce cure or temporary improvement. 1. The first crop of enlarged nodes is removed. This seems to prevent other developments for about 6 months. 2. Radiotherapy of affected tissues is achieved by irradiation or radio-active phosphorus. 3. Cytotoxic drugs are given at the same time. 4. Anaemia is relieved by blood-transfusions. 5. Pain and itching are relieved by aminopryrine or phenylbutazone.

DISEASES OF THE SPLEEN	Primary diseases of the spleen are uncommon. Accessory spleens are present in about 10 per cent of people. Congenital absence can occur. Primary tumours are rare; secondary tumours can occur in generalized malignant disease. Cysts of the spleen occur in hydatid disease. Infarction can occur in any large spleen as a result of the slowness of the circulation through it and in any septicaemia; a septic infarct can be the cause of an abscess. *Perisplenitis*, inflammation of the peritoneal covering of the spleen, is usually due to an infarct. Rupture of the spleen can occur in any large spleen and in infective mono-nucleosis.
Causes of enlargement of the spleen	1. *Infection.* Malaria, acute or chronic, is the commonest cause of splenic enlargement in the tropics. Other infections in which a slight to moderate degree of enlargement can be found are: infective mononucleosis, enteric fever, subacute bacterial endocarditis. 2. *Diseases of blood and lymph-tissue.* Iron deficiency anaemia, pernicious anaemia, hereditary spherocytosis, sickle-cell anaemia, thalassaemia, polycythaemia, leukaemia, lymphadenoma, Banti's syndrome [1]. 3. *Other conditions.* Thyrotoxicosis, hydatid cyst, new growth.

The normal spleen cannot be felt unless, as happens rarely, it is pushed down by something above it. The spleen has to be enlarged about 3 times before it is palpable. The tip is then felt just below the costal margin. In some diseases — such as chronic malaria and myeloid leukaemia — it can become very large, reaching as low as the umbilicus and the right iliac fossa.

Small enlargements are not noticed by the patient. Large enlargements can cause dragging pain and the patient notices that his abdomen is becoming distended. Infarcts in the spleen cause acute pain.

[1] *G. Banti* (1852-1925) Italian pathologist

The surface of the spleen, unless it contains a new growth or a cyst, is smooth. Very typically a notch can be felt in the presenting edge.

BANTI'S
SYNDROME [1]

Other names: congestive spleno-megaly [2], splenic anaemia
This is a disease of uncertain origin. The important feature is an increase in pressure in the portal vein. In most cases the increase appears to be due to a cirrhosis of the liver; why the liver should become cirrhosed is unknown. The increase in pressure leads to (a) enlargement of the spleen, (b) oesophageal varices — varicose veins where the oesophagus joins the stomach; and (c) in one type of the disease a similar ring of veins at the umbilicus and on the abdominal wall. The enlargement of the spleen and bleeding from the oesophageal varices cause anaemia.

Clinical features

The patient complains of vague ill-health, tiredness and sometimes a dragging pain the abdomen (due to the enlarging spleen). His complexion is sallow; spider-naevi [3] appear in his skin.

The spleen is enlarged, sometimes to the umbilicus. Bleeding from the varices can be slight or catastrophic. There is a modest degree of hypochromic anaemia and a leucopenia.

The outlook for life depends on the degree of liver damage. With severe progressive damage the patient is not likely to live more than 5 years. Death is usually the result of a severe haemorrhage, ascites or hepatic coma.

Special tests

Scintillation counting (after percutaneous injection of radio-isotopes into spleen) is a method of studying portal vein circulation.
Oesophagoscopy: to see oesophageal varices.
Barium swallow: to demonstrate varices on X-ray.
RBCs: usually below 4 million per mm³. *Hb:* reduced.
White cells: always reduced below 5,000 per mm³.

Treatment

The basic aim of treatment is to reduce the pressure in the portal vein. It is sometimes possible to anastomose the portal vein to the inferior vena cava or the splenic vein to the left renal vein, so that another communication is produced between the portal and the systemic circulations.

The bleeding from the varices can be stopped by tying them; this may be combined with splenectomy. Blood transfusions and iron are given for anaemia.

[2] *spleno-megaly:* enlargement of spleen
[3] *spider-naevus:* blood-vessels radiating from a central arteriole

6   Diseases of the Kidneys

Any disease of the kidneys and urinary tract is likely to interfere with the basic functions of the kidneys:

1. The excretion of the end-products of metabolism, especially urea, uric acid and creatinine.
2. The maintenance within normal limits of the pH and amount of tissue-fluids.
3. The maintenance of the tissue-fluids at a constant composition, especially the amounts of sodium and potassium in them.
4. The excretion of some drugs and other 'foreign' substances and their break-down products.

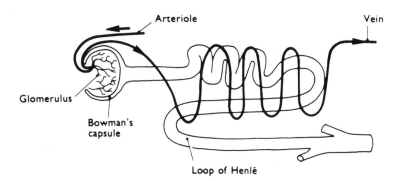

Fig. 34. A nephron.

Each kidney contains about 1 million nephrons. Many of them can be put out of action by disease without interfering very much with kidney function, for there is in each kidney a 'renal reserve' of nephrons that in normal conditions are not working all the time or to their full capacity. However, when this 'renal reserve' is affected, when there are not enough healthy nephrons left to carry out their full function, renal efficiency is impaired and evidence of renal disease appears. Interference with the basic functions causes biochemical changes of great complexity, which produce various clinical features, serious interference with many vital functions, and, in total failure, death.

[4] *pH:* symbol used to express hydrogen-ion concentration; pH above 7 indicates alkalinity, below 7 acidity (in an aqueous medium).

THE URINE   Evidence of disease of the kidneys and urinary tract and of several metabolic diseases can be found in the urine.

Specimen. A fresh specimen is advisable as changes can take place in urine left standing. A sterile specimen is obtained: in men, by a mid-stream specimen; in women, by parting the labia and cleaning them, or by suprapubic aspiration. Passing a catheter to obtain a specimen is unnecessary and dangerous; it can produce a lower urinary-tract infection (urethra and bladder).

Amount. The amount passed in 24 hours varies with the fluid intake and fluid excretion by other means, i.e. in perspiration and faeces.

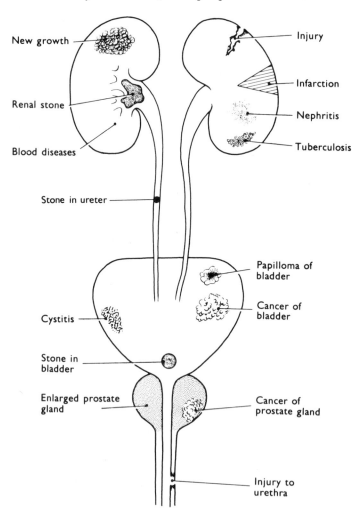

Fig. 35. Common causes of haematuria.

Colour. The colour varies from pale to deep yellow. Abnormal colour can be due to:

(a)   bile pigments which darken it;

(b)   blood which in small amounts makes it 'smoky', in large amounts bright red;

(c) Alkaptonuria, a rare metabolic disease, in which the urine goes dark on standing.

Specific Gravity (SG). This is an indication of the amount of substances dissolved in it. It is usually 1,002-1,032.

Cells. A few red and white blood cells are present in normal urine; the numbers can be much increased in diseases. An *Addis count* is a count of the cells in a counting chamber; an increase or decrease is an indication of the progress of disease.

Sugar. Sugar is not normally present in the urine. It can occur in 2 conditions: (a) diabetes mellitus (b) renal glucosuria.

Ketone bodies. Acetone and acetoacetic acid occur in some metabolic diseases in which fat metabolism is disturbed, especially diabetes mellitus (always in diabetic crisis), starvation, excessive vomiting, acute fevers in childhood.

Blood. Blood is not normally present in the urine. Common causes are:

any infection of kidney or urinary tract

injury to kidney	tumour of kidney
any bleeding disease	stone in urinary tract
papilloma of bladder	enlarged prostate gland

Pus. Pus can occur in any infection of the urinary tract.

Protein. Protein (albumin) occurs in:

(a) any disease of the kidney or urinary tract;

(b) ortho-static proteinuria: this condition occurs only in some young people; protein appears in the urine when they are up and about, and not when they are at rest; it is possibly due to increased pressure in the renal veins which is itself a result of pressure by the liver on the inferior vena cava; it is harmless.

Casts. Casts are small bodies formed by protein which has become solidified in the renal tubules. Hyaline casts (which have no cells in them) are normal. Casts with cells in them (cellular, granular casts) are found in nephritis, nephrosis, renal failure and hypertension.

ACUTE GLOMERULAR-NEPHRITIS

This appears to be an allergic reaction to a streptococcal infection. The patient is usually a child or adolescent with a history of a streptococcal infection of the throat (tonsillitis, pharyngitis, scarlet fever) 1-3 weeks previously.

In acute nephritis the kidneys become swollen and inflamed, the glomeruli being particularly involved in the inflammatory changes. Blood and protein leak out. The renal tubules are less if at all involved and allow the re-absorption of water and salt with the result that the tissues become oedematous.

Clinical features

The illness begins abruptly with fever, shivering, pain in the loins or abdomen, headache and vomiting. Oedema develops, showing first as a puffiness around the eyes. The amount of urine excreted is reduced. The urine contains protein and red blood cells, which give it a 'smoky' appearance, or obvious blood. The blood-pressure is slightly raised.

In about 90 per cent of cases, the patient starts to improve in a few days, his symptoms disappear, he excretes more urine and his oedema disappears. Some patients, however, continue to excrete protein for months.

Complications

Renal failure, hypertension and death within a year.
Persistent albuminuria, with renal failure years later.

| Acute heart failure | Acute pulmonary oedema |
| Infections | Hypertensive encephalopathy. |

Special tests

Urine: protein and red blood cells are present.
Blood urea: normal or slightly raised (normal: 20-40 mg/100 ml). Sodium and potassium are retained. Anti-streptococcal titre is high.

Treatment

1. The patient should go to bed and stay there until free from symptoms. If all clears up except albuminuria, he can be allowed up.
2. During the acute stage, the diet is restricted to water, fruit juice, glucose, cereals, in order to minimize the work done by the kidneys, and should be salt-free, for it is the retention of salt that causes the oedema. With recovery other food should be introduced gradually. Fluid balance is controlled.
3. Procaine penicillin: 600,000 units are given daily to clear up any streptococcal infection.
4. Phenoxymethyl penicillin: 240 mg daily for several years may be ordered, for it can possibly stop any recurrence of the streptococcal infection.
5. Infected tonsils may be removed later, when the patient has recovered.
6. Any subsequent attack of streptococcal infection is treated with antibiotics as soon as possible.

The urine is examined daily for its volume and protein content. The BP is taken daily. The ESR is examined weekly.

ACUTE RENAL FAILURE

Other name: acute oliguric uraemia
This is an emergency in which the glomeruli suddenly cease to function. It can be a result of:
(a)   a very low BP due to shock or severe haemorrhage;
(b)   a crush injury with extensive tissue-damage;
(c)   any severe acute renal disease, sudden interference with urinary excretion, and following intravenous pyelography;
(d)   obstetrical haemorrhage;
(e)   incorrect or mismatched blood-transfusion with free haemoglobin in the blood;
(f)   septicaemia;
(g)   poisoning by heavy metals;
(h)   following surgical operations.

Clinical features

Urinary output diminishes sharply. The blood urea and blood potassium rise steeply; acidosis is produced. The patient becomes sleepy, has nausea and vomits, and passes into stupor or coma. About 50-60 per cent die. If he survives for a few days, the kidneys can start to refunction, excreting large amounts of pale urine, and the patient recovers. In this stage of excessive urine secretion too much potassium and salt can be lost from the blood.

Complications	Bleeding from the gums Purpura Any infection
Special tests	*Urine:* examined daily for urea, sodium, potassium. *Blood:* examined daily or on alternate days for urea, sodium, potassium, chloride, haematocrit value. *ECG:* daily examination, for certain changes in it are an indication of the effects of a high potassium concentration in the blood.
Treatment	The aim of treatment is to keep the patient alive until the kidneys recover. It is advisable that the patient should be where a dialysis unit is available. Fluid and electrolyte loss are replaced. Frusemide in large doses (2-3 g daily) intravenously is given to promote renal flow.

NEPHROTIC SYNDROME

Other name: nephrosis

In this condition an excessive amount of plasma protein (up to 30 g daily) is lost in the urine and oedema produced.

It can occur in:

(a)   subacute glomerular nephritis (sometimes called nephritis type 2), which is sometimes of unknown origin, sometimes a result of acute glomerulo-nephritis, which accounts for more than half the cases;

(b)   diabetes, amyloid disease, thrombosis of the inferior vena cava or a renal vein, systemic lupus erythematosus, poisoning by heavy metals (which damage the renal tubules not the glomeruli).

The result of any of these is a degeneration of the glomeruli. The biochemical changes that follow are complicated. The loss of protein in the urine causes a fall in the amount of plasma protein; this leads to a low osmotic pressure and a diffusion of fluid into the tissues and accordingly the production of oedema. At the same time the fall in blood volume may stimulate the adrenal cortex to secrete an excessive amount of aldosterone, which leads to the retention of salt and fluid and so more oedema.

Clinical features	Oedema is the chief feature. Beginning in the ankles in a patient who is upright or over the sacrum of a patient in bed, it extends into the legs, genitalia, abdominal wall and arms. Ascites and pleural and pericardial effusions occur. Oedema of the lungs, brain and retinae can occur. A secondary thrombosis of a renal vein will produce a further deterioration. The course of the disease is variable, with the amount of oedema varying from time to time. Spontaneous recovery can occur when glomerular damage has been minimal. Treatment by steroids appears to produce a remission in most children but in less than half the affected adults. Usually, after months or years, renal function ceases and the patient dies.
Complications	Any infection, especially pneumonia, pleurisy, peritonitis, cellulitis.
Special tests	*Urine:* shows a gross amount of protein and sometimes red blood cells. *Blood:* blood urea may be normal at first; rises with renal failure (normal: 20-40 mg/100 ml)

Serum potassium may be low (normal: 3.9-5.2 mEq/litre)

Serum cholesterol may be raised (normal: 100-300 mg/100 ml);
the reason for this is unknown. Serum albumin is low.

Renal biopsy: to estimate degree of glomerular damage as an indication of prognosis.

Treatment

Treatment is aimed at restoring the plasma-protein to normal.

1. The patient is confined to bed for a few weeks and the cause treated.
2. *Diet:* high protein (100 g daily) and low salt.
3. *Steroid treatment.* Prednisolone is given in doses of 20-80 mg daily and continued according to the patient's response. How it acts is unknown. If there is no response within a fortnight, it can be discontinued and restarted later. Tolerance can develop.
4. *Diuretics.* Chlorothiazide and other diuretics are used to promote excretion.
5. *Tapping* of ascites or pleural effusion may be necessary.
6. *Potassium* is given if serum potassium is low.
7. *Antibiotics* are given for any infection.

PYELO-NEPHRITIS

This is an infection, acute or chronic, of the renal pelvis, ureters and kidneys. *E. coli* is the usual infecting organism.

Pyelo-nephritis can follow:

(a) a lower urinary tract infection in women,

(b) urinary tract obstruction by a congenital deformity of the renal pelvis or ureter; stasis of urine due to stone in the renal pelvis, ureter or bladder, enlargement of the prostate gland, a new growth in the urinary tract, stricture of the urethra.

The infecting organism can reach the pelvis either by ascending from the urethra and bladder or by the blood-stream. In women a lower urinary tract infection, involving urethra and bladder, can occur after first sexual intercourse (the 'honeymoon cystitis'); although it usually settles down in a few days, there can be recurrences and infected urine can pass backwards up the ureter. In children, too, the act of micturition can force urine up the ureters.

Attacks of pyelo-nephritis are very likely to recur, producing a more or less chronic infection, which can go on to cause fibrous degeneration of the kidneys and a decline in renal function. In some patients the disease is symptomless, the condition being discovered at autopsy.

Clinical features

In an acute attack the patient feels ill, has a raised temperature, complains of pain in his loins and sometimes in the suprapubic region, and has frequency and urgency of micturition. The kidneys may be tender.

Chronic pyelo-nephritis causes intermittent fever, frequency of micturition, and eventually signs of renal failure.

Special tests

Urine: contains pus cells and an excessive number of organisms (urine of healthy people can contain organisms); organisms are tested for sensitivity.

Blood: will show leucocytosis.

X-ray of urinary tract: by intravenous pyelogram for evidence of obstruction, etc; a micturating cystogram may demonstrate urine entering ureters during micturition.

Treatment   In acute pyelo-nephritis the patient is put to bed. As the most likely infecting organism is *E. coli*, an organism found only in acid urine, the urine is made alkaline by giving sodium citrate 3.0 g and sodium bicarbonate 3.0 g 2-hourly, the dose being reduced when the urine becomes alkaline. A course of appropriate sulphonamide is given (e.g. sulphamethizole, sulphafurazole) or ampicillin.

The patient should recover within a few days. If he does not, he is treated with a course of the drug to which the organism has by this time been found to be sensitive.

Recurrent infections indicate that a thorough investigation of the urinary tract should be carried out by intravenous or retrograde pyelography.

An acute lower urinary tract infection is usually cured by a 10-day course of sulphonamide.

Chronic pyelonephritis requires up to 6 months' treatment with courses of an appropriate antibiotic the organism is sensitive to. The patient may require treatment for renal failure.

CHRONIC RENAL FAILURE

This is the result of any progressive renal disease, occurring when the kidneys fail to function adequately. *Uraemia* is the condition produced by renal failure.

The effects of renal failure are:

(a) toxic substances are retained. These are mostly derived from the breakdown of protein in the body and include urea, urates, creatinine, sulphate, phosphate and hydrogen-ion. Measurement of the blood urea is the most convenient way of measuring the degree of this retention.

(b) electrolyte disturbance takes place. A healthy kidney keeps constant the amount of sodium in the blood by adjusting the output to the intake. With renal failure the kidney keeps up a fairly constant excretion. If the patient reduces the amount of sodium taken, he develops a 'sodium leak', losing more than he takes in; and as a result of the lowering of the amount of sodium in the blood, he develops nausea, cramps, hypotension and loss of weight. Potassium loss causes fatigue.

(c) water excretion is disturbed. With renal failure the kidney cannot concentrate urine and in consequence excretes a large amount of diluted urine.

(d) calcium metabolism is disturbed. (e) acidosis can occur.

Clinical features   The onset is usually gradual as more and more nephrons are put out of action. Symptoms do not appear until the blood urea has reached about 150 mg per 100 ml, which is an indication that the GFR (glomerular filtration rate) has fallen below 25 per cent.

The earliest features are (a) the passing of too much urine and having to get up in the night, (b) fatigue and (c) anaemia.

The patient may remain in this state for years. However, with increasing biochemical dysfunction, more serious symptoms and signs appear in many systems:—

(a) *Alimentary system:* dirty tongue; unpleasant breath; hiccoughing, nausea, vomiting, gastro-intestinal bleeding, haematemesis, melaena, diarrhoea.

(b) *Respiratory system:* gasping respiration, Cheyne-Stokes breathing in terminal state.

133   *Diseases of the Kidneys*

(c) *Central Nervous System:* listlessness, drowsiness, twitching, fits, coma.

(d) *Cardio-vascular system:* raised blood-pressure, papilloedema, retinal haemorrhages.

(e) *Skin:* dry, yellow-brown; pruritus; crystals of urea excreted in the sweat form a 'urea frost'.

(f) *Bone:* generalized decalcification.

(g) *Blood:* severe microcytic anaemia which does not respond to treatment.

Special tests *Urine:* low SG; contains protein, red blood cells, casts.
Blood: urea raised much above normal (normal: 20-40 mg. per 100 ml.)

Treatment Treatment is by diet, dialysis and transplantation of kidney; surgical treatment is indicated for any obstruction.

1. Diet (a) to reduce unwanted and dangerous metabolites to a minimum, a special diet is provided in which the protein content is not greater than 18 g daily; additional calories are provided by protein-free bread; (b) to maintain electrolyte and water balance, sodium, potassium and water intake are adjusted to the patient's needs.

By this means life may be prolonged for a long time when renal failure is slight and for a few months when it is severe.

2. Dialysis This acts on the principle of a semi-permeable membrane which leaves large molecules (red blood cells, proteins) in the blood but allows smaller molecules to pass through. In this way unwanted substances can be removed from the blood.

(a) *Peritoneal dialysis* The patient's own peritoneum acts as the semi-permeable membrane. The dialysis fluid is run into the peritoneal cavity; the unwanted solutes in the blood pass into it through the peritoneum; and the fluid is then allowed to run away. The method is simple and does not require an elaborate machine.

(b) *Haemodialysis* This is the method in which an 'artificial kidney' is used. An artery and vein are connected by a cannula so that there is a direct flow between them. At the appropriate time the shunt is connected to the artificial kidney. The blood, to get from artery to vein, now has to pass between cellophane membranes, which act as semi-permeable membranes. Unwanted solutes pass through them into the dialysis fluid which is circulating on the other side of the membrane.

The patient selected is usually 15-50 years old and should be stable and reliable. Treatment is begun in hospital and continued at home when the patient and a reliable adult living with him have both been trained. The number of treatments necessary varies with the patient's degree of renal function and the type of machine; commonly it is done 2-3 nights a week for a total of 28-30 hours a week. Dietary and fluid restrictions have to be continued for the machine is not as efficient as a healthy kidney. About 10 per cent of patients die within the first few months of treatment, but after that time the mortality drops sharply.

Complications of dialysis are:

(a) *Infection:* The shunt can become infected and clotted. Micro-organisms can get into the blood-stream via the shunt. If the patient develops hepatitis, he is likely to become a carrier. Staff can become infected.

(b) *Mental state:* The patient and his assistant are likely to be tense, frightened and annoyed, especially in the early stages.

(c) *Disequilibrium syndrome:* Headache, vomiting, twitching and fits are produced by biochemical imbalances between the various fluid and cellular compartments of the body as a result of the rapid removal of chemical substances from the blood.

(d) *Peripheral neuropathy:* This occurs occasionally, sometimes in a very severe degree.

(e) *Bone disease:* Bones can become decalcified. If this is due to excessive secretion from the parathyroid glands, they are removed.

(f) *Iron-deficiency anaemia:* This is treated by iron given by mouth.

3. Renal transplantation

An effective method of dealing with renal failure should be the transplantation of a kidney. The surgical difficulties have been overcome, but the immunological difficulties remain: the transplant may die, the patient has to take immuno-suppresive drugs and risk infection, complications of prolonged cortico-steroid treatment can occur.

HYPERTENSION DUE TO UNILATERAL RENAL DISEASE

Hypertension is sometimes a result of unilateral renal disease, due to:

atheroma of a renal artery	pyelo-nephritis
renal injury	renal cyst
renal tumour	hydronephrosis
renal infection.	

It is due to an excessive production of renin by the kidney.

Clinical features

The clinical features are those of hypertension.

Special tests

X-ray of urinary tract by intravenous pyelography.
Aortography for evidence of blocking of a renal artery.
Urine collected by ureteric catheter from each kidney for comparison of secretions.
I_{131} *hippuran:* a radio-active substance injected intravenously and each kidney separately monitored to measure its output.

Treatment

Treatment is unsatisfactory. Drugs that lower the BP can be given. If the condition can be shown to be due to narrowing of a renal artery, a plastic operation can be performed. If the other kidney can be shown to be functioning normally and to be healthy, the affected kidney could be removed.

FAILURES OF RENAL TUBULAR FUNCTION

The renal tubules sometimes do not function adequately. This can occur in:

(a) *Fanconi's syndrome:* a rare familial disease in which the tubules fail to reabsorb sugar, amino-acids and phosphates, all of which are excreted in the urine. The condition occurs in childhood, the affected child being dwarfed, developing renal rickets, having polyuria and thirst, and eventually dying of renal failure.

(b) *Renal tubular acidosis:* the tubules are incapable of making the urine acid. An excessive amount of bicarbonate is excreted and this leads to acidosis; an excessive excretion of calcium in the urine causes calcium to be deposited in the kidney (nephro-calcinosis); the serum potassium is low. Affected children do not thrive, vomit, become dehydrated and may die. If the child survives into adult life, renal function sometimes becomes normal. If the disease occurs in adult life, the excessive secretion of calcium produces osteomalacia and renal calcification.

Treatment

Treatment is by giving sodium or potassium citrate and sodium bicarbonate by mouth to try to combat acidosis, and calcium to relieve the calcium deficiency.

7   Disorders of Fluid and Electrolyte Balance

The volume and composition of the body-fluids are controlled by mechanisms within the body and in health are kept constant in spite of wide variations in the intake of fluids and electrolytes. Disease and injury can upset these mechanisms and produce serious physical and chemical changes, sometimes severe enough to cause death.

Terms The following terms are used:

ion: an electrically-charged particle.

anion: an ion with a negative electric charge (chloride, bicarbonate, phosphate, protein, etc.)

cation: an ion with a positive electric charge (hydrogen, sodium, potassium, etc.)

pH: an indication of the concentration of hydrogen (H) ions in a solution and hence the degree of acidity. The normal pH of the plasma is 7.35-7.45 and depends on the proportion of carbonic acid (including dissolved CO_2) to bicarbonate in it.

acidosis: a fall in pH below the normal, as a result of (a) impaired excretion of carbon dioxide (CO_2) or (b) retention of acid or loss of base.

alkalosis: a rise in pH above the normal, as a result of (a) excessive excretion of CO_2 or (b) loss of acid or retention of base.

acid: any substance that gives up hydrogen ions.

base: any substance that receives hydrogen ions — bicarbonate, dibasic phosphate, some amino-acids.

buffer solution: one which resists a change in pH when small amounts of acid or base are added to it.

electrolyte: any base or acid, etc. which when dissolved produces ions.

Na: abbreviation for sodium (Natrium); a sodium atom.

K: abbreviation for potassium (from Arabic — *kali*); a potassium atom.

WATER IN THE BODY All the metabolic activities of the body take place in water. Water forms about 75 per cent of the body of an infant, about 60 per cent of an adult man, and about 55 per cent of an old man. In women, because of the different proportion of fat, the amount of water is about 10 per cent less than in a man. An adult man weighing 70 kilos (11 stones) contains about 50 litres of water. These figures are important when estimates of fluid and electrolyte needs are being calculated.

136

The amount of water gained (which is the sum of both water-intake and water-production) must equal the amount of water lost.

Water gain is mainly from three sources:

(a)   drinking, the amount drunk usually being controlled by thirst,

(b)   eating, as food contains water,

(c)   metabolism, as water is produced by metabolic activities.

Water loss is mainly controlled by the kidneys. Daily, in health, about 180 litres of water pass through the glomeruli of the kidneys, but most of this is promptly reabsorbed in the renal tubules back into the blood-plasma, and only about 1.5 litres of water are excreted as urine.

Some water is also lost in the breath, faeces, sweat and tears.

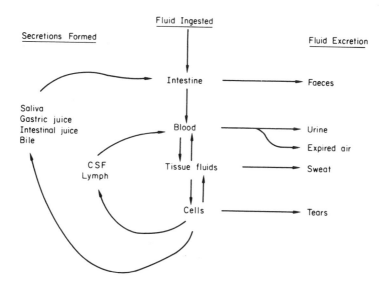

Fig. 36. Diagram of the ingestion, circulation and excretion of fluid.

FLUID COMPARTMENTS OF THE BODY

Water is contained in the body in the following places and proportions:

1. *Intra-cellular Fluid* (ICF). This is fluid inside the cells; the amount contained in this way is about 50 per cent of body-weight.

2. *Extra-cellular Fluid* (ECF). Fluid outside the cells is:

(a)   interstitial fluid: this is fluid in the tissue-spaces, the spaces between cells; it forms about 10 per cent of body-weight.

(b)   blood-plasma: it forms about 5 per cent of body-weight.

(c)   cerebrospinal fluid, fluid in serous cavities, joints, etc.

The ECF is the medium for the transport of chemical substances from one cell to another. The ICF is the medium in which the chemical activities of cells take place.

The important compartments for fluid-balance are the ICF, the interstitial fluid and the plasma of the blood. The distribution of fluids in the body depends on the amount of ions and proteins in these main compartments.

Disorders of Fluid and Electrolyte Balance

Fluid Balance　　　The nurse should appreciate that the chemical exchanges between the ECF and the ICF are complicated and difficult to understand; only the simplest account of them can be given here.

The chemical substances of the body that are important for the control of water-balance between the various compartments are:
1. in the *ICF:* potassium, organic phosphates, proteins, organic acids;
2. in the *interstitial fluid:* sodium, chloride, bicarbonate.
3. in the *plasma:* sodium, chloride, bicarbonate, protein.

The total volume of fluid in the body is determined by the total amounts of sodium and potassium in it.

The amount of intra-cellular fluid is determined by the amount of potassium in the body.

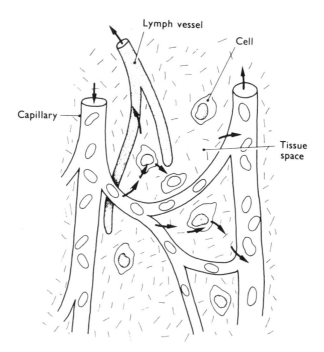

Fig. 37. Diagram to show the exchange of fluids between blood, tissue-spaces, cells and lymph.

The amount of extra-cellular fluid is determined by the amount of sodium in the body, and is also affected by the exchange of fluid between the interstitial and plasma compartments.

In normal conditions the sodium is discharged out of the cells by a mechanism called the 'sodium pump' and potassium is retained in the cells. Although the substances in the ICF and the ECF are different, the osmotic pressures are the same, and this ensures that the correct fluid-balance is maintained.

DISTURBANCES OF　　　Fluid deficiency may be (a) pure water deficiency, (b) mainly electrolyte loss, (c) a
FLUID BALANCE　　　mixture of these.

138

Water deficiency	This is due to a failure of intake of water due to (a) inability to swallow, (b) the patient's being in coma, (c) no water available as in a desert. Even when water is not being taken, there is an inevitable loss of water in the following approximate daily amounts: respiration (600 ml), perspiration (400 ml), urine (500 ml). These losses being of almost pure water, the concentration of the ECF rises. In consequence the osmotic pressure of the ECF become higher than that of the ICF and water passes from ICF to ECF, the fluid-loss being in this way shared by all the body-fluids.
Clinical features	Thirst (in the conscious patient), dry mouth, confusion, coma.
Special tests	Plasma sodium raised Haemoglobin raised.
Treatment	Water by mouth if the patient is conscious and can swallow. Intravenous 5 per cent dextrose is given if he is unconscious or cannot swallow.
Mainly electrolyte loss: *salt deficiency*	The causes of this are: (a) loss from the gastro-intestinal tract: diarrhoea, vomiting, fistulae, intestinal obstruction; (b) excessive use of diuretics; (c) Addison's disease; (d) excessive sweating with inadequate salt intake, as in the tropics and some industrial work. When salt is lost, water is also lost and the volume of the ECF diminishes. But the osmotic pressure remains the same and equal to that of the ICF. Therefore the ICF cannot contribute any fluid to the ECF. This is important because severe diminution of the amount of plasma leads to circulatory failure and renal failure. Lost electrolytes as well as lost water have to be replaced. Giving water alone would cause the ECF to become hypertonic, fluid would pass from the ECF to the ICF, and so the ECF would become even shorter of water.
Clinical features	Weakness, muscular cramps, dry skin, sunken eyes, hypotension, circulatory failure leading to renal failure.
Special tests	Plasma and sodium chloride decreased; plasma proteins raised. Haemoglobin raised.
Treatment	Fluid and electrolyte are replaced by normal saline (flavoured) by mouth or normal saline with glucose given intravenously. A fluid-balance chart is kept. The estimation of salt-deficiency is difficult. Plasma-electrolyte levels are used as a guide to treatment, which is continued until protein and electrolytes are normal.
Fluid excess *(over-hydration)*	This can be due to: (a) an excess of water alone, due to over-secretion of ADH (the anti-diuretic pituitary hormone); (b) a retention of sodium in renal failure, which causes a passive retention of water. The excessive fluid is shared equally by the intra- and extra-cellular spaces.
Clinical features	Oedema, cardiac failure if the plasma compartment is overloaded with fluid, convulsions, coma.
Special test	Plasma electrolytes decreased.
Treatment	The cause is treated. Diuretics are given to relieve oedema. Dialysis may be necessary if renal failure develops.

DISORDERS OF POTASSIUM	An excess of potassium in the blood can be due to:

DISORDERS OF POTASSIUM

Hyperkalaemia

An excess of potassium in the blood can be due to:
1. Acute renal failure
2. Diabetic coma
3. Circulatory failure
4. Addison's disease

   Even when the amount of potasssium in the blood is normal or high there can be a dangerous shortage of it in the cells.

Clinical features

Muscle weakness and an abnormal ECG can occur as a result of the excessive amount of potassium in the blood.

Hypokalaemia

This means an abnormally low level of potassium in the plasma, but what is more important is that there is an abnormally low level of potassium in the cells of the body. The causes are:
1. Loss of potassium from the gastro-intestinal tract by diarrhoea or vomiting.
2. Loss through the kidneys as a result of (a) a prolonged use of diuretics without potassium supplements being given by mouth to the patient, or (b) the diuretic phase of acute renal failure, i.e. when recovery from failure is taking place.
3. When prolonged glucose-saline therapy is being given without potassium supplements.
4. After the treatment of diabetic coma with insulin.

Clinical features

These are apathy, drowsiness, confusion, excessive secretion of urine, thirst, paralysis, abdominal distension, paralytic ileus [5]. Muscular weakness and an abnormal ECG can occur as when there is too much potassium in the blood.

Treatment

1. *By mouth*:   orange and other fruit juices (which are rich in potassium); Slow K (which contains potassium chloride) or effervescent potassium.
2. *By intravenous injection*: potassium chloride in saline-glucose is given with care. The urine output and the electrolytes are checked.

ACID-BASE BALANCE

The pH of the extra-cellular fluid is normally between 7.3 and 7.5.

   Acids. Carbon dioxide and acids, which are both produced by metabolism, tend to lower the pH and have to be excreted. Carbon dioxide is ultimately excreted by the lungs and the acids by the kidneys.

   Base. If there is too much base, the rate and depth of respiration are reduced, with the result that carbon dioxide is conserved in the blood, and the healthy kidney excretes bicarbonate and conserves hydrogen ions.

   The buffer systems of the body maintain the pH of the blood within normal limits by temporarily coping with an excess of acid or base. But they cannot overcome the effects of a very large excess of either nor overcome the effects of respiratory or renal failure; and a failure of these compensatory mechanisms leads to acidosis or to alkalosis.

[5] *paralytic ileus:* paralysis of intestine leading to dilatation and obstruction

ACIDOSIS	This is a fall in pH below the normal. It can be (a) *respiratory acidosis* due to a failure to excrete carbon dioxide or (b) *non-respiratory acidosis* due to either a gain of acid or a loss of bicarbonate.
Respiratory acidosis	This condition develops when carbon dioxide is not excreted by the lungs in adequate amounts as a result of a failure of respiratory function, as can occur in: chronic bronchitis and emphysema status asthmaticus paralysis of the muscles of respiration barbiturate poisoning
Clinical features	In addition to the features of the original disease, the patient is likely to develop dyspnoea, cyanosis, confusion and unconsciousness.
Non-respiratory acidosis	*Gain of acid* can occur in; diabetic ketosis acute and chronic renal failure (when hydrogen ions are not excreted) after some operations, e.g. uretero-colostomy (transplantation of the ureters into the colon) hard physical exercise *Loss of bicarbonate* can occur in: diarrhoea renal tubular acidosis (the kidneys cannot reabsorb bicarbonate in the tubules after it has been excreted by the glomeruli)
Clinical features of non-respiratory acidosis	These are usually fatigue, increased respiration and unconsciousness.
Treatment	The cause is treated. Fluid and electrolyte imbalance is corrected. Buffer bases can be replaced by sodium bicarbonate solution or sodium lactate solution.
Lactic acidosis	In this condition there is an accumulation of lactic acid in the blood. It can occur (a) as a familial disorder in children with neurological diseases, (b) in uraemia, diabetes, liver disease, leukaemia, alcoholism, (c) without known cause. It is measured by estimation of the blood-lactate level.
Treatment	Biochemical abnormalities are corrected if possible.
ALKALOSIS	This is a rise of pH above the normal. It can be (a) *respiratory alkalosis* due to loss of carbon dioxide through the lungs or (b) *non-respiratory alkalosis* due to loss of acid or gain of bicarbonate.
Respiratory alkalosis	*Loss of carbon dioxide* becomes excessive as a result of hyperventilation, in which the patient breathes too deeply and too quickly. This can occur in: salicylate poisoning brain damage anxiety hysteria
Non-respiratory alkalosis	*Loss of acid* can be due to (a) vomiting or (b) gastric aspiration, in both of which there is removal of the acid gastric juice from the stomach. *Gain of bicarbonate* can be due to (a) an excessive intake of bicarbonate, e.g. in the treatment of a peptic ulcer, or (b) as a complication of potassium deficiency.
Clinical features	The usual features are drowsiness, paraesthesiae (tingling, pins and needles, etc.), tetany and fits.
Treatment	The cause is treated. Fluid and electrolyte imbalance is corrected.

8 Diseases of the Alimentary Tract, Liver and Pancreas

The alimentary tract has several functions, and the diseases of the tract — they are many — can in various ways affect these functions.

The *mouth* is concerned with chewing and the mixing of food with saliva. Lack of teeth, aching teeth and ill-fitting dentures can interfere with these functions and prevent proper mastication. The interior of the mouth can develop fungal and other infections. The tongue is normally moist and clean; if a patient is dehydrated, the tongue becomes dry; in renal failure or acute abdominal disease it becomes coated with fur; and in deficiency of vitamin B complex and some anaemias it becomes bright-red and smooth.

The *oesophagus* is the organ for the transmission of masticated food from the mouth to the stomach. Diseases of the oesophagus, by interfering with this function are likely to cause difficulty in swallowing, pain and vomiting.

The *stomach* is concerned with the digestion of food. Common diseases are gastritis, ulcer and carcinoma. Interference with its functions is likely to cause at first loss of appetite, nausea, flatulence and abdominal discomfort; and with progression of the disease, the patient is likely to develop vomiting, abdominal pain and loss of weight.

The *small intestine* is concerned with the digestion and absorption of foodstuffs. The part of the duodenum nearest to the stomach is likely to suffer the development of an ulcer similar to the ulcer that occurs in the stomach. Gastro-enteritis [6] will produce abdominal pain, vomiting, diarrhoea and loss of fluid. Mal-absorption syndromes follow a failure of the small intestine to absorb essential foodstuffs, minerals and vitamins. In typhoid fever the Peyer's patches of lymph-tissue in the small intestine are liable to become inflamed, to bleed and to burst into the peritoneal cavity. Tumours of the small intestine are uncommon.

The *large intestine* is concerned with the onward passage of the contents of the intestine, the absorption of water from them, and their conversion into faeces. Diseases of the large intestine (the most common are colitis, carcinoma and diverticulitis) are likely to cause diarrhoea, blood and abdominal pain or discomfort.

The *liver* has many metabolic activities. It is concerned in the metabolism of carbohydrate, fat and protein, and in the destruction of red blood cells. It is particularly liable to be affected by infections, by degenerative changes, and by car-

---

[6] *gastro-enteritis:* inflammation of the stomach and intestine

cinomatous growths secondary to carcinoma elsewhere in the body. Jaundice is a common sign of disease of the liver.

The *pancreas* has two functions. The first of these is the production of pancreatic juice, which is necessary for the digestion of food. This function is likely to be disturbed by an acute or chronic inflammation of the pancreas. The second function is the secretion of insulin, lack of which produces the symptoms and signs of diabetes mellitus, and of glucadon.

Diseases of the Alimentary Tract

DISEASES OF THE MOUTH
STOMATITIS

Stomatitis is inflammation or degeneration of the mucous membrane of the mouth and occurs in various forms.

(a) *Catarrhal Stomatitis* occurs in poorly nourished children, in heavy smokers and drinkers, in severe illness, and when the teeth are carious and the mouth is neglected.

The mouth is painful and tender. The mucous membrane is red, the tongue furred and the breath often offensive.

It is prevented by adequate oral hygiene in health and disease, by adequate nourishment, and by the avoidance of tobacco and alcohol. It is treated by an adequate diet, by stimulating the flow of saliva with chewing-gum, and by mouth-washes of hydrogen peroxide.

(b) *Thrush* is an infection of the mouth with a fungus *Candida albicans.* It occurs in badly nourished and neglected children, in severe chronic illness in adults, and as a complication of treatment by cortico-steroids and some antibiotics.

It appears as ulcers covered with white sloughs.

It is prevented by adequate oral hygiene and by proper care in childhood, and is treated by swabbing with nystatin twice a day until it clears up.

(c) *Aphthous stomatitis* occurs as multiple, small, painful ulcers in the mucous membrane. It can be a complication of any severe illness, can be due to a *trichomonas* infection, or can occur in people who are apparently in good health.

Treatment

Treatment is by amethocaine lozenges to relieve the pain. Metronidazole (Flagyl) is given by mouth (swallowed) when it is due to *trichomonas* infection.

GLOSSITIS

Glossitis is inflammation or degeneration of the mucous membrane of the mouth; it can be part of a general stomatitis.

(a) *Nutritional glossitis* is due to a failure of absorption of a vitamin of the B group (as in pernicious anaemia) or due to an iron-deficiency anaemia. The tongue is painful, tender and raw, and if the condition becomes chronic the papillae are lost off its surface, which becomes smooth and shiny. It clears up when the basic condition is adequately treated.

(b) *Syphilitic glossitis* can occur as a primary chancre, as 'mucous patches' in the secondary stage, and as a gumma (a hard, painless lump) in the tertiary stage (see p. 49).

(c) *Leucoplakia* occurs in the tongue due to syphilis or other infection or injury from jagged teeth. It appears as smooth, white patches, painless at first, becoming painful later when fissures develop in them. It can become malignant.

DISEASES OF THE OESOPHAGUS
PEPTIC OESOPHAGITIS

In this condition there is inflammation and ulceration of the epithelium of the oesophagus as a result of a leak upwards of gastric juice. This happens most commonly when there is a hiatus hernia, i.e. a hernia of the fundus of the stomach through the oesophageal opening in the diaphragm into the chest. The juice starts to digest the epithelium, which cannot resist it.

Clinical features

Many people with a hiatus hernia have no symptoms. With the development of oesophagitis the patient complains of retro-sternal pain. Unlike a very similar pain, that of angina pectoris, this pain is brought on not by exertion but by stooping or lying down. The patient is likely to call the pain 'heart-burn'. Sometimes gastric juice comes up into the mouth. The pain may occur at night and is relieved by sitting up in bed. If the oesophagus is ulcerated, bleeding is likely and can cause anaemia.

Special tests

Oesophagoscopy: the inflammation and ulceration are visible through an oesophagoscope. *X-ray:* a barium meal is given and the patient placed in a head-down position to demonstrate the hiatus hernia of the stomach and the flow of barium into the oesophagus.

Treatment

1. The patient is advised to avoid stooping and to sleep with the upper part of his body propped up or the head of the bed raised on blocks.
2. Meals should be small.
3. Antacid tablets are sucked; in severe cases the full medical anti-peptic ulcer treatment is given.
4. Anaemia is treated with iron or if necessary a blood-transfusion.
5. If these measures fail the patient can be operated on and the gap in the diaphragm closed.

CANCER OF THE OESOPHAGUS

This cancer occurs usually in late middle or old age, in men more often than women. Its high incidence in men engaged in the alcohol trade (e.g. publicans, barmen, brewers) suggests that alcoholic inflammation of the oesophagus may be a predisposing factor. The usual site is in the middle third.

Clinical features

The patient has difficulty in swallowing, slight at first but getting worse, for solids at first and later for all food and drink. He feels that food is held up at one spot, which he can often localize fairly accurately with a finger-tip on the chest-wall. Complete obstruction develops in about 8 months. Regurgitation of food begins a few weeks after the swallowing disability is first noticed. Wasting is rapid. Lymph-nodes draining the part become invaded by cancer cells. Cough, hoarseness and difficulty in breathing are caused by pressure on the trachea by the growth itself or by enlarged lymph-nodes; ulceration of the growth makes the breath offensive. Death usually occurs within 6-12 months of the onset.

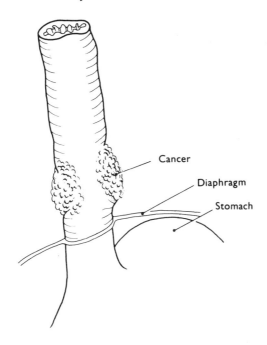

Fig. 38. Cancer of the oesophagus, causing constriction and obstruction to the passage of food.

Complications

Perforation into trachea, bronchi or pleural cavity
Bronchopneumonia, gangrene of lung, empyema
Starvation.

Special tests

Oesophagoscopy: the cancer can be seen through an oesophagoscope and a specimen of the growth removed for histological examination.
X-ray: a barium swallow indicates the site of obstruction and the dilatation of the oesophagus that occurs above it.

Treatment

Treatment is unsatisfactory.
(a) *Surgery:* the growth is occasionally removable; a oesophago-gastrostomy is performed, joining the divided oesophagus to the stomach.
(b) *Radio-therapy:* if removal is not possible, radio-therapy is given; the results are not very good.
(c) *Dilatation* of a fibrous growth may be attempted; it is sometimes possible to leave a permanent dilator in place.

ACHALASIA OF THE OESOPHAGUS

In this condition there is an inability of the lower oesophageal sphincter to relax adequately after a swallow and an absence of normal oesophageal peristalsis. The condition occurs in both sexes and at any age. The oesophagus becomes dilated and food accumulates in it. It can occur in vitamin B group deficiencies. There is a degeneration of the nerve-cells in the oesophageal wall through which the normal movements are controlled.

Clinical features The onset can be sudden or gradual. The patient has difficulty in swallowing and retro-sternal discomfort. The condition is made worse by emotional upsets, and because of the obvious difficulty the patient may be unwilling to eat away from the privacy of home. Loss of weight does not occur.

Complications Pneumonia or lung abscess, due to spilling over of food into the trachea. Cancer of oesophagus.

Treatment An inhalation of octyl nitrite gives temporary relief. The muscle can be divided down to the mucous membrane (Heller's operation). Dilatation under radiological control gives good results in about 75 per cent of cases.

CORKSCREW OESOPHAGUS *Other name:* oesophageal dyskinesia [8]
An elderly patient complains of difficulty in swallowing. A barium-swallow shows that the contractions of the oesophagus have a corkscrew-like twist and that there is no proper peristalsis. Treatment is by surgical division of the muscle-coat of the affected part.

DISEASES OF THE STOMACH AND DUODENUM PEPTIC ULCER A peptic ulcer can occur in: (a) the stomach, (b) the duodenum, (c) on either side of a gastro-intestinal anastomosis and (d) in the lower end of the oesophagus and in a Meckel's diverticulum, [9] in both of which places gastric mucous membrane can be present and can secrete gastric juice.

A peptic ulcer can be acute or chronic.

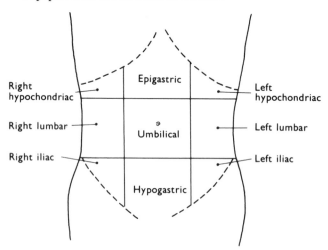

Fig. 39. The regions of the abdomen.

Acute ulcer An *acute ulcer* is the less important condition, for usually it heals without causing

[8] *dyskinesia:* faulty contraction
[9] *Meckel's diverticulum:* this congenital abnormality, present in about 2 per cent of people, is a diverticulum from the ileum about 2 inches long and about 2 feet from the caecum.

Chapter 8

symptoms. There may be a single ulcer or there may be several ulcers at the same time. Multiple superficial ulcers can develop in the upper two-thirds of the stomach in patients who have suffered severe stress from trauma, major surgical operations (especially cardiac operations) or severe sepsis. Aspirin, alcohol, prednisone and indomethacin can cause ulcers.

Chronic ulcer

A chronic peptic ulcer can occur in the pyloric region or on the lesser curvature of the stomach and, most commonly of all, in the first and second parts of the duodenum. An ulcer is the result of a local digestion of the mucous membrane of the

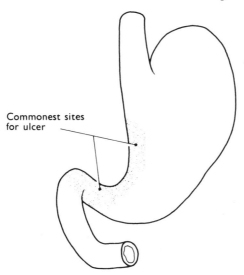

Commonest sites for ulcer

Fig. 40. The stomach and duodenum showing the commonest sites for a peptic ulcer.

stomach or duodenum by gastric juice. Normally gastric juice does not digest the mucous membrane, possibly because of the layer of mucus over it. The causes of a peptic ulcer are not clear, Among the factors involved are:

1. *Acid secretion:* in a duodenal ulcer there is an excessive secretion of acid by the gastric mucous membrane apparently as a result of over-activity of the vagi nerves. In a gastric ulcer, however, acid secretion is average or low.

2. *Age:* gastric ulcers are most common in middle and old age.

3. *Sex:* duodenal ulcers are much more common among men than women; gastric ulcers occur equally in both sexes according to some studies, or rather more commonly in men according to others. Ulcers are rare in pregnancy, a phenomenon that suggests a hormonal factor is involved.

4. *Family history:* there is often a family history of ulcers.

5. *Blood group:* more ulcers occur in people of blood group 0 than any other group.

6. *Social state:* gastric ulcers are more common in people of the lower socio-economic groups and duodenal ulcers are said to be an 'executive disease' of people in professional, executive and managerial positions. Other studies, however, have suggested that duodenal ulcers occur equally in all classes.

7. *Mental state:* a psychosomatic factor has been sought, ulcers being said to develop in people whose outwardly expressed aggression, hard work, ambition and

rigidity hide a personality that is basically childish and dependent.

8. *Steroid therapy:* can cause ulceration or make it worse.

Clinical features

The clinical features of a chronic peptic ulcer are characteristic. Attacks of pain, vomiting and water-brash (the filling of the mouth with saliva) are likely to occur over periods of weeks or months with long periods of freedom from symptoms.

The *pain* is usually felt in the epigastrium, occasionally in the back, chest or lower abdomen. If the ulcer is in the stomach, it comes on 30-60 minutes after a meal. If the ulcer is in the duodenum, it comes on 2-3 hours after a meal, and often

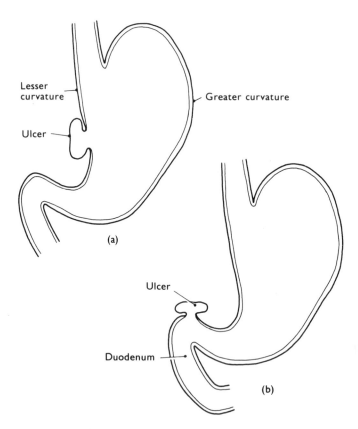

Fig. 41. An ulcer of (a) the stomach and (b) the duodenum.

wakes the patient up in the middle of the night, although, curiously, it does not occur just before breakfast. The pain is relieved by food and by vomiting.

Vomiting is common in patients who have severe pain or who have pyloric obstruction. It usually relieves the pain.

The patient usually points to the epigastrium as the site of the ulcer. There may be some 'guarding'[1] of the abdominal muscles over the ulcer.

Some ulcers heal spontaneously with a cessation of all clinical features. Ulcers

[1] *guarding:* local increase in muscle-tone.

tend to be made worse by stress and infections. Sometimes there is no obvious reason for an improvement or relapse.

Zollinger-Ellison syndrome is an association of a fulminating peptic ulcer with massive secretion of acid by the stomach and tumours of the islets of the pancreas and of other endocrine tissue.

Complications

1. *Haemorrhage.* An ulcer bleeds if the ulceration involves a blood-vessel. Bleeding can be slight or severe. The blood may be vomited (haematemesis) or appear in the stools. If bleeding is profuse, the patient feels week, has nausea, can vomit blood and faint; the pulse-rate increases and the blood-pressure falls.

2. *Perforation.* Perforation occurs in about 10 per cent of ulcers; 90 per cent of perforations are of duodenal ulcers. The ulceration extends completely through the wall of the stomach or duodenum and allows the contents to escape into the peritoneal cavity; occasionally the perforation is into another organ, such as a loop of intestine. The patient's condition becomes extremely serious. He collapses, sweating profusely and perhaps vomiting. He experiences agonizing pain in the upper abdomen. Sometimes the pain is referred to the tip of a shoulder, because of the innervation of the diaphragm by cervical nerves (via the phrenic nerve) whose sensory distribution is to the shoulder. The patient's abdominal wall is held in 'board-like' rigidity. After this very acute onset the patient's symptoms may diminish for a time as the acidity of the gastric juice is neutralized, but his condition relapses as general peritonitis sets in. The death-rate from perforation is 5-10 per cent.

3. *Pyloric obstruction.* This can be due to (a) oedema and muscular spasm produced by an ulcer in its active state and (b) fibrosis due to the healing of a chronic

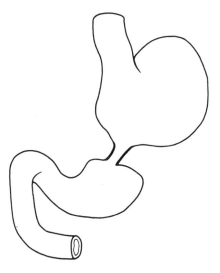

Fig. 42. An hour-glass constriction of the body of the stomach following the healing of an ulcer and the contraction of fibrous tissue.

ulcer. The patient develops vomiting and gastric distension. 'Splashing' of the stomach contents can be demonstrated. Wasting and dehydration can follow.

4. *Cancer.* Cancer develops rarely in gastric ulcers and never in duodenal ulcers.

149   *Diseases of the Alimentary Tract, Liver and Pancreas*

Special tests	1. *X-rays:* a chronic ulcer can almost always be demonstrated by a barium meal. Acute ulcers cannot usually be seen.

Special tests

1. *X-rays:* a chronic ulcer can almost always be demonstrated by a barium meal. Acute ulcers cannot usually be seen.
2. *Gastroscopy:* an ulcer in the body of the stomach can be seen; an ulcer in the pyloric canal or duodenum cannot be seen.
3. *Gastric secretion test:* Pentagastrin (Peptavlon) is used in a gastric secretion test, being given by injection or infusion.
4. *Occult blood in stools:* test is often positive.

Treatment

1. *Bed-rest.* The patient should stay in bed for 2-4 weeks and is allowed up only if symptoms have improved. With proper bed-rest the pain almost always stops. Sitting in front of a TV set is not bed-rest. Seeing visitors and answering the telephone are forbidden.

2. *Smoking* should be forbidden as stopping smoking promotes the healing of an ulcer.

3. *Diet.* Small frequent meals are usually given, for they relieve symptoms, although there is evidence that they increase the secretion of gastric juice. A glass of milk between meals can be taken. In severe cases milk can be given as a drip through an intragastric tube. A 'bland' diet, low in roughage, is recommended, but there is no need for a strict diet and food-fads once the acute phase is over.

4. *Antacids* are given to reduce the acidity of the gastric juice and so relieve pain. They do not hasten the healing of an ulcer, would have to be taken in enormous doses if complete neutralization were attempted, and in large doses have serious side-effects. Sodium bicarbonate, magnesium oxide, magnesium hydroxide, and calcium carbonate can be given in doses of 5 g hourly during the acute phase, followed by magnesium trisilicate in doses of 0.5-2.0 g 3-4 times a day.

5. *Carbenoxolone sodium* (a drug obtained from liquorice) is given in doses of 50-100 mg 3 times a day after meals. It aids the healing of a gastric ulcer (possibly by stimulating the formation of mucus in the stomach), but not of a duodenal ulcer. Side-effects are hypertension, sodium retention and oedema. Some other forms of liquorice may not cause fluid-retention.

6. *Spasm of gastric muscle* is relieved by vagus-paralysing drugs, e.g. tincture of belladonna 4-8 ml often given as a single dose at night, or atropine sulphate 250 mcg-2.0 mg by mouth. Gastric secretion is reduced.

7. *Anxiety* is relieved by a sedative such as phenobarbitone in doses of 30-120 mg. or a tranquiliser such as chlorpromazine in doses of 15-50 mg. daily in divided doses or chlordiazepoxide.

8. *Surgical treatment* is given for:
(a) persistent ulcers that are not cured by medical treatment,
(b) haemorrhage, severe or repeated,
(c) perforation,
(d) cancer of the ulcer,
(e) A jejunal ulcer following gastro-jejunostomy,
(f) stenosis of the pylorus.
(g) Zollinger-Ellison syndrome.

   Gastric ulcers are treated surgically by partial gastrectomy; the ulcer and the ulcer-bearing area of the stomach are removed and either a gastro-enterostomy is done or the gastric stump is anastomosed to the duodenum.

Duodenal ulcers are treated by either (a) vagotomy (division of the vagi nerves) in order to reduce the secretion of gastric juice; this is combined with a drainage operation (either a gastro-jejunostomy [1] or a pyloroplasty [2]) in order to allow the gastric contents to leave the stomach more readily, as the vagotomy also stops persistalsis of the stomach, or (b) partial gastrectomy to remove the acid-secreting part of the stomach, combined with gastro-jejunostomy or pyloroplasty.

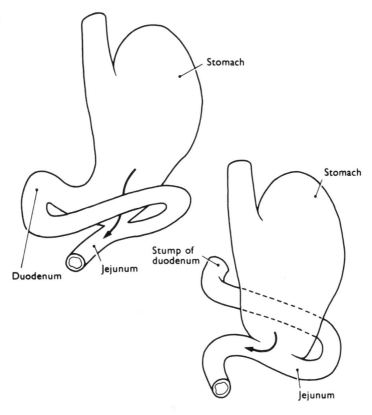

Fig. 43. (a) A gastro-enterostomy and (b) A partial gastrectomy.

Before any of these operations the patient should (a) be forbidden to smoke, (b) have any necessary dental treatment, (c) have blood checked for anaemia, which if present is treated, and (d) be given large doses of vitamin C to correct any deficiency.

Treatment of Complications

1. *Haemorrhage:* The patient is put to bed. Morphine sulphate 15 mg is given subcutaneously or intramuscularly to allay anxiety. The pulse and BP are taken every 15 minutes. If haemorrhage is severe or persistent, blood transfusions are given and then if necessary a partial gastrectomy, vagotomy with pyloroplasty, or direct suture is performed.

[1] *gastro-jejunostomy:* an opening between stomach and jejunum
[2] *pyloroplasty:* operation on pylorus of stomach to allow better exit for gastric contents

Diseases of the Alimentary Tract, Liver and Pancreas

2. *Perforation:* The stomach is emptied by a naso-gastric tube. Morphine is given to relieve pain. Fluid electrolyte balance is checked. Operation is then performed, the ulcer being closed or a partial gastrectomy carried out.

If an operation cannot be performed, the following treatment is given:
(a) continuous suction of gastric contents,
(b) maintenance of water and electrolyte balance,
(c) antibiotics to prevent peritonitis.

3. *Pyloric stenosis:* Pre-operative treatment for 7-10 days: daily gastric lavage, vitamin C in large doses, fluid and electrolyte balance maintained by intravenous saline with potassium. Operative treatment: a partial gastrectomy or gastro-enterostomy.

4. *Cancer:* Partial gastrectomy if possible is performed.

Post-Operative Conditions

1. *Jejunal ulcer.* This is an ulcer that occurs on the site of a gastro-jejunal anastomosis. The clinical features are similar to those of a gastric ulcer. The usual history is that the patient has had a period of relief from symptoms for days to months after a gastro-enterostomy. Another complication of such an ulcer is a gastro-jejunal-colic fistula in which the jejunum becomes attached to the colon and perforates into it.

The ulcer is usually visible on gastroscopy but not on X-ray. Such an ulcer can heal spontaneously. Others may heal following vagotomy and the subsequent diminution of gastric secretion.

2. *Ulcer of gastric remnant.* This is an ulcer on the gastric side of a gastric-jejunostomy. There is usually not a very high secretion of gastric juice, and the ulcer usually heals with medical treatment.

3. *Dumping Syndrome.* This condition can follow gastrectomy, but it can also occur in people with an ulcer who have not been operated on and also in otherwise healthy people. The syndrome consists of weakness, faintness, fullness in the epigastrium, sweating and sometimes diarrhoea. An early form comes on immediately after a meal, a late form 1-1½ hours later. Its cause is obscure. One theory is that the rush of food into the jejunum causes an attraction of tissue-fluid into the jejunum and this produces a reduction in blood-volume, which reduction is the immediate cause of the symptoms. Another is that it is due to hypoglycaemia due to an over-production of insulin. Patients subjected to it should lie down after a meal, and if it is due to hypoglycaemia take some sugar.

4. *Post-vagotomy syndrome.* Following vagotomy there is both a reduction in gastric secretion and delayed emptying of the stomach owing to lack of peristalsis. The patient feels full and belches and may have diarrhoea. Pyloroplasty relieves any gastric retention.

CANCER OF THE STOMACH

Cancer of the stomach is a common condition, but it is said to be decreasing in Britain and the U.S.A. Its cause is unknown. It is more common in men than women and in people of blood group A. It is an uncommon complication of a gastric ulcer.

Sites of occurrence are:
1. in the pyloric region, where it is likely to cause pyloric obstruction;
2. in the body of the stomach, where it can occur as a large, fungating and ulcerating mass;

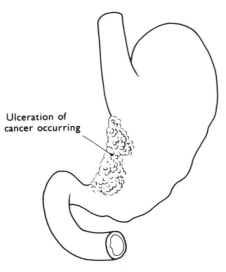

Ulceration of
cancer occurring

Fig. 44. Cancer of the
stomach.

3. as a generalized cancer with much fibrous tissue, producing a thick-walled narrow 'leather-bottle' stomach.

Clinical features Indigestion is the first symptom; and any indigestion occurring in a person over the age of 45 and not clearing up within a fortnight should be investigated as a possible cancer of the stomach. The patient goes on to complain of loss of appetite, abdominal discomfort and nausea. There may be blood in the vomit (haematemesis) or in the stools. Anaemia is slight to severe. In early days there are usually no physical signs; with the development and spread of the cancer a hard mass is felt in the upper abdomen. Lymph-nodes become invaded; secondary growths can cause enlargement of the liver and jaundice.

By this time the patient has severe abdominal pain, more vomiting, and loses weight rapidly. The outlook is usually poor, for most patients do not come early enough for treatment and the condition is by then inoperable. The expectation of life from the onset of symptoms is about 12 months.

Complications Haemorrhage. Perforation into peritoneal cavity.

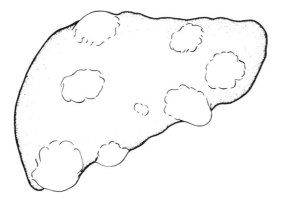

Fig. 45. A liver with
multiple secondary growths
(as can occur in carcinoma
of the stomach, etc.).

153   *Diseases of the Alimentary Tract, Liver and Pancreas*

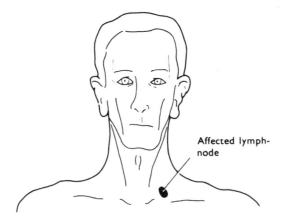

Affected lymph-node

Fig. 46. A common site for a secondary tumour from a cancer of the stomach.

Metastases in peritoneum, lymph-nodes, liver, prostate, bone, brain, ovaries. A cancerous node just above the left clavicle is typical.

Special tests

1. *Gastric contents:* contains pus red blood cells and sometimes fragments of tumour-tissue; absence of hydrochloric acid in less than half the cases.
2. *X-ray of stomach* following a barium meal is likely to show irregular filling or interruption of peristaltic waves.
3. *Gastroscopy:* a cancer can usually be seen; a specimen is removed for histology.
4. *Blood:* there is usually some anaemia (hypochromic); raised ESR.

Treatment

A gastrectomy is performed if possible, but the presence of 'secondaries' indicates that it is too late for surgery.

ACUTE GASTRITIS

This is an acute inflammation of the stomach and is due to:
(a) excessive alcohol consumption;
(b) aspirin, which is likely to cause erosion of the mucous membrane, haematemesis and blood in the stools.
(c) food poisoning, usually a staphylococcal gastro-enteritis;
(d) an irritant poison, e.g. arsenic;
(e) influenza, peptic ulcer, cancer of the stomach.

Clinical features

The patient has abdominal discomfort and pain. He feels nausea and vomits. He may complain of giddiness. An associated enteritis produces lower abdominal pain and diarrhoea. If the cause is removed, the condition usually clears up.

Treatment

The patient should go to bed and stay there until better. He is given a milk diet and mild sedation. Blood-transfusions may have to be given for a severe haemorrhage.

CHRONIC GASTRITIS

This is a chronic degeneration of the gastric mucous membrane. It is uncommon in people under 40 years. It occurs in pernicious anaemia. In other patients it is due to prolonged alcohol or aspirin consumption; it is often associated with gastric ulcer, cancer of the stomach, and iron-deficiency anaemia. Some cases have been regarded as examples of an auto-immune condition (see Chapter 12).

The mucous membrane atrophies. The condition is usually untreatable for the destroyed mucous membrane does not regenerate.

Chapter 8

DIARRHOEA	Diarrhoea is the condition in which unformed stools are passed several times a day or more frequently. It is not a disease in itself but a symptom of disease or disorder. Among the causes are:

Irritation of bowel	Purgatives	Excessive roughage in diet
	Food allergies	Irritant poisons

Infections	Gastro-enteritis	Bacterial food-poisoning
	Bacterial dysentery	Gastric influenza
	Typhoid and paratyphoid fever	Tuberculosis of bowel

Parasites	Amoebic dysentery
	Giardia lambia infections[4]

Defective absorption from bowel	Steatorrhoea	Regional ileitis
	Pancreatic disease	

Gastric conditions	Achlorhydria	Carcinoma of stomach
	following gastrectomy or vagotomy	

Diseases of colon	Acute colitis	Ulcerative colitis
	Carcinoma of colon	Diverticulitis

Psychological factors	Fear, anxiety
	Traveller's diarrhoea (plus infection, change of diet and excretory habits)

Clinical features Loose stools are passed with undue frequency, and the patient has abdominal discomfort, pain or discomfort. In a severe diarrhoea he collapses, sweats profusely, and has a rapid pulse and low BP.

Complications Loss of fluid, dehydration
Loss of electrolytes, especially potassium, leading to coma and death
Loss of blood-proteins, causing oedema
Malabsorption of essential food factors.

Special tests *Stools:* for organisms, parasites, poisons, fat content.
Rectal examination and signmidoscopy: to exclude carcinoma of colon and diverticulosis.
X-ray: barium enema for evidence of ulcerative colitis, carcinoma of colon, diverticula

Treatment 1. The patient should go to bed and stay there until the diarrhoea has stopped. Warmth to the abdomen helps to relieve pain. If infection is suspected, barrier nursing is instituted.
2. The cause of the diarrhoea is investigated and treated.
3. The following *drugs* may be given:

[4]*giardia lambia:* a parasite of the small intestine

(a) *Lomotil:* (a proprietary preparation containing diphenoxylate hydrochloride with atropine): used to reduce excessive movements, does not have an anti-infective action. Dose for an adult: 5.0 mg 3-4 times a day.

(b) An appropriate sulpha drug, e.g. *sulphadimidine* or *sulphadiazine* in doses of 3 g followed by 1-1.5 g every 4-6 hours.

(c) *Kaolin:* to absorb gases and poisons, in doses of 17-75 g.

(d) *Opium:* to relieve pain, e.g. tincture of opium in doses of 0.25-2.0 ml.

4. *Diet* should be of milk at first and free from roughage for some time later.

5. *Fluids and electrolytes* are given by intravenous drip in severe cases.

CONSTIPATION

Constipation is said to exist if the residue of food taken on one day has not begun to be excreted within the next three. That a person's bowels are opened once a day is usually a matter of habit, training and convenience, and perfectly normal people may have their bowels opened several times a day or only once or twice a week. Constipation can therefore be held to be present when a person retains his faeces for much longer than his normal period. Usually the condition is self-adjusting.

Constipation can be due to:

(a) lack of opportunity to open the bowels at a convenient time,

(b) lack of food in the under-nourished or lack of roughage to stimulate mass peristaltic movements in the colon,

(c) mental illness: depression, anorexia nervosa, dementia,

(d) physical illness: hypo-thyroidism, fever,

(e) retention of faeces in the rectum, in infancy or old age.

(f) pain from anal fissure, haemorrhoids

Complications

Anal congestion, haemorrhoids.　　　　　Anal fissure

Faecal impaction, at extremes of age.

Treatment

Constipation is prevented by training in correct bowel habits with opportunity for unhurried emptying in a warm lavatory if possible; by taking vegetable and fruit to provide adequate roughage in the large intestine; by taking fluids; by taking exercise daily. Haemorrhoids and anal fissure should be treated. If a patient is used to taking a purge and it is not doing any harm, there is no reason why it should not be continued.

The following purges can be used:

(a) *magnesium sulphate:* 5-15 g as an occasional purgative, or in smaller doses in chronic constipation.

(b) *cascara sagrada:* the mildest of the irritant purgatives; dry extract: 100-250 mg; liquid extract 2-5 ml.

(c) *liquid paraffin* 10-30 ml; useful for softening faeces in elderly, but can interfere with absorption of fat-soluble vitamins, leak out of anus, and cause pulmonary complications if it gets into the lungs.

(d) *agar:* 4 g used to increase bowel contents.

(e) *Beogex:* a suppository which liberates carbon dioxide in the bowels; useful in elderly and post-operatively.

(f) *bisacodyl:* as a suppository or by mouth 5-10 mg; useful in elderly.

Very hard faeces may have to be softened by an olive oil enema and removed by an ordinary enema. Manual removal is sometimes necessary.

MALABSORPTION SYNDROME

This condition is characterized by a failure of the intestine to absorb from the diet an adequate amount of the essential foodstuffs, vitamins and minerals. Such poor absorption can occur in a number of conditions:

(a) coeliac disease,

idopathic steatorrhoea,

tropical sprue

(b) pancreatic disease, because of a reduction of fat - splitting enzyme in the pancreatic juice and therefore increased excretion of fat in the stools.

(c) liver and gall-bladder disease, where there is a lack of bile-salts and therefore incomplete absorption of fat from the intestine.

(d) regional ileitis,

tuberculous enteritis,

following operations: gastrectomy, gastro-enterostomy, formation of a blind-loop of bowel (which interferes with bacterial action in the intestine).

The following are likely to occur:

Failure of fat absorption: in coeliac disease, steatorrhoea, tropical sprue, producing very fatty stools and emaciation.

failure of iron absorption: hypochromic anaemia.

failure of folic acid and vitamin B_{12} absorption: macrocytic anaemia (pernicious anaemia type).

failure of vitamin K absorption: purpura[5], epistaxis[6], menorrhagia[7]

failure of vitamin D absorption: rickets, osteomalacia.

failure of calcium absorption: tetany

failure of vitamin B group absorption: glossitis, dermatitis, pigmentation.

failure of potassium and salt absorption: fatigue, prostration, mental disturbance, coma, death.

Various combinations of these effects can be seen. Children affected fail to thrive and can remain permanently stunted.

Treatment

The cause of the condition is ascertained and appropriate treatment given. Measures are taken to increase the amount of missing substances in the diet or to administer them where possible by routes other than the alimentary tract.

IDIOPATHIC STEATORRHOEA

Other names: coeliac disease [8] when it occurs in children; non-tropical sprue.

The cause of this disease appears to be a sensitivity to gluten, a protein found in wheat and rye; in some patients the cause is unknown.

[5]*purpura:* haemorrhagic spots in the skin
[6]*epistaxis:* nose-bleeding
[7]*menorrhagia:* excessive menstrual flow
[8]*coeliac:* referring to the abdomen, from a Greek word for cavity

Clinical features	The first signs usually appear in childhood when the child starts to eat bread or cake. He loses his appetite, develops diarrhoea, and fails to thrive. The abdomen is distended. The stools are large, pale and offensive; they float in water and are not easily flushed down the lavatory pan. Vitamin absorption is disturbed, and there may be defective absorption of iron and vitamin B_{12}. The condition persists into adult life, but is much relieved by dietary restriction when it is due to gluten-sensitivity.
Complications	Avitaminosis · · · · · · · · · · · · · · · · · · Anaemia Infections · Stunted growth
Special tests	*Stools*: contain excessive amount of fat *Xylose tolerance test:* a dose of 25 g. of xylose is given by mouth. It is excreted unchanged in the urine; if it has not been absorbed from the intestine, there is a reduction of the amount excreted to less than 5 g. in 5 hours. *Jejunal biopsy:* likely to show loss of normal villi. *X-ray:* Barium meal to show pattern of intestinal mucous membrane.
Treatment	When the disease is due to gluten-sensitivity, the patient should be placed on a gluten-free diet; special flour is obtainable. Additional vitamins should be given and anaemia corrected. Cortico-steroids may be given to try to stimulate a regrowth of intestinal mucous membrane.

REGIONAL ILEITIS

Other name: regional enteritis, Crohn's disease[1]

This is a disease of unknown cause characterized by areas of chronic inflammation in the small intestine and sometimes in the large intestine as well. Affected areas are swollen, oedematous and ulcerated, and inflamed loops of bowel become attached to one another or to the abdominal wall with fistulae occurring between attached parts. Stenosis of the bowel can occur. It occurs at all ages, with a peak of incidence in young adults and another in old women. Young patients tend to have disease of the small intestine and old patients of the large intestine.

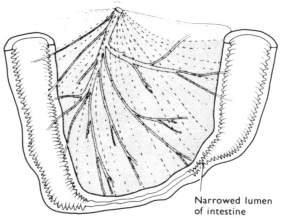

Fig. 47. A loop of small intestine in regional ileitis showing narrowing of lumen as a result of the formation of fibrous tissue.

Narrowed lumen
of intestine

[1] B.B. Crohn (1884 –   ): American physician

Clinical features	The patient has abdominal pain, colic and diarrhoea. A tender lump of matted intestines is felt in the lower abdomen. A fistula may discharge on to the abdominal wall. The condition can become mistaken for appendicitis or tuberculosis of the bowel. Fever, loss of weight, iron-deficiency anaemia and ulceration of the mouth are common. The fingers may become clubbed. The disease runs a continuous course and can be fatal.
Special tests	*X-ray:* a barium meal followed into the small intestine is likely to show narrowed segments with dilated segments proximal to them. *Stools:* blood and pus may be present. *Blood:* likely to show slight to moderate anaemia, leucocytosis and a raised ESR.
Treatment	Medical treatment is by: (a) bed-rest for weeks or months, (b) a diet free from roughage, (c) azathioprine 4 mg per kg for 10 days and 2 mg per kg thereafter, (d) cortico-steroids. Surgical treatment is by removal of affected segments.

IDIOPATHIC PROCTOCOLITIS	*Other name:* Ulcerative colitis This is a chronic inflammation of the colon of unknown origin. The usual age of onset is 20-40; it can occur in children and in people over 60. It is rare in Africa and Japan. The mucous membrane of the colon and rectum becomes inflamed, ulcerations appear in it, and the mucous membrane is eventually destroyed.
Clinical features	The disease runs a very prolonged course with ups and downs, with attacks separated by periods of partial or complete remission. Attacks can last from one week to several months and remissions for several years. Common symptons are: (a) diarrhoea, with the passing of many semi-solid stools, (b) the stools contain blood, pus and mucus; massive haemorrhages can occur, (c) attacks of abdominal pain and discomfort; the colon may be palpable and tender, (d) fever, weakness, anaemia, emaciation, mal-absorption of protein and vitamins. Attacks can vary in severity from very mild to fulminating and fatal.

Complications	*Acute:* perforation of colon acute dilatation of colon
	Chronic: stricture of colon intestinal obstruction
	           polypoid growths cancer of colon
	           fatty degeneration of liver infection or cancer of the bile-ducts

Special tests	*Sigmoidoscopy:* the inflamed and ulcerating outline to the colon and in chronic fibrosed cases a narrow 'drain-pipe' colon. *Stools:* Blood and pus are present. Microbiological examination is made to exclude bacterial infection and amoebic dysentery. *Biopsy:* A specimen of rectal mucous membrane is taken for microscopic examination. *ESR:* raised.
Treatment	*Mild disease.* A patient with mild disease can lead a normal life and have ordinary food. Drug treatment is by: (a) sulphasalazine 0.5 g three times a day, increased quickly to 1.0 g three times a

day. The drug is taken after meals to avoid dyspeptic side-effects or given as an enteric-coated tablet. Other side-effects are headache, malaises, rashes and anaemia (b) corticosteroids given as a suppository or retention enema self-administered (c) iron by mouth to correct anaemia.

Severe disease. A patient is admitted to hospital. He is given a high calorie diet with a high protein content. Milk restriction may improve the condition. Corticosteroids are necessary: the usual one given is prednisolone 40 mg daily. Corticotrophin gel in a single daily dose of 60-120 units by intramuscular injection is given to patients who do not respond to prednisolone. Iron, blood, electrolytes and fluid may be essential as replacement therapy.

Very severe disease. Surgical removal of the colon may be necessary after a short course of intravenous corticosteroids and replacement therapy.

Chronic disease. Surgical removal of the colon may be advised when symptoms do not improve with medical treatment.

Surgical treatment

Total or sub-total colectomy and the establishment of a permanent ileostomy is performed for (a) very acute disease not responding to medical treatment and (b) long-standing disease where there is involvement of the whole colon and a risk of cancer. If the patient has been having cortico-steroid drugs, the dose is increased during the operative period and then gradually decreased.

IRRITABLE BOWEL SYNDROME

Other names: Irritable colon, spastic colon, mucous colitis.

This is a symptom-complex of uncertain cause. Factors involved are stress, depression, and lack of fibre in the diet; it has followed dysentery. It can occur in children and adults; there may be a family history.

Clinical features

These include alteration in bowel-habits: constipation, diarrhoea, or a combination of both; the passing of much flatus; abdominal discomfort, pain or distension. The stools may consist of pellets like rabbits' droppings. The patient may otherwise feel well, or suffer from anxiety, depression and insomnia. In some patients the condition becomes chronic.

Treatment

This is by reassurance, the removal of stress-producing conditions, and eating faecal-bulk producing food, including whole-meal bread, bran and green vegatables.

DIVERTICULOSIS AND DIVERTICULITIS

Diverticulosis is a condition in which numerous small projections of mucous membrane are present in the wall of the colon, usually the descending and sigmoid colon. It occurs in about 30 per cent of people over 65. Predisposing conditions are obesity, constipation and an excessive use of purgatives. The diverticula do not produce symptoms unless they become inflamed.

Diverticulitis is inflammation of these diverticula, which is brought about by the accumulation of faeces in them. The patient complains of acute abdominal pain in the left side — hence the name of 'left-sided appendicitis'. There may be guarding of the abdominal wall; the inflamed colon can sometimes be felt. There is thickening of the peritoneum over the inflamed diverticula, and adhesions can form between them and adjacent organs, especially the bladder with the production of frequency of micturition.

Varicose veins are common in patients with diverticulosis, and it is suggested that both have a common cause.

Complications Perforation of diverticulum, local abscess or general peritonitis.
Fistula between colon and bladder. Intestinal obstruction. Anaemia.

Special tests *X-ray:* a barium enema shows the diverticula.
Stools: Mucus, blood and pus may be present.

Treatment Medical treatment is by bed-rest, warmth to the abdomen, courses of antibiotics, and liquid paraffin. A faecal bulk-producing diet is taken. Surgical treatment is necessary for intestinal obstruction, perforation of the bowel, peritonitis, abscess and fistula formation.

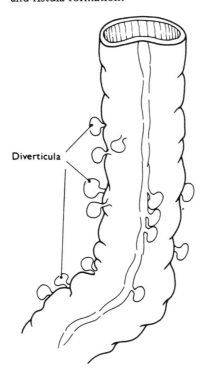

Diverticula

Fig. 48. Diverticulosis of the descending colon.

MEGACOLON This is a condition in which the colon is enormously enlarged, in part or in whole. In *Hirsch-prung's disease* (which is one type of it) there is for some unknown reason an absence of nerve-cells and fibres in the wall of the colon. The disease is rare, occurring about once in 30,000 births; 9 out of 10 cases are boys. The affected part of the colon is narrow and does not transmit the normal peristaltic waves and the part of the colon on its proximal end (i.e. nearer the small intestine) becomes enormously enlarged. Another type of the disease is attributed to constipation and faecal impaction in the rectum in infancy.

Diseases of the Alimentary Tract, Liver and Pancreas

Clinical features	As Hirschprung's disease is congenital, signs appear in the first days or weeks of life. The bowels do not work properly; stools are usually soft, but hard masses may be passed; constipation may be relievable only by enemas. The abdomen becomes distended as a result of the accumulation of faeces and gas, and the diaphragm is pushed upwards. Many patients die in childhood; but if the patient does survive into adult life, the abdomen is less distended and although the diaphragm is high in the chest there is little impairment of cardiac or pulmonary function; the only feature may be constipation.
Complications	Volvulus[2] may occur but usually rights itself.
Special test	*X-ray:* a barium enema shows the narrow part of the colon with the distended part beyond it.
Treatment	The only treatment that is effective is surgical removal of the affected section and anastomosis of the cut ends. If symptoms are mild, treatment of constipation is all that is necessary.

DISEASES OF THE PERITONEUM
ASCITES

Ascites is free fluid in the peritoneal cavity. It can be due to:-
(a) heart failure   (b) renal failure   (c) peritonitis,
(d) cancer of the peritoneum   (e) cirrhosis of the liver,
(f) obstruction of the portal vein,
(g) escape of bile following liver-biopsy, operation or rupture of the gall-bladder.
    The ascitic fluid can be clear, turbid when due to infection, blood-stained when due to cancer.

Clinical features	The abdomen becomes enlarged. The abdominal wall is pushed forward, the umbilicus pushed inside out; with further pressure the flanks are pushed out. The diaphragm is pushed up, causing embarrassment to the heart and lungs. The abdomen is dull to percussion except over the bowel. A 'thrill' can be felt if one side of the abdomen is tapped sharply with the finger-tips while the other hand is held flat against the opposite side.
The enlargement of the abdomen can be wrongly attributed to obesity, pregnancy, distended bowel, an ovarian cyst, a large pancreatic or mesenteric tumour, or a large hydronephrosis.
Treatment	Treatment of the cause is indicated. When ascites us due to heart or kidney disease, the fluid is got rid of by diuretics and other appropriate methods. If the ascites is causing severe discomfort or is embarassing heart or lungs, paracentesis is necessary: under aseptic conditions a trocar is inserted into the peritoneal cavity (either in the midline between umbilicus and pubes or in the flank) and the fluid allowed to escape. The escape must be gradual for a sudden drop in pressure can cause rupture of distended veins within the abdomen.

CHRONIC PERITONITIS

Chronic peritonitis is produced by tuberculosis, by cancer, by talc powder off surgeons' gloves. In *Pick's disease*[3] (which is often due to tuberculosis) a chronic peritonitis can be associated with constrictive pericarditis; in *Concato's disease*[4] the pleura, pericardium and peritoneum are all involved.

[2] *volvulus:* a twisting of the bowel on itself, producing obstruction
[3] F. Pick: German physician (1867-1926)
[4] L.M. Concato: Italian physician (1825-1882)

Some young or middle-aged people develop a recurrent peritonitis which may be of allergic origin. Ascites and oedema of the feet occur. The condition can go on for years, and for much of the time the patient is otherwise in good health. Paracentesis is necessary from time to time.

CANCER OF THE PERITONEUM

Cancer of the peritoneum is almost always secondary to cancer elsewhere – usually in the alimentary tract, the ovary or the breast. Cancer cells invade the peritoneum by scattering within the peritoneal cavity, by direct spread, or by invasion along lymph-vessels or blood-vessels.

Clinical features

These are those of the original disease plus the signs of peritoneal disease. Tumours may be felt inside the abdomen; the omentum may be a thick rolled-up bar of matted fibrous tissue and cancer cells; and the umbilicus may be infiltrated by cancer. Ascites is produced; it can be blood-stained. Adhesions or growths can cause intestinal obstruction. The patient goes rapidly downhill and dies within 6 months.

Treatment

Treatment can only be palliative by opium, morphine and pethidine to relieve pain and anxiety, and by paracentesis to relieve ascites.

Diseases of the Liver
JAUNDICE[5]

Jaundice is due to an increase in the amount of bilirubin in the blood. Bilirubin is produced by the breakdown of the haemoglobin of red blood cells, which after a life of about 120 days are destroyed in the reticulo-endothelial cells of liver, spleen and bone-marrow. The bilirubin circulates in the blood and reaching the liver is excreted by liver-cells into the bile-ducts.

The types of jaundice are:

1. Haemolytic jaundice

This is due to an excessive destruction of red blood cells and the production of more bilirubin than the liver can cope with. It happens in haemolytic and sickle-cell anaemias, in some infections (especially malaria), and when an incompatible blood-transfusion has been given.

The jaundice is slight because the increase in bilirubin is slight and lemon-yellow because of the combination of haemolysis and anaemia.

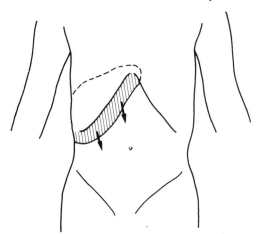

Fig. 49. Enlargement of the liver.

2. Hepato-cellular jaundice

This, the commonest type of jaundice, is due to damage to liver-cells (which are rendered incapable of transferring bilirubin from blood into the bile-channels) and

[5]*jaundice:* from Old French: *jaunisse* – yellow

sometimes and to a lesser degree to stagnation in the bile-channels and reabsorption from them of any bile that has been formed.

Common causes are:

(a) infections: infective hepatitis, infective mono-nucleosis, septicaemia, yellow fever, lepto-spirosis;

(b) drugs: arsenic, alcohol, chloroform, chlorpromazine (Largactil), cincophen, gold, thiouracil, etc.

3. Obstructive jaundice   Any obstruction in the common bile-duct dams up the bile which is then re-absorbed via the lymph-vessels into the blood. Common causes are:

(a) an impacted gall-stone;

(b) cancer: of the head of the pancreas, of the liver, of a lymph-node that presses on the bile-duct;

(c) chronic pancreatitis.

Clinical features   Jaundice is seen first in the conjunctivae, then in the mucous membrane of the mouth, then in the skin of the face, then in the rest of the skin. In severe chronic jaundice the colour can turn from yellow to green and xanthomata (patches of cholesterol) can form.

The patient complains of malaise, loss of appetite, a metallic taste in the mouth and itching.

In obstructive jaundice and when there is re-absorption in hepato-cellular jaundice, the absence of bile from the bowel causes the stools to be pale, clay-coloured and offensively smelling. Bleeding from any cut is likely to be prolonged because vitamin K absorption from the bowel is impaired when there is a shortage of bile and when damaged liver-cells, as in hepato-cellular jaundice, cannot produce prothrombin.

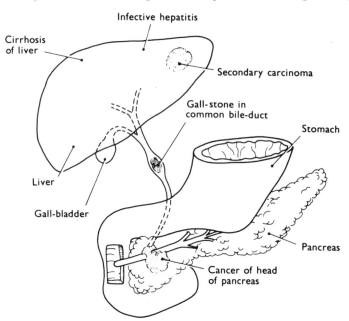

Fig. 50. Common causes of jaundice.

Chapter 8

As bilirubin is excreted by the kidneys from the blood, the urine with increasing jaundice darkens to deep brown or black.

A sudden painless jaundice preceded by loss of appetite and any desire to smoke or take alcohol in a young adult is usually due to a virus infection; attacks of intermittent jaundice with abdominal colic in middle age are usually due to a gall-stone in the bile-duct; a severe jaundice in later life associated with pain radiating to the back is usually due to cancer.

Special test *Blood:* serum bilirubin is raised (normal: 0.1-0.4 mg per 100 ml). *Van den Bergh reaction:* a *direct positive reaction* indicates that jaundice is likely to be due to liver damage or an obstruction; an *indirect positive reaction* indicates that jaundice is likely to be due to haemolytic anaemia.

Treatment Treatment of jaundice is that of the cause. Itching is relieved by taking alkaline baths, by applying carbolic acid 1 in 40 solution, and by taking anti-histamine drugs by mouth; it is quickly relieved by removal of an obstruction causing the jaundice.

CIRRHOSIS OF THE LIVER This condition is a degeneration of the liver with necrosis of cells, loss of normal liver structure, nodules of regeneration and replacement of damaged tissue by fibrous tissue. The condition is progressive and irreversible. The common causes are:
(a) chronic alcoholism, partly as a result of low protein-intake;
(b) malnutrition and dietary deficiencies from other causes;
(c) acute infective hepatitis;
(d) congestive heart failure;
(e) biliary obstruction and infection;
(f) haemochromatosis.

Clinical features These are a mixture of the results of (a) hepato-cellular failure and (b) portal hypertension.
(a) *Hepato-cellular failure,* a failure of the liver cells to carry out their normal functions, is the cause of:
Malaise, loss of appetite, loss of weight, indigestion, flatulence, furred tongue, fatigue.
A low-grade fever.
Foetor hepaticus: an offensive smell, detectable on approaching the bed.
Slight jaundice.
'Spider naevi': naevi of tiny vessels radiating from an arteriole; occur on chest, neck, face and upper arm.
Erythema of thenar and hypo-thenar eminences and on pads of fingers.
A 'flapping tremor' of the out-stretched hands.
Hiccuping, yawning, abnormal behaviour, excitement, drowsiness, coma, death.
(b) *Portal hypertension:* an increase of pressure in the portal veins due to fibrosis in the liver, is the cause of:
Enlargement of the spleen.
Varicose veins at the places where the portal veins anastomose with the general

systemic veins: at the lower end of the oesophagus, at the anus (with the production of haemorrhoids), at the umbilicus.

Ascites (fluid in the peritoneal cavity).

The *course* of the disease is progressive and death is likely within 2-3 years from haematemesis, an infection or liver-failure. In some young heavy drinkers the illness, running a rapid course, kills within a year. Hepatic coma is often fatal, and if with treatment a patient does recover he is likely to suffer another attack before long.

Complications   Haematemesis, from a ruptured varicose vein at the lower end of the oesophagus.
　　　　Infections, usually pneumonia or tuberculosis.
　　　　Primary carcinoma of liver in 5 per cent of patients.
　　　　Peripheral neuropathy.

Treatment   1. The patient must become teetotal.
2. A balanced diet is taken, unless signs of coma are developing, when the protein intake is reduced.
3. *Hepatic failure* is treated as follows:
(a) *active cirrhosis:* by cortico-steroids and azathioprine (an immuno-suppresive agent).
(b) *ascites and fluid retention:* by diuretics (too vigorous treatment can cause encephalopathy and electrolyte disorder).
(c) *haemorrhage from oesophageal varices:* by vasopressin and surgery.
(d) *encephalopathy:* by correction of its causes, withdrawal of protein from diet and by purgation, neomycin to aid bacterial decomposition of protein in the bowel, correction of electrolyte imbalance, and glucose intravenously if the patient is unable to swallow.
(e) *restlessness and noisiness:* by sodium phenobarbitone or diazepam intra-muscularly.

CANCER OF THE LIVER   This usually occurs as multiple secondary growths from a primary growth in the alimentary tract or other part of the body; a primary growth is rare; a secondary sarcoma can occur from a primary growth in bone and elsewhere.

Clinical features   The patient has discomfort or pain in the right hypochondrium. The liver enlarges and the growths can often be felt as hard rounded lumps with a central depression where degeneration is taking place. Jaundice follows pressure on the bile-duct and ascites follows pressure on the portal vein or secondary growths in the peritoneum.

Treatment   This can only be palliative, with the relief of pain and the removal of ascitic fluid.

INFECTIVE HEPATITIS   See p. 19-20

ACUTE YELLOW ATROPHY OF THE LIVER   This is an acute failure of liver function sometimes seen in acute infective hepatitis, eclampsia [6] and drug-intolerance. There is a wholesale degeneration of liver-cells, a shrinking of the liver and a collapse of function. The patient develops jaundice, purpuric haemorrhages in the mucous

[6] *eclampsia:* a toxic state causing convulsions in pregnancy or labour.

Chapter 8

membranes, and internal haemorrhages; becomes confused; passes into coma and is likely to die. The only treatment that can be given is intravenous glucose.

CONGENITAL HYPER-
BILIRUBINAEMIA

Other name: chronic benign intermittent jaundice

There are several conditions in which the patient is liable to suffer intermittent attacks of jaundice as a result of failure of the enzyme-systems necessary for the transport of bilirubin through liver cells. Patients are usually young males and have a family history of the condition. Recurrent attacks of slight jaundice occur, with dyspepsia and fatigue. The liver and spleen are not enlarged. The condition is harmless; no treatment is required.

Diseases of the Pancreas

ACUTE PANCREATITIS

Other name: acute necrosis of the pancreas

This is an acute abdominal disease (often mimicking an upper abdominal surgical emergency), with patches of necrosis, haemorrhage, infection and suppuration in the pancreas. It is due to destruction of pancreatic tissue by pancreatic enzymes following obstruction in the duodenal ducts and their rupture under increased pressure. Causes are:

(a) a flow of bile up the pancreatic duct, which can happen when bile-duct and pancreatic-duct have a common opening into the duodenum and this opening becomes blocked, e.g. by spasm of the sphincter of Oddi or by a gall-stone;

(b) gall-bladder disease, with gall-stones and infection of the biliary tract;

(c) chronic alcoholism; following a drinking bout or heavy meal;

(d) oestrogen-containing oral contraceptives;

(e) Coxsackie virus infection.

Clinical features

The patient has excruciating pain in the upper abdomen and can collapse. He starts to vomit — gastric contents at first, then bile — and the vomiting is likely to continue. The abdomen becomes distended and the abdominal wall rigid; occasionally the swollen pancreas can be felt. Pyrexia and slight jaundice can develop. Very severe cases are often fatal.

Complications

Peritonitis, chronic pancreatitis, diabetes mellitus.

Special test:

serum amylase usually very high (normal 80-180 units per 100 ml).

Treatment

1. The patient is admitted into hospital.
2. Fluid and electrolyte loss (due to the vomiting) is restored by intravenous saline or plasma.
3. Pethidine 100 mg or morphine 15-20 mg are given to relieve pain.
4. No food or drink is given by mouth.
5. Antibiotics are given to control infection and prevent peritonitis.
6. Surgical drainage is performed if an abscess forms.

CHRONIC PANCREATITIS

This occurs as a result of acute pancreatitis and of gall-bladder disease and sometimes without obvious cause. Chronic inflammatory and fibrous changes make the pancreas large and hard.

Clinical features There may be a history of attacks of acute pancreatitis or of gall-bladder disease. Fibrous constriction of the common bile duct causes a painless, chronic, deepening jaundice. The liver and gall-bladder may be enlarged. If pancreatic function is seriously diminished, there is interference with the absorption of fats, with the development of steatorrhoea and emaciation.

The disease can be painless or marked by attacks of upper abdominal and left-sided pain lasting for a few days and recurring at intervals of weeks or months. Calcification of the pancreas can develop and be visible on X-ray examination.

Complications Diabetes mellitus if the islets of Langerhans are involved.
Peptic ulcer.

Treatment Treatment is not very effective, unless the patient has an infected gall-bladder and has it removed. The diet should be low in fat and the patient should avoid alcohol. Pain is relieved by propantheline bromide 15 mg Morphine may be required in severe attacks.

CANCER OF THE PANCREAS The usual site is in the head of the pancreas. Pressure on the common bile duct causes a progressive obstructive jaundice. The stools become pale and fatty, and the patient wastes rapidly. Severe pruritus makes the patient's life a misery. If he is eating meat, undigested meat fibres are found in the stools owing to the lack of pancreatic digestive enzymes. Cholecystenterostomy (the gall-bladder being drained into a loop of small intestine) relieves the jaundice and itching and improves the digestion of fat; but the course of the disease is usually rapid and death likely within 6 months.

9 Metabolic and Deficiency Diseases

Metabolism is the sum of all chemical and physical processes going on in the body. These very complex changes can be upset in any disease, but in most they are slight. In other conditions metabolism can be seriously disordered. Such a severe metabolic disorder can be the result of :

(a) a gene-abnormality as a result of which there is a failure of some biochemical reaction, as in phenylketonuria;

(b) an endocrine abnormality, which itself may be the result of a gene-abnormality. In diabetes mellitus there is a dangerous under-secretion of insulin;

(c) over-eating causing the production of obesity in societies where food is readily available in large quantities;

(d) starvation;

(e) any very severe illness;

(f) the action of some drugs;

(g) in any disorder of fluid and electrolyte balance (see Chapter 7).

Deficiency diseases are due to a lack of essential foodstuffs from the diet. Starvation can be due to a lack of food or to some peculiarity or abnormality in an individual as a result of which he does not take adequate amounts of food; a severe and chronic lack of protein has serious effects. Other deficiency diseases are due to lack of essential minerals (e.g. iron) or of vitamins from the diet: these are most likely to occur in the under-developed countries, but they can occur anywhere as a result of poverty, ignorance or mental disorder. Certain addictions (e.g. to alcohol) can lead to a person taking an inadequate amount of food or to failure of absorption of food from the bowel; other absorption failures can be due to disease of the small intestine (see malabsorption syndrome).

OBESITY This is the condition in which there is an excessive storage of fat in the subcutaneous tissues, omentum and other fat-storage areas of the body, an excess to a degree that interferes with any normal function of the body. It is a common disorder of Western societies where ample food is available for human consumption.

The factors concerned in the production of obesity are:

1. *Food intake.* There is an excessive consumption of food or alcohol, a consumption above that of the body's requirements. The excessive consumption is of carbohy-

drates, which are cheap and readily available in enticing forms. The villains are sugar, sweets, chocolates, bread, cake, potato and alcohol.

2. *Lack of exercise.* The affected person has not taken enough physical exercise daily, and as he gets fatter he takes less.

3. *Emotional problems.* Some worried people take to the bottle, others eat big meals or nibble constantly.

4. *Endocrine factors.* These are uncommon. They include hypothyroidism, pituitary disturbances, and disturbances of sex-hormone secretion. Obesity can be a result of pregnancy.

Clinical features   Fat people have a lot of weight to carry round. They become less inclined to take physical exercise, dislike the heat, sweat easily, and die before their time.

Complications   1. Coronary disease and anginal attacks: due to fatty deposits in and on the myocardium and to the extra work the patient has to do in carrying the fat everywhere he goes.

2. Hypertension and athero-sclerosis.

3. Diabetes mellitus (but obesity may be a sign rather than a cause of diabetes).

4. Gall-stones.

5. Arthritis of hips and knees: due to excessive weight-bearing.

6. Gout.

7. Skin infections (e.g. below breasts).

Treatment   Treatment is difficult. To slim, a person has to be determined and persistent. He has to resist his own inclinations to over-eat and the enticements given to him by his family and friends to share the pleasures of the table. A fat person who is to slim satisfactorily will almost certainly have to follow for the rest of his life a regime that is easy to break. Many do break it and the relapse-rate is high.

1. *Diet.* The patient must eat less. Most specialists are agreed on what he should eat less of, but differ in the precise applications. In general the following principles apply:

(a) *Carbohydrates.* There must be a sharp reduction in the consumption of carbohydrates. The patient should take no sugar as such; he must sharply reduce his consumption of bread, cake, sweets, chocolate, beer, cereals, potato, and any preparation of them.

(b) *Protein.* He can take ordinary amounts of protein: lean meat, eggs, fish, cheese.

(c) *Fats.* Opinion is divided over fat consumption: some would allow ordinary amounts, others would reduce them.

The patient keeping to this diet is likely to lose several pounds promptly and then to lose weight slowly. But the temptations to default are great, and the slightest weakness in some patients causes them to put on weight again very quickly.

2. *Exercise.* The patient must be encouraged to take some moderate physical exercise daily — to walk to work rather than drive, to walk upstairs rather than take the lift, to garden, go for daily walks, swim, play golf. The amount of calories consumed in this way is small, but some exercise appears an essential aid to loss of weight as a result of diet-restriction.

3. *Weighing.* The patient should weigh himself daily or once a week and keep a record of his weight-loss. He should know what his desirable weight is and should aim at reaching it and keeping at it.

4. *Drugs.* A number of appetite-reducing drugs are on the market. They are unnecessary for the patient who has the strength of will to keep to the appropriate regime.

MAXIMUM DESIRABLE WEIGHTS

(naked weights: if weighed in shoes and clothes add 10 lb for a man, 6 lb for a woman; heights without shoes)

MEN

ft	in	small frame		medium frame		large frame	
		st	lb	st	lb	st	lb
5	3	8	6	9	2	10	0
5	4	8	9	9	5	10	2
5	5	8	11	9	9	10	6
5	6	9	3	9	13	10	13
5	7	9	7	10	4	11	4
5	8	9	11	10	8	11	8
5	9	10	2	10	12	11	12
5	10	10	6	11	3	12	3
5	11	10	10	11	8	12	8
6	0	11	0	11	13	12	13
6	1	11	5	12	4	13	4
6	2	11	9	12	9	13	9

WOMEN

ft	in	small frame		medium frame		large frame	
4	11	7	0	7	9	8	7
5	0	7	1	7	12	8	10
5	1	7	6	8	1	8	13
5	2	7	9	8	5	9	3
5	3	7	12	8	9	9	7
5	4	8	2	9	0	9	11
5	5	8	6	9	4	10	1
5	6	8	10	9	8	10	5
5	7	9	0	9	12	10	9
5	8	9	5	10	2	11	0
5	9	9	9	10	4	11	5
5	10	9	13	10	8	11	11

DIABETES MELLITUS

Diabetes[7] mellitus[8] is a disorder of metabolism involving carbohydrate, fat, protein, water and electrolytes, and characterized mainly by a raised blood-sugar and the excretion of sugar in the urine.

[7] *diabetes:* from Greek: *diabainein* – to pass through
[8] *mellitus:* Latin: *mellitus* – honey

Metabolic and Deficiency Diseases

It is a result of a failure of the beta cells of the islets of Langerhans in the pancreas to secrete enough insulin or possibly in some cases a failure of tissues to respond to a normal secretion of insulin. Only occasionally are the islets seen to show any degenerative changes. The cause is unknown. One suggestion is that diabetes mellitus is a late result of infection of the pancreas by a Coxsackie virus.

Diabetes may be 'latent': the patient does not have any signs or symptoms of the disease, but he has an abnormal blood-sugar curve and is a candidate for the disease. From surveys that have been made in various populations, it is reckoned that for every known case of diabetes there is one unknown case whose symptoms are mild and one latent one whose symptoms have not appeared. In a latent diabetic the disease may be rushed into a frank one if the patient becomes pregnant, develops an infection, has a serious injury or suffers an emotional crisis.

Heredity: there is a high incidence of the disease in certain families, and identical twins have been known to develop it at the same time. Genetic factors are likely to be important only in young patients.

Age: it can develop at any age; the highest incidence is in the 60-70 age-group. There is a marked difference in the severity and course of the disease in early life and in later life (see below).

Weight. patients who develop the disease over the age of 40 have usually been over-weight, and in them the disease has been attributed to the metabolic strain the pancreas has undergone in producing extra amounts of insulin to cope with an excessive intake of carbohydrate.

Sex: the disease occurs in both sexes. A woman with latent diabetes may give birth to an over-weight baby.

Clinical features

These vary with the age of onset and severity of the disease.

In the *Growth-Onset, Ketotic or Juvenile Form* (in which no insulin at all may be produced):
(a) the patient is young;
(b) diabetes is likely to be severe;
(c) fat metabolism is disturbed and ketosis likely;
(d) diet by itself is inadequate to control the disease, oral anti-diabetic drugs are ineffective, and insulin is required.

In the *Mature-Onset, Non-Ketotic or Adult Form* (insulin being produced but in inadequate amounts:)
(a) the patient is middle-aged or old;
(b) he is probably obese;
(c) diabetes is likely to be mild;
(d) fat metabolism is less disturbed and ketosis unlikely;
(e) a complication of diabetes may be the first sign;
(f) diet may be adequate to control the disease, with or without an oral anti-diabetic drug; insulin is not likely to be required.

Common symptoms are:
(a) *polyuria:* the patient is excreting sugar in the urine; to get rid of the sugar he has to excrete more water;

(b) *severe thirst* and *dehydration* follow this excessive excretion of water;

(c) *loss of weight* and *muscular weakness* in young patients;

(d) *increased appetite;*

(e) *ketosis:* in young, severely affected diabetics, there is an interference with fat metabolism with the result that ketone bodies are increased in the blood and excreted in the urine; the patient becomes drowsy and ill, his breath smells of new-mown hay, he is heading for a diabetic crisis.

(f) *restless legs.* (See p.254.)

(g) any of the *complications* of the disease.

Complications	Complications are common and sometimes the first sign of the disease.
1. Diabetic crisis (coma)	This is most common in the juvenile type and rare in the adult type. It is due to ketosis and the result of interference with fat metabolism. It can be the result of emotional disturbances, lack of treatment, inadequate treatment, carelessness in the administration of insulin, an infection, an infarction or an injury. The onset is slow, over hours or days. The patient becomes confused, drowsy and passes into a coma. The new-mown hay smell of acetone is present in his breath. Respiration is deep and slow and 'air-hunger' develops. The pulse has a small volume, the BP is low. The skin is dry. The urine contains sugar and ketones. Untreated, the crisis is likely to end in death.

Aketotic diabetic coma is a form of diabetic coma in which there is severe dehydration without ketosis. It occurs in older patients more often than in younger, and in many of them diabetes has not previously been diagnosed. Its cause is uncertain: it is possibly a reaction to drinking large amounts of sugar-containing drinks in order to quench thirst. The patient loses large amounts of water via the kidneys and by vomiting and diarrhoea, passes gradually into coma, and may have fits. The blood-sugar is very high – often over 1,000 mg per 100 ml; the urine and blood do not however, contain more than small amounts of ketones, the breath does not smell of acetone, and the patient does not over-breathe. About 50 per cent of patients with this kind of coma die.

A hypoglycaemic coma may be mistaken for a diabetic crisis, for both occur in diabetics. But a hypoglycaemic coma is the result of too little sugar in the blood, caused by an overdose of insulin or by not taking enough carbohydrate to 'cover' the proper dose, or by taking excessive exercise. The onset is rapid; the patient sweats profusely; the pulse is bounding, the BP normal or raised; there is no acetone in the breath; respiration is rapid and shallow. the urine may contain sugar but not ketones.

2. Athero-sclerosis	The arteries of a diabetic are particularly liable to show degenerative changes. The cerebral and coronary arteries may be among those involved. Gangrene of the feet can occur.
3. Degenerations of the eye	Blindness can be the result of the development of cataracts or of degenerative changes in the retina. A diabetic patient is up to twenty times more likely to

173   *Metabolic and Deficiency Diseases*

become blind than a non-diabetic person. Diabetic retinopathy, once established, gets worse even though the blood-sugar is controlled. Diabetic retinitis is one of the commonest causes of blindness in the western world.

4. Kidney disease   Diabetics can have albuminuria and have a particular degeneration of the glomeruli of the kidneys called the Kimmelstiel-Wilson lesion, which can result in oedema, a rising BP, and degeneration of the eyes. Pyelonephritis is common.

5. Neuropathy   Diabetics are prone to develop degeneration of the peripheral nerves, with pains, cramps, weakness, loss of tendon-reflexes, and little or no sensory loss. Painless ulcers can occur. The neuropathy improves with adequate treatment of the diabetes.

Special tests
1. Urine   (a) SG above 1025 (due to the sugar in it).
(b) Tests for Glucose:-
   (i) *Clinistix stick.* Tip of stick is dipped in urine. If glucose is present, the tip turns blue usually within 1 minute. The test is specific for glucose and is a guide to the degree of glucosuria.
   (ii) *Hema-Combistix.* This stick is dipped in the urine. The four reagents on it provide information on pH, glucose, protein and blood.
   (iii) *Clinitest method.* 5 drops of urine are placed in test-tube with dropper provided. Dropper is rinsed and 10 drops of water are added. One Clinitest tablet is dropped into the tube. Effervescence and boiling occur. 15 seconds after boiling has stopped, the colour is compared with colour-chart provided. Any reducing substance (glucose is the commonest) causes the colour to change through green (0.5 per cent) to orange (2 per cent).
(c) Tests for ketone bodies:
   (i) *Acetest method:* A tablet of Acetest is put on a clean white surface and 1 drop of urine on the tablet. A mauve colour develops if ketones are present; depth of colour is a rough indication of the amount present.
   (ii) *Nitroprusside test:* 10 ml. of urine are saturated with ammonium sulphate (saturation is reached when no more will dissolve). 3 drops of sodium nitroprusside are added and then 2 ml. of strong ammonia. If ketones are present, solution turns a deep permanganate (purple-red) colour.
   (iii) *Ferric chloride test.* Urine is put in a test-tube and ferric chloride 10 per cent added. If aceto-acetic acid (a ketone) is present, the solution becomes reddish-purple. Salicylates produce the same colour in boiled as well as unboiled urine.

2. Blood   *Glucose tolerance test.* The patient must have been taking ordinary amounts of carbohydrate for a week before. He must have had no food since the night before. Blood is taken for a 'fasting blood-sugar'. He drinks 50 G of glucose dissolved in 100 ml. of water. Specimens of blood are taken every ½ hour for 2½ hours.
   A patient with diabetes is likely to show: (a) a fasting blood-sugar above the normal (normal: 70-120 mg/100 ml); (b) a raised blood-sugar curve; (c) the blood-sugar not returned to normal level within 2 hours. A patient with latent or slight diabetes shows a moderately raised blood-sugar and a slow return to normal.
   Dextrostix is a stick which, dipped into blood, is a guide to the amount of glucose in the blood; it is especially useful in making a rapid diagnosis of hypoglycaemia.

Treatment   Treatment is aimed at:
1. enabling cells to utilize glucose
2. keeping the blood-glucose and blood-cholesterol and lipid values within normal limits

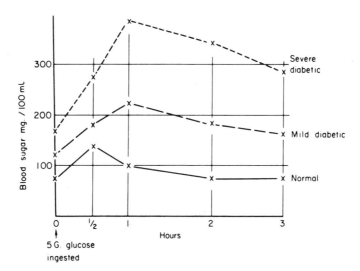

Fig. 51. Typical blood-sugar curves after the ingestion of 5 G of glucose in a normal person, in a mild diabetic and a severe diabetic.

3. the prevention of ketosis
4. the maintenance of weight, health and strength and, for children, growth.
5. the prevention of complications

A patient with diabetes should carry a card with his name and address and a statement that he is a diabetic.

Treatment varies with the form of diabetes.

(a) Growth — onset, ketotic or juvenile form

This form of diabetes is likely to be controlled only by insulin. The patient takes an ordinary diet — one appropriate to his age and needs — and is given daily injections of insulin in doses adequate to fulfil the 4 aims of treatment given above. *Insulin* has to be given by injection because it is a protein and if it were taken by mouth it would be broken down by the gastric juice into useless amino-acids.

Insulin is available as:

(a) *soluble insulin[9]* : this form of insulin acts quickly, being effective within 20 minutes, but it does not act for long and ceases to be effective 4-6 hours after injection. An overdose causes hypo-glycaemia. It is necessary for the treatment of severe diabetics, unstable diabetics, ketosis, diabetic crisis, and when patient has an infection or has to have an operation.

(b) *slowly acting insulin:* there are several kinds of these — protamine zinc insulin (PZI), ultralente (IZS crystalline). They do not start to act for 4-6 hours and thereafter are effective for up to 24 hours.

Insulin is commonly prescribed as soluble insulin and a slowly acting insulin together. The patient gives himself the prescribed amount before breakfast. The soluble insulin controls the diabetes for the first few hours until the slowly acting one takes over; in severe diabetes a second dose of the soluble insulin may be required later in the day. Soluble insulin and PZI should not be mixed in the same syringe, but they can be given from two syringes through the same needle, only one puncture being necessary.

[9] *soluble insulin:* in U.S.A. this type of insulin is called *regular insulin*

Metabolic and Deficiency Diseases

(b) Mature — onset, non-ketotic or adult form	The patient with this form of diabetes is likely to be over-weight and is placed on a reducing diet. His weight is measured and his urine examined at least once a week. If the glucosuria disappears, no treatment other than continued dieting is necessary. If the glucosuria persists, he is given an oral anti-diabetic drug. If, as sometimes happens, oral anti-diabetic drugs cannot control the diabetes, insulin is given.
Oral anti-diabetic drugs	Some drugs can control diabetes when given by mouth. They belong to three groups: (a) the sulphonyl-urea group (which appear to act by stimulating into activity what beta cells in the pancreas are still capable of some secretion); (b) the diguanide group (which possibly act by stimulating the chemical changes involving glucose in the cells of the body): (c) the sulphonamide-pyrimidine group.
	These drugs are used for diabetics whose diabetes has begun in adult life, who are not grossly overweight and whose diabetes is not satisfactorily controlled by diet alone. For some patients a combination of drugs from each group is necessary. These drugs are useless and indeed dangerous for diabetics whose illness has begun in early life; there is some evidence that they produce cardiovascular disease.
Sulphonyl-urea group	Chlorpropamide: 100-500 mg daily; it is effective for about 24 hours and has to be taken 2 or 3 times a day.
	Tolbutamide: 500 mg-1.0 g; it is effective for up to about 10 hours and has to be taken 2-3 times a day.
	Glibenclamide: 2.5-20 mg in a single daily dose.
Diguanide group	Metformin: 500 mg-1.0 g three times a day.
	Phenformin: 25-50 mg.
Treatment of complications 1. Diabetic crisis	1. The patient is admitted into hospital and nursed in the semi-prone position until the stomach has been emptied.

1. The patient is admitted into hospital and nursed in the semi-prone position until the stomach has been emptied.
2. Intravenous treatment is given according to the analysis of the blood:
(a) soluble insulin, intravenously at first, later intramuscularly; prescribed dose is likely to be 100-200 units; a continuous low-dose intravenous infusion of insulin can be given;
(b) saline and fluid: up to 8 litres of isotonic saline in 12 hours;
(c) when there is severe acidosis, isotonic sodium bicarbonate (or isotonic sodium lactate solution) in place of half of the isotonic saline solution,
(d) dextrose 5 per cent solution,
(e) potassium chloride 1 g to each 500 ml of glucose solution;
(f) blood or plasma for shock.
3. The blood-concentration of glucose, potassium and bicarbonate is measured at least every 2 hours until the patient recovers consciousness.
4. Gastric aspiration is performed to prevent the inhalation of vomit.
5. An enema is given if the patient is severely constipated.
6. Antibiotics are given to prevent or stop infection.
7. Oral feeding is begun when the patient is conscious, water and salt deficit has been remedied and the patient has ceased to show ketosis. Feeds should be frequent and small, and each should contain 25 g carbohydrate as sugar, fruit juice, milk or milk-preparations. Soluble insulin is given to prevent ketosis and glucosuria.
8. A return is made to a full diet and insulin soluble and slow-acting.

The treatment of *aketotic coma* is by insulin and large amounts of fluid given as hypotonic saline intravenously and water by intragastric tube.

2. Hypoglycaemic crisis

Mild hypoglycaemic crisis, with the patient able to swallow, is stopped by taking 2-3 lumps of sugar.

Severe hypoglycaemic crisis, with the patient unable to swallow is treated by an intravenous injection of glucose 50 ml of a 50 per cent solution or by glucose given by gastric tube. Glucagon 1 mg is given intramuscularly in emergencies.

3. Vascular disease and gangrene

Atherosclerosis cannot be stopped; but it is hoped that adequate treatment of the diabetes will retard its progress. In patients likely to develop gangrene, particular care is paid to the feet; nail-cutting and the care of corns are important procedures; to avoid burns the patient should wear bed-socks rather than have a hot-water bottle. The services of a chiropodist are advisable. If the patient develops gangrene, amputation of the foot or leg becomes necessary.

4. Infections

Infections must be treated promptly and adequately by the usual methods. It is likely that the patient will require a larger dose of insulin and if this is not given there is a danger that he will be precipitated into a diabetic crisis.

5. Eye disease

Photocoagulation of newly diseased blood-vessels may improve vision.

GLUCOSURIA

Glucosuria is not necessarily pathological. It can occur in the following conditions as well as in diabetes mellitus.

1. Renal glucosuria

The normal renal threshold for glucose is 180 mg/100 ml; when the blood-glucose exceeds 180 mg per cent, glucose appears in the urine. The threshold tends to be lower in young adults and higher in old people. Some people have an abnormally low renal threshold; the condition is sometimes called renal diabetes. In some people renal glucosuria may precede frank diabetes.

2. Alimentary glucosuria

There may be a temporary glucosuria after a large intake of carbohydrate with the blood-glucose rising above the renal threshold.

3. Emotional glucosuria

Emotional conditions can cause over-secretion by the adrenal glands and hence a breakdown of glycogen stores and the excretion of glucose. Glucosuria from this cause is common in students before examinations.

HYPER-INSULINISM

An excessive secretion of insulin can be due to: (a) an adenoma, a non-malignant tumour, of the pancreas, (b) cancer of the pancreas, or (c) an over-growth of the islets of Langerhans. The blood-sugar is lowered.

Clinical features

A patient is likely to have attacks of sweating, disturbance of consciousness and mood-change; with further lowering of the blood-sugar he can have a fit. The condition is likely to be mistaken for a neurosis, a psychosis, epilepsy or other neurological disease.

Special test	*Blood:* in attacks the blood glucose falls to below 40 mg per 100 ml
Treatment	Intravenous glucose is given during an attack. An adenoma of the pancreas is removed surgically; carcinoma of the pancreas can be treated only palliatively; for overgrowth of pancreatic tissue, a sub-total pancreatectomy is performed.
GLUCAGONOMA SYNDROME	A tumour of the alpha-2 cells of the islets of Langerhans of the pancreas produces an excessive amount of glucagon and a syndrome characterized by redness and blistering of the skin, stomatitis and loss of weight. Most patients also have diabetes mellitus.
Treatment	Surgical removal of the tumour.
HAEMOCHROMATOSIS [1]	*Other name:* bronze diabetes This is a rare genetically-determined disorder of iron metabolism, in which there is an excessive absorption of iron from the alimentary tract and a deposit of it in the tissues. The skin becomes pigmented a dirty bronze colour, as a result of the deposit in it of iron and melanin. The liver, spleen and pancreas show a heavy deposit of iron. The pancreas becomes fibrosed and a mild diabetes results. The liver becomes fibrosed and portal cirrhosis develops. Arthritis and calcification of cartilage can occur.
Treatment	Attempts are made to get rid of the excess iron by means of a chelating agent[2], desforrioxamine B. Venesection of 300 ml of blood daily helps. Diabetes is treated by diet and oral anti-diabetic drugs.
PORPHYRIA	The porphyrins are chemical substances involved in haemoglobin (in red blood cells), myo-haemoglobin (in muscle-fibres) and cytochrome C (necessary for cell-respiration). Disturbances of porphyrin metabolism are: (a) *congenital:* due to a recessive gene; porphyrins are deposited in the skin (causing a light-sensitivity dermatitis and over-growth of hair), lavender-coloured teeth, brown-coloured bones, an enlarged spleen, and port-wine coloured urine. *Treatment* is by the avoidance of sunlight and by splenectomy. (b) *acute:* possibly due to a dominant gene; in adult life occur attacks of abdominal pain, vomiting, constipation, peripheral neuritis, hallucinations and delirium. Patients are hyper-sensitive to barbiturates and taking one may precipitate an attack. *Treatment* is by sedation (barbiturates are not used) and the relief of pain. (c) *cutaneo-hepatic:* patient is hyper-sensitive to barbiturates or sulphonamide or other drugs, which can precipitate attacks of blistering of the skin by sunlight, friction or heat, and of jaundice and sometimes cirrhosis of the liver. *Treatment* is by the avoidance of anything known to precipitate an attack. (d) *secondary porphyria:* the result of bone-marrow damage by lead, arsenic, phosphorus and some drugs; attacks of abdominal pain, vomiting, constipation and peripheral neuritis occur.
GOUT	This is usually an 'inborn error' in the metabolism of purine. Purine does not occur in nature, but is part of the basic structure of several substances known as purine bodies of which uric acid is one. In gout the blood uric acid content is raised and crystals of sodium urate are deposited in and around the synovial cavities of joints. The metatarso-phalangeal joint of the big toe is the one usually affected, but other joints in the feet and hands can be involved. Gout is usually an inherited condition, more than half the cases having a family history. It is much more common in men than women; it can occur as early as

[1] *haemochromatosis:* Greek: *haima* – blood; *chroma:* colour
[2] *chelating agent:* drug that converts a heavy metal into a form in which it can be excreted

puberty, but the first attack is usually at 30-40 years. Affected people may be addicted to a consumption of heavily fortified wines, such as port and sherry. It can occur as a complication of some blood diseases; polycythaemia and leukaemia.

Clinical features   An attack of acute gout usually begins suddenly, but it may be preceded by some gastro-intestinal disturbance. The patient wakes up with agonizing pain in one of his big toes. The toe is swollen, inflamed and extremely tender; the condition may be mistaken for an acute cellulitis. The patient is unable to put his foot to the ground. He runs a slight temperature. Identical attacks can occur in other joints. An attack should subside quickly with treatment, and slowly without it. Between attacks the patient may be perfectly well; but if he has frequent attacks he is likely to develop chronic gout.

In *chronic gout* the patient develops a chronic arthritis of the involved joints and bursitis. Tophi, which are permanent deposits of sodium urate crystals, are deposited in the ears and around joints and in tendon sheaths; they can be seen and felt.

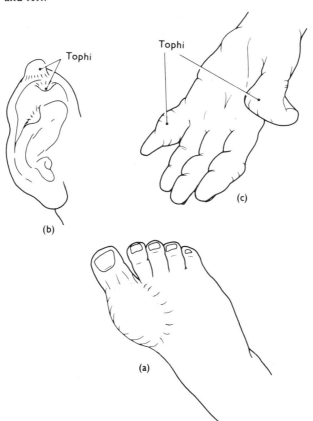

Tophi

Tophi

(b)

(c)

(a)

Fig. 52. The foot in acute gout. (b) Tophi on the ear in chronic gout. (c) Multiple tophi on the hands in severe gout.

Complications   Urinary calculi: leading to hydronephrosis, pyonephrosis, renal failure.
    Coronary disease.   Obesity.   Chronic arthritis.

Special tests	*Blood:* during attacks the uric acid is raised above normal (normal: up to 6 mg/100 ml in men, up to 5 mg/100 ml in women), ESR is raised and leucocytosis occurs.
	X-ray: in chronic gout, tophi produce punched-out patches of decalcification in bones and signs of osteo-arthritis.
	Joint fluid: uric acid crystals are found in aspirated fluid.

Treatment: acute gout

1. The patient stays in bed with the affected joint protected from jarring by cotton wool and a cradle.

2. He is given either (a) colchicine in doses of 0.5 mg every 2 hours until relieved of pain or until he develops diarrhoea or vomiting, and then 0.5 mg three times a day for several days; or (b) phenylbutazone, 600-800 mg on first day, reduced on subsequent days to 200-300 mg daily, or (c) indomethacin 150 mg daily for 3-5 days.

3. Between attacks the patient should (a) abstain from drinking fortified wines, (b) not eat liver, kidney, sweetbreads, fish-roe and meat extracts, which are rich in purine bodies, and (c) take fluids freely.

4. Uric acid excretion is promoted, acute attacks prevented and complications avoided by taking regularly either (a) probenecid (Benemid) 500 mg, 3-4 times a day with colchicine 1 mg daily, (b) sulphinpyrazone (Anturan) 200-400 mg daily or allopurinol 200-600 mg daily. in divided doses. Probenecid and sulphinpyrazone have no effect on acute attacks, but prevent them by increasing the excretion of urates by the kidneys. The uric acid level in the blood is estimated from time to time to check that the dose is appropriate.

HEPATO-LENTICULAR DEGENERATION

Other name: Wilson's disease

This is a rare genetically determined disease in which there is a disturbance of copper meta-bolism. A deficiency of caeruloplasmin, a protein responsible for the transport of copper in the blood, occurs; excessive amounts of copper are absorbed from the alimentary tract and deposited in the liver and in the basal ganglia and cerebral cortex. The patient develops cirr-hosis of the liver and degeneration of the parts of the brain in which the copper is deposited.

Clinical features

The biochemical disturbance is present at birth and signs appear in childhood. Cirrhosis of the liver is always present but sometimes not very apparent. Some patients have attacks of haematemesis or ascites; some develop jaundice and may die in hepatic coma before signs of brain damage appear.

Brain damage is shown by tremor and rigidity. The tremor is usually coarse and slow, with flapping of the hands and nodding of the head. Tonic and choreic movements can appear. The patient has a fixed, smiling expression and difficulty in speaking. Damage to the cerebral cortex is revealed by irritability, childishness and a decay of intellectual functions leading to dementia.

A deposit of copper around the periphery of the cornea forms a visible brown ring called a Kayser-Fleischer ring.

Treatment

Penicillamine (by mouth) and dimercaprol (BAL) are chelating agents which increase the excretion of copper by the kidneys. An alternation of low and high protein diets increases the excretion. Mushrooms, spinach, cocoa, liver, nuts and shell-fish, which have a high copper content, are avoided. An enteric-coated capsule of potassium sulphide 20 mg with each meal renders copper insoluble and prevents its absorption.

If a vitamin in the necessary amounts is lacking for long enough from the diet, certain clinical features will be produced. In countries where people are well nourished, vitamin deficiency is not very common but can be due to (a) ignorance of the need to take the foods that contain necessary vitamins, (b) food faddism, (c) chronic alcoholism, (d) drug addiction, (e) malabsorption syndromes, (f) poverty and (g) some types of institutional feeding. More than one kind of vitamin deficiency may occur in a person at the same time and he is then likely to show a combination of various clinical features.

Vitamin A deficiency

Sources of vitamin A: liver, butter, vitaminized margarine, cheese, eggs and fish-liver oil.

Occurrence: Africa, India, China, Middle East; hardly ever in the Western World.

Features of deficiency

(a) poor night vision (vitamin A forms part of the molecule of visual purple);
(b) xerophthalmia (dryness and thickening of the conjunctiva and inflammation of cornea);
(c) thickening of the horny layers of skin.

Treatment

Cod liver oil, shark liver oil and red palm oil are used to prevent and treat this deficiency.

2. Thiamine (vitamin B_1) deficiency

Sources of vitamin B_1: liver, kidneys, eggs, pork, ham, beans, peas, nuts, husks of rice.

Occurrence: Beri-beri is the condition produced by this deficiency. It occurs mostly in the Far East, where polished rice, from which the husk has been removed, is the staple article of diet; it occurs in chronic alcoholics and food-faddists.

Clinical features

(a) The patient develops a peripheral neuritis with paraesthesiae[3], painful calves, muscular paralysis, foot-drop, wrist-drop, ataxia[4], muscle-wasting and loss of tendon-reflexes.
(b) Acute congestive heart failure can develop quickly or slowly, with feeble heart-action, rapid pulse, dyspnoea, generalized oedema, effusions into pleural, pericardial and peritoneal cavities, and a large tender liver. Sudden death can occur.
(c) Confusion, ataxia, double vision, squint.

Treatment

Thiamine chloride 50 mg is given daily by mouth; in severe cases 100 mg of it is injected intravenously, followed by a further dose of 50 mg intravenously and thereafter 50 mg daily by mouth.

The diet is adjusted to include thiamine-containing foods.

3. Riboflavine deficiency

Sources of riboflavine: milk, cheese, eggs, green vegetables, liver and yeast.

Occurrence: It occurs most commonly in Africa and Asia; but it can occur in patients with the malabsorption syndrome, in those who have been on wide-spectrum antibiotics for a long time, or who have been having intravenous glucose only for a long time. Lack of it is likely to be associated with lack of thiamine.

[3] *paraesthesia:* sensations of tingling, burning, etc.
[4] *ataxia:* incoordination of muscular activity, affecting the gait

Clinical features	(a) glossitis, stomatitis; (b) seborrheic dermatitis of the face, chest, scrotum and vulva; (c) degeneration of the cornea
Treatment	This is by food containing riboflavine.
4. Nicotinamide (vitamin B$_7$, nicotinic acid) deficiency	*Source of nicotinamide:* cereals, meat, liver, yeast. *Occurrence:* Pellagra is the condition caused by this deficiency. It occurs commonly where maize is the staple article of diet, for maize contains the vitamin in a form in which it is not liberated for use in the body. It also occurs in mal-absorption syndromes and chronic alcoholism.
Clinical features	(a) dermatitis on exposed parts, the skin becoming reddened, scaling and then becoming deeply pigmented and cracking; (b) glossitis, tongue becoming swollen and magenta-coloured and sometimes fissured and ulcerated; stomatitis; fissures at the corner of the mouth; (c) abdominal discomfort and diarrhoea (diarrhoea can cause potassium deficiency). (d) mental disturbance, depression, dementia.
Treatment	Nicotinamine amide or nicotinic acid 100-200 mg is given by mouth for mild cases. For severe cases they are given intravenously in a dose of 300-400 mg for 4 days, followed by smaller amounts for 10 days. The diet is adjusted appropriately.
5. Vitamin B$_{12}$	(a) Megaloblastic anaemia, (b) subacute combined degeneration of cord.
6. Ascorbic acid (vitamin C)	*Sources of ascorbic acid:* fresh fruit and vegetables, especially oranges, tomatoes, blackcurrants, watercress, rose hips. It is destroyed by excessive or prolonged heating. *Occurrence: Scurvy* is the condition produced by deficiency of vitamin C. It is most likely to occur (a) in infants whose mothers do not know that infants require orange or rose-hip juice to provide them with vitamin C not present in dried or condensed milk; (b) in old people living by themselves and not taking fresh fruits and vegetables; (c) and people in institutions where food is cooked hours before a meal and then kept warm.
Clinical features	(a) listlessness, fatigue; (b) gums become swollen and livid and bleed; breath is offensive; (in people without teeth the gums appear normal); (c) small purpuric haemorrhages into skin; bruising; anaemia; (d) sub-periosteal haemorrhages and severe pain (may be mistaken for fracture or for poliomyelitis if infant is not using the limb); (e) delayed normal healing; (f) sudden death.

Treatment　Scurvy is prevented by taking fresh fruit or vegetables daily or ascorbic acid 25-50 mg in tablet form. Mild cases will recover with this; severe cases require 250 mg 4 times a day for several days in order to saturate the tissues.

7. Vitamin D deficiency: Rickets, Osteomalacia (a) Rickets

Sources of vitamin D: liver, butter, vitaminized margarine, cheese, eggs, fish-liver oils.

　Occurrence: Rickets is produced in infancy by shortage of vitamin D and osteomalacia in adult life. It is likely to occur in infants where there is lack of vitamin D and of calcium in the diet and where smoke and smog keep out sunlight.

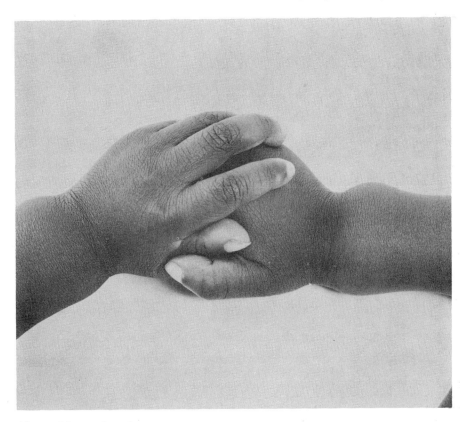

Fig. 53. Swollen epiphyses in rickets (photograph by Dept. of Audio-Visual Communication, St. Mary's Hospital Medical School)

Clinical features　(a) irritablity and restlessness;
(b) enlarged epiphyses at ends of long bones and at costo-chondral junctions (where bone of rib is united with costal cartilage), where a line of bumps called a 'rickety rosary' is formed;
(c) softening and bending of long bones, especially of arm bones when child tries to support himself and leg bones when he tries to walk, with production of bow legs;
(d) bossing of frontal and parietal bones causing a 'hot cross bun' effect;
(e) muscles become flabby from loss of muscle-tone;
(f) abdominal distension, chronic diarrhoea;
(g) anaemia of hypochromic type (iron-deficiency);

　　　　　　　Metabolic and Deficiency Diseases

(h) chronic catarrh,

(i) tetany if serum calcium is low.

Untreated the disease runs a long course, to right itself as the growing child starts to eat a more varied diet. Some of the deformities may persist, some clear up. Rickets is not fatal, but it can be a serious complication of other diseases of infancy. Deformation of pelvis can cause difficulty in childbirth.

Special tests *X-ray* of bones shows lack of calcium and abnormal growth at epiphyses.

Prevention is by an adequate diet. If the mother's diet is adequate, a breast-fed child will get an adequate amount of vitamin D up to the age of 3-4 months, and thereafter will require vitamin D supplements by cod-liver oil to provide vitamin D 400 international units daily up to the age of 2 years. Sunlight, by manufacturing vitamin D in the skin, and exercise in the open air are required. As the child is weaned, care must be taken that his food includes animal fats. The diet should include milk up to 1 pint daily for the first two years of life.

Treatment (a) an adequate diet.

(b) Vitamin D (calciferol) 3,000-5,000 international units daily;

(c) exercise in the open air; sunlight or artificial sunlight.

Over-dosage with vitamin D produces nausea, vomiting, muscular weakness, and calification of blood-vessels and kidneys.

(b) Osteomalacia This is due to vitamin D shortage in adult life. It is more common in the East than in the Western World. It is the result of either dietary deficiency or malabsorption. In adult life there is a continuous process of bone-remodelling, and when vitamin D is short the normal protein structure of bone does not become adequately calcified.

Clinical features The patient complains of fatigue, pain in bones, and muscular weakness. Tetany can occur if the plasma sodium is very low. Swellings at the costochondral junctions, fractures, deformities of bone and collapse of vertebral bodies can occur. Deformities of the pelvis can lead to difficulties in child-birth.

Special tests *X-ray of bones:* (a) decalcification of bone is seen only when 50 per cent of the calcium has been lost; (b) Looser's zones are thin lines of increased translucency which are sometimes mistaken for fractures.

Prevention The disease can be prevented by an adequate diet and the treatment of malabsorption.

Treatment Vitamin D is given in doses of 2,000-3,000 units daily. Calcium lactate is taken daily. An adequate diet is given.

8. Vitamin K deficiency *Sources of vitamin K:* (a) green vegetables and other foods, (b) synthesis in the bowel by bacteria.

Occurrence: vitamin K deficiency can occur (a) in infancy during the first few

days of life when the stock of it absorbed from the mother is used up and synthesis in the bowel has not been established;
(b) when bile is absent from the alimentary tract,
(c) in steatorrhoea.

Clinical features Vitamin K being necessary for the formation of prothrombin, deficiency of it causes a fall in the amount of prothrombin in the blood. Haematuria and other haemorrhages occur. A severe haemorrhage can be fatal.

Prevention To prevent deficiency in the newly-born, the mother can be given vitamin K 2 mg daily during the last week of pregnancy.

Treatment Vitamin K is given by mouth in doses of 2-5 mg daily. In obstructive jaundice it is not absorbed from the bowel and has to be given by intramuscular injection.

PROTEIN DEFICIENCY Protein deficiency occurs: (a) when the intake of protein is inadequate for essential functions and (b) when the supply is adequate but the patient cannot utilize protein because of a mal-absorption syndrome, cancer of the oesophagus or stomach, a severe infection or after severe injury.

Clinical features The patient becomes dull, apathetic and hungry. He loses weight and his muscles waste, and in consequence he becomes easily tired. His heart is small, his pulse slow, his BP low.

Treatment Adequate amounts of protein are supplied and any cause is treated.

Kwashiorkor (malignant malnutrition) This is a disease of children due to severe protein deficiency. It occurs in Africa and other parts of the world where protein is short and carbohydrates are the main food. Sufferers from it are likely also to have vitamin deficiency and infections by bacteria or parasites.

Patients show physical and mental retardation, muscle-wasting, anaemia, under- or over-pigmentation of the skin, gastro-intestinal disorders, and fatty or fibrous degeneration of the liver. Untreated, many patients die.

Treatment is by the controlled administration of protein (in severe cases by protein hydrolysates intravenously), by the restoration of water and electrolyte balance, and by iron or blood-transfusion for anaemia. Infections must be treated appropriately.

10   Diseases of the Endocrine Glands

The endocrine glands produce secretions called hormones, which pass out of the cells of the gland directly into the blood-stream and, circulating throughout the body, have effect upon tissues. The endocrine glands are:

the pituitary	the thyroid
the parathyroids	the adrenals
the pancreas	
the testis	the ovary

The pituitary gland, through its secretions, has a general control of the secretions of other endocrine glands. Some glands have other functions as well: the pancreas produces pancreatic juice, the testis produces sperm, the ovary produces ova.

A disease of an endocrine gland causes an over-secretion or an under-secretion of its hormone or of one or more of its hormones if it produces several. But an endocrine gland does not function alone: it affects the secretion of hormones in other glands. The clinical picture of one of these diseases is therefore likely to reflect both the over-secretion or under-secretion of the gland primarily affected and also the effect of this on the secretions of other glands.

Diseases of the Pituitary Gland

Diseases of the pituitary gland affect its production of hormones. The *anterior lobe* produces 6 hormones; one of them controls the growth of the body, the others control the activities of the thyroid gland, the adrenal cortex, the testis, the ovary and the corpus luteum; and any disorder of the anterior lobe is likely to affect their activities. The *posterior lobe* produces ADH (anti-diuretic hormone) and one other hormone, oxytocin.

Diseases of the pituitary gland are likely:

(a) to increase the secretion of a particular hormone by an over-growth of the cells producing it,

(b) to decrease the secretion of other hormones by hormone action or by pressure on the cells producing them,

(c) when there is a pituitary tumour, to increase intra-cranial pressure and to press on the optic chiasma and the 3rd, 4th and 6th cranial nerves, which run close to the gland.

The gland is functionally linked with the *hypothalamus,* the part of the brain immediately above it and to which it is connected by a stalk; and any disease on

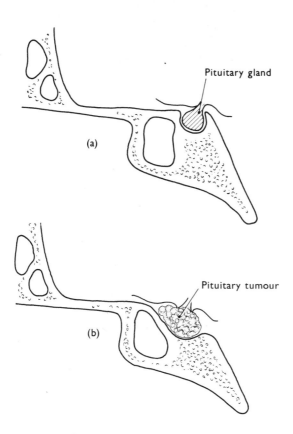

Fig. 54. (a) A normal pituitary fossa. (b) A dilated pituitary fossa with erosion of bone, due to a tumour of the pituitary gland.

mal-functioning of the hypothalamus is likely to affect the production of pituitary hormones.

The diseases of the pituitary gland are:

Hyper-pituitarism (over-production)
    acromegaly
    gigantism
    chromophobe adenoma
    basophil adenoma
Hypo-pituitarism (under-production)
    pituitary infantilism
    Frohlich's syndrome
    Simmond's disease
    diabetes insipidus

HYPER-PITUITARISM: ACROMEGALY AND GIGANTISM

Acromegaly is due to over-production of the growth-hormone and is characterized mainly by over-growth of tissues. Gigantism is due to over-production in early life before growth has ceased and causes excessive height, sometimes in association with acromegaly.

Diseases of the Endocrine Glands

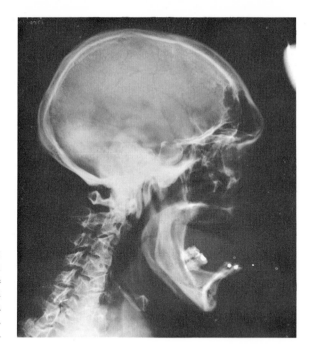

Fig. 55. The head in acromegaly with diagram of X-ray to show the thickened skull and ballooned pituitary fossa (by permission of St. Bartholomew's Hospital).

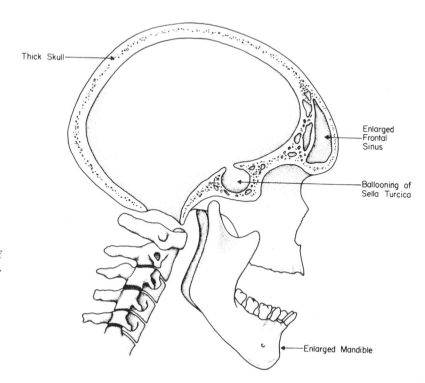

Thick Skull

Enlarged Frontal Sinus

Ballooning of Sella Turcica

Enlarged Mandible

Fig. 55A. Line drawing of the previous X-ray.

Chapter 10

The over-production of the hormone is due to an increase in the number of acidophil (alpha) cells, the ones that produce that hormone. Sometimes there is a general increase in the size of the gland, sometimes the cells are grouped together to form a tumour, an adenoma. The disease develops slowly over years, with long periods when it is apparently stationary.

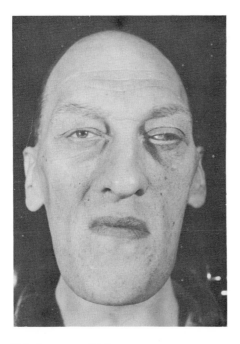

Fig. 56. Acromegaly (from *Samson Wright's Applied Physiology;* courtesy Dr. J. D. N. Nabarro).

Clinical features
1. Due to excessive secretion of the growth hormone

Skin becomes thick.
Features become large and coarse, especially lips, nose and tongue.
Both jaws enlarge; lower jaw sticks out; dentures do not fit.
Feet and hands enlarge; patient takes larger sizes in shoes and gloves.
Chest becomes bigger.
Spine develops kyphosis [5].
Voice becomes husky (due to enlargement of larynx)
Height becomes excessive, in giantism.

2. Under-secretion of other hormones

Amenorrhoea.   Impotence.
Persistent lactation in both sexes.

3. Pressure symptoms

Pressure on optic chiasma: defects in visual fields, blindness.

Pressure on 3rd, 4th, 6th cranial nerves: squint, double vision.

Pressure on hypothalamus: drowsiness, excessive amounts of urine, thirst.

Increasing intra-cranial pressure: headache, vomiting.

[5] *kyphosis:* curvature of the spine backwards

Diseases of the Endocrine Glands

4. Pituitary apoplexy	Attacks of headache, sudden loss of vision, impaired consciousness: due to acute degeneration in a pituitary tumour.
5. Symptoms of uncertain origin	Increased basal metabolic rate. Sweating. Exophthalmos[6]. Hypertension. As the disease progresses the patient becomes enfeebled. The outlook is poor.
Special tests	*X-ray of skull:* ballooning of pituitary fossa, erosion of bone forming it or a 'double floor' due to unequal growth of an asymmetrical tumour. *Blood:* radio-immune assays of growth hormone, thyroid-stimulating hormone, follicle-stimulating hormone, and luteinizing hormone.
Treatment	Treatment is by radio-therapy or surgical removal of the tumour. Subsequently patients may require 'replacement therapy': thyroxine, cortisone, fludro-cortisone (to aid sodium retention), oestrogens for women, androgens for men, insulin or tolbutamide for patients who develop diabetes mellitus, and vasopressin tannate in oil for patients who develop diabetes insipidus. Treatment is unsatisfactory; complete remission is unlikely.
CHROMOPHOBE ADENOMA	This is a tumour of the chromophobe[7] cells of the anterior lobe, cells which are small and do not stain with dyes. A tumour of them can occur at any age and produce: (a) pressure on the optic nerve and olfactory tracts, partial and later complete blindness, interference with the sense of smell; (b) increased intracranial pressure, severe headache, vomiting; (c) pressure on the hypothalamus, sleepiness, obesity, passing excessive amounts of urine, thirst, hypo-thermia[8], low BP, scanty body-hair, loss of sexual desire, atrophy of breasts, disturbances of menstruation; (d) pressure on the other cells of the gland and so eventually hypo-pituitarism.
Special tests	*X-ray of skull:* ballooning of pituitary fossa and erosion of bone forming it.
Treatment	Treatment is by radio-therapy and surgery, but the results are not good.
HYPO-PITUITARISM PITUITARY INFANTILISM (LORAIN TYPE)[9]	This condition is due to a failure of the pituitary gland in childhood; it can be due to pressure on the gland by tumour or cyst. The child, failing to grow, becomes a dwarf. Epiphyses do not unite and the secondary sexual characteristics do not appear. *Treatment* is by intramuscular injections of human growth-hormone until normal height is reached. Thyroid hormone, adrenal corticoids, and testosterone (for boys) and oestrogens (for girls) may be required.

[6] *exophthalmos:* protrusion of the eyeballs
[7] *chromophobe:* colour-avoiding
[8] *hypo-thermia:* abnormally low temperature
[9] *P.J. Lorain* (1825-75): French physician

FROHLICH'S SYNDROME [1]	*Other name:* dystrophia adiposo-genitalis In this condition the child puts on weight and fails to develop sexually, the sex organs remaining infantile and functionless. The basic lesions may be in the hypothalamus and not in the gland itself; the obesity may be more due to over-eating than to glandular dysfunction.
SIMMONDS'[2] DISEASE	This condition is due to degeneration of the pituitary gland. It can occur as a result of a severe ante-partum[3] or post-partum[4] haemorrhage, sometimes of an infarction, sometimes of pressure from an adjoining tumour. There is a complete failure of hormonal secretion by the gland.
Clinical features	The patient loses her appetite and sometimes, but not always, loses weight. She becomes very tired. Pallor of the skin is very noticeable. The breasts, uterus and vagina shrink; and sexual desire is lost. Amenorrhoea occurs. The axillary and pubic hair fall out, and some of the hair of the scalp. Hypotension and hypoglycaemic attacks can occur. The patient can go into coma for no apparent reason and is likely to die in such a coma.
Special tests	Urine: reduced excretion of 17-keto-steroids (normal: men:- 8-20 mg/24 hours: women:- 6-18 mg/24 hours). Glucose tolerance test: flat curve.
Treatment	The best treatment is for the patient to become pregnant again, for another pregnancy can stimulate growth of pituitary tissue; but owing to the sexual degeneration this is not often achieved. Cortisone in doses of 25-50 mg by mouth daily or methyl testosterone in doses of 20-50 mg sublingually should improve the patient's condition.
DIABETES INSIPIDUS	In this disease a failure of the hypothalamus-pituitary mechanism decreases the production of anti-diuretin. Anti-diuretic hormone (ADH), one of the two hormones of the posterior lobe of the gland, is responsible for the re-absorption of water as it passes through the distal part of the renal tubules. If anti-diuretin is not present in adequate amounts the kidneys do not reabsorb water and there is an excessive secretion of a very dilute urine. Causes of damage to the hypothalamus-pituitary mechanism are: pressure or destruction by a tumour, operations on that area, fracture of the base of the skull, meningitis and encephalitis.
Clinical features	The patient passes large amounts (up to 20 litres or more a day) of very dilute urine

[1]*A. Frohlich* (1871-1953): Austrian neurologist
[2]*M. Simmonds* (1855-1925) German physician
[3]*ante-partum:* before birth   [4]*post-partum:* after birth

(SG 1,002-1,004). He becomes in consequence very thirsty and if he did not drink copiously to compensate for the water lost he would become dehydrated.

Treatment Pitressin tannate in oil can be given by intra-muscular or subcutaneous injection in doses of 0.5-1.0 ml every 1-3 days; or lysine vasopressin, which is effective for short periods, as a nasal spray. Chlorothiazide, an oral diuretic, helps to suppress thirst.

Diseases of the Parathyroid Gland

The parathyroid glands produce parathormone, a hormone that (a) liberates calcium from bone into the plasma and (b) regulates the amount of inorganic phosphorus excreted by the kidneys. In these ways it controls the amounts of calcium and phosphorus in the blood. In diseases of the parathyroid glands there is either an increase or a decrease in the amount of parathormone produced.

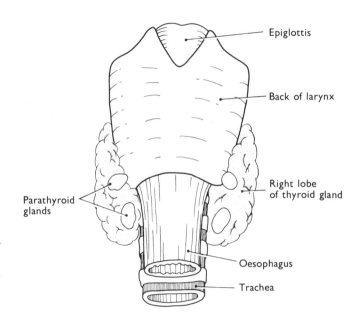

Fig. 57. Posterior view of the larynx and thyroid gland to show the usual position of the parathyroid glands.

HYPER-PARATHYROIDISM In this condition there is an abnormally high secretion of parathormone as a result of the growth of one or more tumours (adenomas) of parathyroid tissue. This condition is much more common in women than in men. The tumours can be tiny or large enough to be felt easily in the neck. As a result of excessive secretion by the tumour-cells:

(a) more phosphorus is excreted by the kidneys; there is an increase of phosphorus in the urine and a decrease of it in the blood;

(b) there is a rise of calcium in the blood and secondary to that rise an increase in the amount excreted by the kidney.

Over-growth of parathyroid tissue can be due to renal failure.

Chapter 10

Clinical features	The excessive amount of calcium in the blood causes weakness, hypotonia[5], loss of appetite, difficulty in swallowing, nausea, vomiting and constipation. It can occur in an 'apathetic' form — with apathy, depression, loss of weight, muscle-wasting and heart-failure.

The excessive excretion of calcium can cause renal calculi, composed of calcium oxalate or phosphate. Renal colic is sometimes the first sign of the disease. With large stones, renal function suffers. Some bones (usually the femur and tibia) can develop patches of fibrous tissue.

Complications

Generalized osteitis fibrosa   Pathological fractures
Infection of urinary tract   Uraemia
Peptic ulcer (reason unknown).

Special tests

Serum inorganic phosphorus: lowered (normal: 2.5-4.5 mg/100 ml)
Serum calcium: raised (normal: 8.7-10 mg/100 ml)
Urine calcium: usually above 200 mg excreted/24 hours.
X-ray of kidney: for renal stones.
X-ray of bones: for osteitis fibrosa.

Treatment

The tumour is removed surgically.

**HYPO-
PARATHYROIDISM**

In this condition there is a decreased production of parathormone, which can happen if the parathyroid glands happen to be removed during thyroidectomy. There is an increase of the amount of phosphorus in the blood because the renal tubules reabsorb it, and there is less calcium in the blood.

Clinical features

Tetany is produced. Tetany is a condition in which nerves are hyper-excitable. It occurs in:
(a) any condition in which there is a low serum calcium: hypo-parathyroidism, rickets, osteomalacia, malabsorption syndrome, chronic renal failure.
(b) in alkalosis:
any severe persistent vomiting, severe diarrhoea, excessive intake of alkalis, hyperventilation.

In tetany the patient complains of numbness and tingling in the fingers and toes and around the lips. He gets painful cramps and muscular contractions. When the hands and feet are involved in the cramp it is called carpo-pedal spasm: the position of the hands is typical — the fingers are extended at the inter-phalangeal joints and slightly flexed at the metacarpo-phalangeal joints.

The patient can develop attacks of nausea, vomiting and abdominal pain. He can get attacks of laryngeal spasm, 'crowing' on inspiration, and have dyspnoea[6], cyanosis[7] and fits.

Increased intra-cranial pressure can occur, producing headache and papilloedema

[5] *hypotonia:* reduced muscle tone
[6] *dypsnoea:* difficult breathing
[7] *cyanosis:* blueness of skin and mucous membranes

Calcification of the small intra-cerebral arteries is sometimes seen on X-ray examination.

The hair becomes coarse and falls out. The nails become brittle. If the patient is a child, malformations of developing teeth can occur.

Special tests

Chvostek's sign: can be positive in tetany: a spasm of the facial muscles occurs when the facial nerve is tapped on in front of the ear. It can occur in people who have not got tetany.

Trousseau's sign: in tetany constricting the arm produces the characteristic spasm of the muscles of the hand and forearm.

Serum calcium: reduced (normal: 8.7-10 mg/100 ml)

Serum inorganic phosphorus: raised (normal: 2.5-4.5 mg/100 ml)

Treatment

Tetany is treated with calcium given intravenously, e.g. calcium gluconate 10-30 ml of a 10 per cent solution in 1,000 ml of normal saline. Subsequently calcium is given intramuscularly or calcium lactate 4 g, 6 times daily by mouth with vitamin D until the serum calcium has risen to normal. Maintenance doses are then given.

Diseases of the Thyroid Gland

Diseases of the thyroid gland are likely to affect its production of thyroxine, increasing or decreasing it. The production of this hormone is controlled by a hormone of the anterior lobe of the pituitary gland, and thyroid function is therefore likely to be affected by disease of that gland.

The diseases of the thyroid gland are:

hyperthyroidism malignant exophthalmos
cretinism myxoedema
goitre thyroiditis

HYPERTHYROIDISM

Other names: thyrotoxicosis, exophthalmic goitre, Graves' disease

This disease is produced by an excessive secretion of thyroid hormones. Its cause is unknown. Usually there is a generalized overactivity of the whole gland, but in about 5 per cent of cases the condition is due to a toxic adenoma in the gland. Most of the clinical features can be attributed to the excessive secretion, but the eye signs cannot. The disease can be familial. Its onset is sometimes associated with mental stress or with trauma, but the association may be a coincidence. The personality of the patient who develops the disease is said to be one in which the patient is driven by ambitions he cannot achieve. He may have shown neurasthenic symptoms or had attacks of manic excitement. In a woman it can be produced by a hydatidiform mole.

Clinical features

The onset may be rapid or slow, the attack mild or severe. The thyroid gland is usually enlarged and firmer than normal. A general enlargement is said to be associated with neurological and eye signs; a nodular enlargement is said to be associated with heart disease.

The patient becomes tired, cannot walk as far as he could and finds going up and downstairs particularly fatiguing. He loses weight in spite of having a good appetite. He sleeps poorly. He sweats excessively and may have pruritus. Menorrhagia[8] or amenorrhoea can occur.

The heart-rate is increased and often irregular. The bowels are moved frequently

[8] *menorrhagia:* excessive menstruation

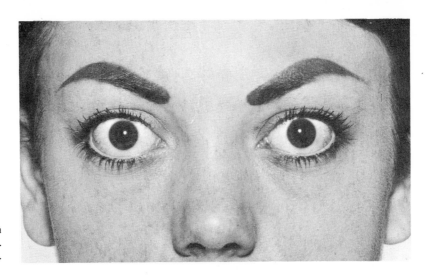

Fig. 58. Hyperthyroidism (by permission of St. Bartholomew's Hospital).

and diarrhoea may develop. The patient is likely to show a fine rapid tremor of his fingers and tongue. The eye signs that can occur are: prominence of the eyes, dilatation of the pupil, retraction of the upper lid and sometimes the lower, a lagging of the lid, and a reduction in blinking.

The patient is irritable, impatient, anxious and restless. Poor sleep is made worse by anxiety-dreams and nightmares. Attacks of hypomania or hysteria can occur. Thyroidectomy may relieve a mental attack or precipitate one. The patient may boil over into a 'thyroid crisis', in which be becomes acutely ill and may die. Such a crisis can be produced by operating on an inadequately prepared patient.

Complications 'Thyroid heart', with tachycardia, atrial fibrillation and congestive heart failure.
Enlarged spleen and lymph-nodes.
Osteo-porosis[9] : rib and other fractures, collapse of vertebral body.
Thyrotoxic myopathy: degeneration of muscles, weakness, death.

Special tests Basal metabolic rate: raised.
Blood: protein-bound iodine concentration in serum raised above 8.0 micrograms per 100 ml
Uptake of radio-iodine by gland: usually above 60 per cent.

Treatment Treatment is by:
(a) antithyroid drugs, given for at least one and usually two years. A large dose is given for a month and then a small maintenance dose. Treatment is regulated according to the patient's pulse rate and weight. Toxic effects are rare; the serious one is agranulocytosis. Drugs in use are

	Initial dose mg/day	Maintenance dose mg/day
methyl thiouracil	300	50-100

[9] *osteo-porosis:* reduction of calcium in bone, atrophy of bone

	Initial dose mg/day	Maintenance dose mg/day
propylthiouracil	150	25-50
carbimazole	30	5-10
methimazole	30	5-10
potassium perchlorate	800	200-400

(b) radio-active iodine (I^{131}). It is given by mouth and taken up by the thyroid cells, which it then destroys. Results are not apparent for 2-3 months. The chief complication is hypothyroidism. It is usually given to old or frail patients and those for whom antithyroid drugs have not been effective. It is contra-indicated in pregnancy
(c) subtotal thyroidectomy: about 95 per cent of the gland is removed; the posterior parts of each lobe are left in order to provide some thyroid secretion and to leave the parathyroid glands intact.

A *thyroid crisis* is treated by:
(a) propranolol 40 mg 6-hourly by mouth or 2 mg intravenously: to reduce sympathetic overactivity; or reserpine 2.5 mg 6-hourly: as a sedative
(b) hydrocortisone 100-300 mg intravenously: to reduce stress and oppose any adrenal insufficiency
(c) sodium iodide 1-2 g intravenously: to prevent the production of thyroxine
(d) methylthiouracil 1000 mg or carbimazole 100 mg: to reduce hormonal secretion
(e) intravenous glucose and then glucose-saline: to prevent dehydration and provide a source of energy
(f) oxygen: for anoxia
(g) tepid sponging and ice-packs: for hyperpyrexia.

MALIGNANT
EXOPHTHALMOS

This condition occurs more often in men and usually in middle life. It is possibly due to some abnormal pituitary secretion. The thyroid gland is not much enlarged and the usual signs of hyperthyroidism are not very pronounced. What is obvious is the extreme protrusion of the eyeballs. With this protrusion the patient is likely to have oedema of the eyelids, photophobia[1], excessive tear formation, inability to move the eyeballs, and corneal ulceration. The patient may eventually develop optic atrophy and go blind.

Complications

Pre-tibial myxoedema: purple-pink patches of myxoedematous tissue over the tibiae and elsewhere.
Clubbing of the fingers.

Treatment

There is no satisfactory treatment for this condition. If ulceration of the cornea threatens, the eyelids may have to be stitched together.

HYPO-THYROIDISM
CRETINISM

Cretinism is a form of hypo-thyroidism occurring in early childhood. It is due to lack of the thyroid hormone caused by an inadequate supply of iodine to the child during intra-uterine and early post-natal life. It is common in those parts of the world where endemic goitre occurs and there is a deficiency of iodine in soil and water and hence in the diet, but its incidence has been greatly reduced by adding iodized salt (salt with additional iodine) to the diet. Rarely it is due
[1]*photophobia:* dislike of light

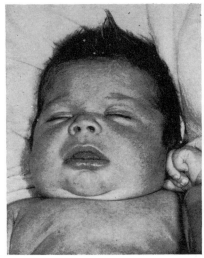 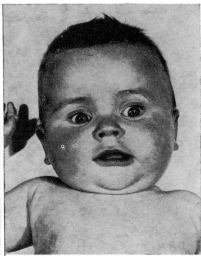

Fig. 59. Cretinism (a) before and (b) after treatment by thyroxine (from Jolly H. (1968) *Diseases of Children*, 2nd ed. Blackwell Scientific Publications).

(a)   (b)

to congenital absence of the gland or to a failure of the gland to produce the hormone. It can follow an inflammation of the gland or antithyroid drugs given in pregnancy.

Clinical features

Cretinism is not often diagnosed at birth, but it is usually obvious within a few months of birth. As a baby the cretin is lethargic and apathetic, cries little, sleeps a lot, is a poor feeder and is constipated. Untreated he is mentally retarded and dwarfed. He is late in sitting and standing; he does not learn to speak but makes noises in a hoarse croak. His skin is thick and dry; his temperature is subnormal and his pulse slow. His tongue is large and protruding. His features are coarse, and his brittle, scanty hair grows low on his forehead. His neck is thick, with supraclavicular pads of fat. He has a large abdomen and an umbilical hernia. He is anaemic and has hypotonic muscles.

Special tests

Basal metabolic rate: low
Blood cholesterol: may be raised (normal: 100-300 mg per 100 ml).

Treatment

Treatment must be begun at once. The longer treatment is delayed the more likely is the child to remain mentally and physically retarded. Thyroxine sodium is given in doses of:
For infants: 12.5 mcg daily, increased by 25 mcg every 2 weeks until effects are produced.
For children: 50-225 mcg daily.
Mental improvement should be apparent soon and in most patients there is a marked physical improvement. In spite of apparently adequate treatment judged by the physical improvement, some cretins do not show much mental improvement. Treatment has to be continued for life.

MYXOEDEMA Myxoedema is due to a failure of thyroid function in later life. It can occur in (a) a juvenile and (b) an adult form. In juvenile myxoedema the thyroid gland fails to produce an adequate amount of its hormone or for some unknown reason is completely destroyed. Symptoms vary with the age of the child and the degree of hypo-thyroidism: the usual history is one of normal physical and mental development for a time, and then a cessation or retardation of growth, a decline in intelligence, and the development of constipation and the signs of myxoedema.

Adult myxoedema is more common. More women are affected than men. Its cause is unknown, except when it follows surgical removal of the gland, radio-iodine treatment, or an attack of thyroiditis. The thyroid gland degenerates, fails to produce an adequate amount of its hormone, and has its secreting cells replaced by fibrous tissue.

Clinical features The patient becomes tired, constipated and obese; she feels the cold very much.

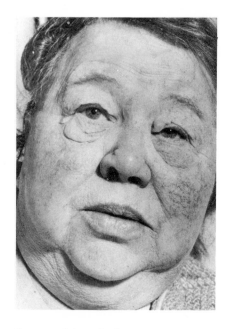

Fig. 60. The face in myxoedema (from Passmore R. & Robson J.S. (Eds) *A Companion to Medical Studies*, Vol. 3, Blackwell Scientific Publications).

She complains of aching pains in the back and legs and of stiff joints. She becomes deaf. Her skin becomes dry and scaly. Her face is typical: it is bloated with myxoedema, with bags under the eyes; the lips are thick, the eyebrows are sparse, the complexion is yellow and the hair falls out. The knees and the small joints of the hands and feet can become swollen. The patient may complain of tingling and other abnormal sensations. The median nerve may become compressed in the carpal tunnel. Bones may become decalcified.

The patient's voice becomes a hoarse croak and she snores thunderously. She may develop generalized oedema. Menorrhagia or amenorrhoea can occur. If the patient passes into a 'myxoedema coma' she is very likely to die in it.

The patient becomes dull and retarded, her memory deteriorates, she cannot grasp ordinary affairs. Some patients develop a psychosis — the 'myxoedema madness' — with delusions of persecution, hallucinations, confusion and violent outbursts.

| *Complications* | anaemia | carpal tunnel syndrome |
| | pericardial effusion | coronary and cerebral atheroma |

Special test — *Blood cholesterol:* almost always 250 mg or more/100 ml (normal: 100-300 mg/100 ml)
P.B.I. (plasma-protein bound iodine): low

Treatment — Thyroxine sodium is given daily in doses of 150-300 mcg daily. There should be a rapid return to health. Maintenance doses must be continued for life.

GOITRE

Any enlargement of the thyroid gland is called a goitre[2]. One type of enlargement is the simple goitre, seen most commonly in adolescent girls, in whom a gradual enlargement occurs for no clear reason. *Endemic goitre* occurs in some parts of the world — especially where there is a shortage of iodine in the soil and water and hence in the diet; where iodine is displaced by excess of fluorine or by other substances; where people eat certain substances (such as cabbage stalks) which contain a toxic substance. Endemic goitre is associated with cretinism. It has disappeared in those parts of the world (such as Switzerland and the USA) where iodine is added to the salt, but in some parts of the world 'iodinization' of salt is not possible.

Goitres can enlarge so much that they produce pressure — symptoms by pressing on the trachea, the larynx and the recurrent laryngeal nerve (running upwards from the vagus between the trachea and oesophagus to supply the larynx) producing hoarseness and difficulty in swallowing. A retro-sternal[3] goitre, which cannot expand forwards, is particularly likely to cause pressure-symptoms.

Some goitres become nodular and are particularly likely to cause toxic cardiac complications.

Complications
1. Thyrotoxicosis.
2. 'Thyroid heart' with rapid heart action; atrial fibrillation; congestive heart failure.
3. Malignant disease: rare.

Treatment
The simple goitre usually disappears in time. Thyroxine sodium can be given until the stimulus that has produced the overgrowth has passed off. For endemic goitre, potassium iodide is given in doses of 5 mg daily for many months.

Surgical removal of the goitre is advised if pressure signs appear, if thyrotoxicosis or atrial fibrillation appear, if malignant disease is suspected, or if the goitre is large and unsightly.

THYROIDITIS

There are several conditions to which the name of thyroiditis has been given; most of them are rare.

[2] *goitre:* from Latin: *guttar* — throat
[3] *retro-sternal:* behind the sternum

Acute thyroiditis can occur after mumps or an upper respiratory tract infection, and there is a *subacute thyroiditis* of unknown origin. In thyroiditis the gland becomes swollen and tender, the patient has a temperature and feels ill. The length of an attack can vary from days to weeks, and relapses are common. Recovery is usual, but myxoedema can develop afterwards if the secreting cells of the gland are extensively damaged.

Treatment is by bed-rest, analgesics, and in severe cases cortisone.

Diseases of the Adrenal Glands

The cortex of the adrenal gland, acting under the influence of a pituitary gland hormone, secretes several hormones, which are steroids concerned with the retention in the body of salt and water, with virilization [4], and with the conversion of tissue-proteins into glucose. The medulla secretes adrenaline and nor-adrenaline.

The diseases of the adrenal glands are:

Addison's disease.   Cushing's syndrome.
aldosteronism.   phaeochromocytoma.

ADDISON'S DISEASE [5]

Other name: adrenal cortical insufficiency

This disease can be caused by anything that profoundly decreases hormone-secretion by the adrenal cortex. Both adrenals have to be affected. The adrenals can be affected in this way by a primary atrophy of the gland (possibly an auto-immune reaction – see Chap. 12), invasion of the glands by a secondary cancer or by leukaemia, by tuberculosis, or by haemorrhage into the glands during a very severe illness. The disease usually begins at 30-50 years. Body chemistry is seriously affected. The amount of sodium chloride excreted by the kidneys is increased, and this produces a decrease in the amount of sodium and chloride in the blood and an increase in the amount of potassium. There is a decrease in the excretion in the urine of 17-ketosteroids, a product of the adrenals.

Bilateral adrenalectomy is sometimes performed for Cushing's syndrome or in association with removal of the ovaries for breast cancer with secondary deposits, and this would produce adrenal cortical insufficiency if appropriate treatment with cortisone were not begun immediately.

Clinical features

Except when due to haemorrhage into the glands, the onset is slow as a rule; occasionally an 'adrenal crisis' is the first sign. Tiredness and weakness are the first symptoms, and as a result of the salt-loss and hormone-deficiencies the patient becomes weaker and weaker. Nausea and vomiting occur. The patient becomes abnormally pigmented with a light brown to black darkening of the skin especially in the creases, in any scar, and in the parts that normally are pigmented. Irregularly shaped patches of pigment occur on the lips and mucous membrane of the mouth. The temperature is below normal and the pulse-rate raised. There is a gradual circulatory failure, with a blood-pressure falling to below 100 mm of mercury. There is in consequence a poor production of urine, an increase in the amounts of urea and other substances in the blood. Hypo-glycaemia is common.

Complication

An *adrenal crisis* can be produced by any stress – an infection, an anaesthetic, an

[4] *virilisation:* change to the characteristics of the male
[5] *T. Addison* (1793-1860): English physician

infarction, a surgical operation, a fracture, exposure to cold. The patient's symptoms suddenly become much worse; he vomits, collapses and is likely to go into a coma and die.

Special tests

Serum sodium reduced (normal: 135-147 m. Eq/1)
Serum potassium increased (normal: 3.3-5.2 m. Eq/1)
17-ketosteroids in urine decreased (normal: men: 8-20 mg/24 hours; women: 6-18 mg/24 hours).

Treatment

The hormone deficiency is remedied by giving: cortisone 25-50 mg daily or fludro-cortisone 0.2-0.4 mg daily.

Common salt is given by mouth to replace that lost, and carbohydrates are given in amounts adequate to prevent hypoglycaemia.

A *crisis* is treated by:

(a) putting the patient to bed,

(b) giving hydrocortisone 100-250 mg intravenously in normal saline with glucose saline 10 per cent to follow,

(c) followed by hydrocortisone 100 mg intravenously 8-hourly or cortisone acetate 100 mg intramuscularly.

(d) penicillin injections if the patient has an infection.

The patient should carry a card with his name, address, nature of his illness, and treatment advised in an emergency.

CUSHING'S
SYNDROME[6]

Other name: adreno-cortical hyperfunction

In this condition there is an over-production of cortisone by the adrenal glands. It may be due to an adrenal tumour or to a pituitary tumour's action on the adrenals. It is more common in women than men. It can occur after prolonged treatment with large doses of cortico-steroids.

Clinical features

Body-fat is redistributed: the face, neck and trunk become fat; the limbs become thin or appear thin in contrast. The face becomes bloated or 'moon-shaped'. Purple streaks called striae appear on the skin of the abdomen, buttocks and thighs. Patients bruise easily. Acne is common.

Sugar appears in the urine and diabetes mellitus can develop.

Osteo-porosis, decalcification of bone, may be present. Kyphosis appears and sometimes the vertebral column becomes shorter because vertebral bodies collapse. Patients complain of backache and tiredness.

Female patients develop amenorrhoea and may show virilization with growth of hair on the face, enlargement of the clitoris, deepening of the voice, and a development of masculine interests.

Special tests

17-ketosteroids in urine: increased above 20 mg/24 hours as a result of breakdown of cortisone in body.

[6] *H.W. Cushing* (1869-1930): American neuro-surgeon

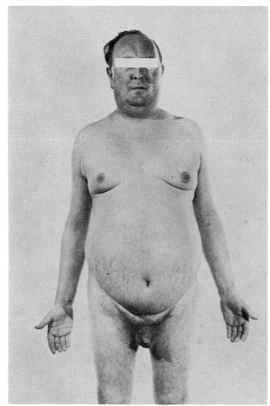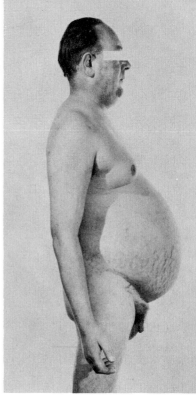

Fig. 61. Cushing's syndrome, showing red moon-face, obesity, abdominal striae, and thin arms and legs (from *Samson Wright's Applied Physiology;* Courtesy Dr. J. D. N. Nabarro).

Treatment The pituitary gland is irradiated or surgical removal of an adrenal tumour is performed. If the condition is due to enlargement of both glands, bilateral adrenalectomy is performed, and to offset the absence of adrenal secretion the patient has to take cortisone by mouth for the rest of his life.

ALDOSTERONISM In this condition a tumour of the adrenal cortex secretes excessive amounts of aldosterone. An excessive secretion of this hormone can also occur in cirrhosis of the liver with ascites, in nephrosis, in stenosis of the renal artery and in congestive heart failure. Excessive amounts of potassium are excreted by the kidneys and the blood-potassium level falls. The patient complains of weakness, of passing excessive amounts of urine and of thirst. Hypertension can occur.

Treatment is by removal of the adrenal tumour or by treating any other cause.

PHAEOCHROMOCYTOMA This is a rare tumour of the adrenal medulla. There is an excessive secretion of adrenaline and nor-adrenaline. The patient develops hypertension and has attacks of anxiety, tremor, weakness, dizziness, sweating and headache.

Treatment is by removal of the tumour.

The Testes

The testes can fail to grow to adult size, fail to produce sperm or to produce an adequate number, and fail to produce testosterone, the testicular hormone.

Failure of the testis to develop can be due to congenital malformation, to a chromosome abnormality, to a failure of the testes to descend, to injury or to infection. It can be due to a failure of the pituitary gland, which from its anterior lobe produces the hormone that stimulates testicular development.

Eunuchoidism is due to a failure of testicular development occurring before puberty. The boy grows tall and lanky, under the influence of the growth hormones. The external genitalia remain small and the secondary sexual characteristics do not develop. As the larynx keeps its infantile shape, the voice does not 'break' and remains high-pitched.

If testicular failure develops after puberty, the external genitalia become small and the patient complains of fatigue, loss of sexual desire and lack of initiative.

A *male climacteric* has been described occurring over the age of 60. It is due to testicular failure in later life; the patient becomes tired and anxious, lacks sexual desire and becomes impotent; he may develop muscular wasting.

Treatment

Testosterone preparations are given by intramuscular injection. When this has been found to be effective, testosterone can be given in subcataneous pellets; such pellets are effective for 6-8 months and can then be repeated. A failure of the testis to descend should be remedied surgically, if possible before puberty.

The Ovaries

The ovaries, acting under the influence of hormones from the pituitary gland, secrete oestrogens from the cells of the graafian follicles and oestrogens and progesterone from the cells of the corpus luteum.

A failure of oestrogen production can be the result of a chromosome abnormality or of infection, or injury of the ovaries or destruction of them by a new growth. When this happens before puberty the secondary sexual characteristics do not develop. The uterus, vagina and breast do not develop; menstruation does not occur; the pubic and axillary hair grows sparsely or not at all; epiphyses do not fuse and X-rays reveal a retarded bone-age.

A failure of *progesterone production* produces a failure of the luteal phase of the menstrual cycle (from ovulation to the onset of menstruation). The patient is likely to have menorrhagia or frequent periods.

Virilization — a shift towards male characteristics — can be produced by excessive secretion of androgens from the adrenals or rarely by an ovarian tumour.

Menstruation is in many women associated with emotional cyclical changes, which are likely to be the result of hormonal changes. *Premenstrual tension* occurs regularly in some women, who for a few days before the onset of menstruation experience a build-up of tension, anxiety, irritability, feelings of frustration and discontent; the whole syndrome vanishes when menstruation begins.

Pregnancy — in spite of the emotional problems it arouses, in spite of its hazards, in spite of its metabolic disturbances — does not often precipitate an illness. Women who accept the female role feel particularly happy, and some neurotics and psychosomatics are actually improved by becoming pregnant. Some women, however, become irritable, tense and emotionally unstable, some develop peculiar appetites.

The *menopause*, the cessation of menstruation at 40-55 years, is rarely a cause of severe illness. With the cessation of the production of oestrogens and progesterone, some women experience irritability, nervousness, 'hot flushes' and tremor. Other conditions that might be precipitated are an excessive hair growth on the face, obesity, arthritis, pruritus vulvae and atrophic vaginitis[7]. The menopause itself is rarely a cause of mental illness. Although it is customary to attribute to the 'change of life' any mental disorder occurring in a woman over 40, other factors are usually found to be responsible.

[7] *vaginitis:* degeneration or inflammation of the vagina

11   The Inheritance of Disease

Inherited diseases are the result of abnormalities of genes.

An individual being the result of the fusion of ovum with sperm, all that he inherits are in these cells. The genes are the elements that decide inheritance. They are arranged along the chromosomes, structures within the nucleus of each cell; and there are thought to be about 100,000 genes on each chromosome.

In man the chromosomes number 46 :

44 non-sex chromosomes (also called autosomes)

2 sex-chromosomes.

The 44 non-sex chromosomes are identical in males and females.

In females the 2 sex-chromosomes are the same and are called XX.

In males there is 1 X chromosome (identical with that in females) and 1 Y chromosome, a very much smaller one.

Thus, in every non-sex (somatic) cell in a female there are 44 somatic and 2 X chromosomes and in every male non-sex cell there are 44 somatic, 1 X and 1 Y chromosome. The sex-cells in both, because of problems of division, are different in some stages.

There are thus about 4,600,000 genes on the chromosomes of each cell. Each gene is believed to be responsible for one enzyme-reaction in the body (an enzyme-reaction is a reaction that makes a change in chemical composition), and by controlling all the enzyme reactions, the genes control all the chemical changes in the body.

Genes can be faulty; there can be too many of them or too few of them. They can also be affected by 'environment', i.e. by anything that affects them from outside, e.g. radiation; but here we are concerned only with the inevitable changes that arise from genes unaffected by any environmental change.

If a gene is faulty, the enzyme-reaction for which it is responsible does not take place. This results in:

(a) a build-up of chemical substances at the chemical level just before the reaction for which the gene is responsible;

(b) the chemical substances along the line after the block do not develop.

It is by these chemical changes that faulty genes are identified.

Very many chemical reactions in the body can be affected, and many disorders produced. Among these are:

phenylketonuria

renal glycosuria
hepato-lenticular degeneration
haemophilia
Christmas disease

Chromosome abnormalities

Chromosome abnormalities can be detected by examining chromosomes under the microscope. Cells from parts of the body (usually the blood and the skin) are cultured (i.e. grown) under special conditions in the laboratory and are stopped in the act of dividing into two. Each chromosome as it divides splits from each end; the

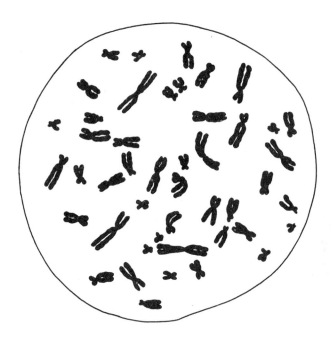

Fig. 62. Normal human chromosomes as they appear in the nucleus of a cell. Each chromosome is in the act of dividing into two; the point at which they have not yet divided is the centromere.

centromere is the spot, somewhere along its length, which is the last place to split. Chromosomes come in different sizes; and by their size and the position of the centromere, they are sorted into pairs and numbered 1-22; the X and Y chromosomes can also be identified. In the nucleus of the cell, the chromosomes are jumbled up; but for examination, they are photographed, enlarged, cut out of the photograph and arranged in pairs. It is then possible to see any gross abnormalities.

Chromosome abnormalities arise during cell division. In somatic cells, each chromosome divides into 2; each nucleus divides into 2; and each cell divides into 2. As a result of these changes each cell has the right number of chromosomes (46 for man).

In the sex cells the division is different at one stage, because each ovum and each sperm has to finish up with 23 (not 46) chromosomes; so that when sperm meets ovum the right number of 46 is produced by their union. Special abnormalities can occur as a result of this special kind of division.

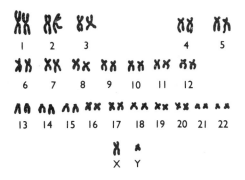

Fig. 63. The chromosomes in this figure have been placed in pairs, decided by length and position of centromere. The chromosomes X and Y are the sex chromosomes and their presence shows this is from a male. In a female there are two X chromosomes and no Y.

About 1 in 40 conceptions results in a chromosome abnormality. Some of these are so severe in their effects that the foetus cannot live and an abortion occurs. About 1 in 200 live births is a baby with a chromosome abnormality.

The abnormalities that can occur include:

(a) too many chromosomes,

(b) part of a chromosome has become lost in the processes of division,

(c) part of a chromosome is *translocated*, i.e. becomes attached to another chromosome.

(d) *mosaicism* is present, i.e. not all the cells are abnormal or show the same abnormality, some can be normal.

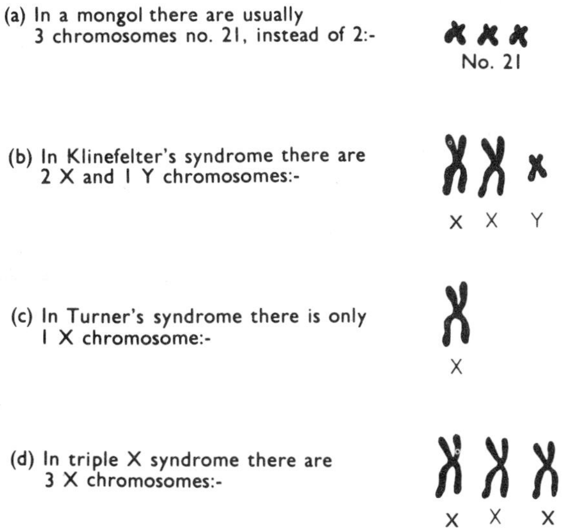

(a) In a mongol there are usually 3 chromosomes no. 21, instead of 2:-

No. 21

(b) In Klinefelter's syndrome there are 2 X and 1 Y chromosomes:-

X   X   Y

(c) In Turner's syndrome there is only 1 X chromosome:-

X

Fig. 64. Some chromosome abnormalities.

(d) In triple X syndrome there are 3 X chromosomes:-

X   X   X

Among the conditions that can result are:

1. *Mongolism.* All or some of the cells in this condition have 47 chromosomes, there being usually 3 chromosomes No. 21; translocation and mosaicism can occur.

2. *Klinefelter's syndrome.* In this condition (which can occur only in males) each cell has 2 X chromosomes and 1 Y chromosome. Affected men are thin, with poor

         The Inheritance of Disease

sexual development, small testes, infertility and female-breast development.

3. *Turner's syndrome.* In this condition (which can occur only in females) there is only 1 X chromosome instead of 2. Affected women are short, have a webbing of the skin extending from the neck onto the shoulders, and have a failure of development of the ovaries.

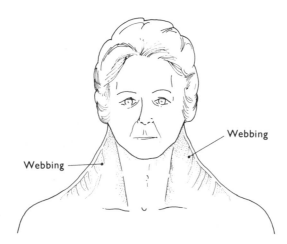

Webbing

Webbing

Fig. 65. Webbing of the neck in Turner's syndrome.

4. *Triple X (Super-female) Syndrome.* Affected females have 3 X chromosomes instead of 2. They are usually of normal physical appearance, but can be mentally retarded.

5. *Cancer cells and leucocytes in leukaemia.* These cells frequently show chromosome abnormalities not present in the healthy cells of the same body.

Inheritance

The inheritance of characteristics, good and bad, is decided on mendelian principles (named after Mendel, the monk who worked them out). Inheritance can be by:

(a) dominant genes.

(b) recessive genes,

(c) sex-linked genes.

(a) Dominant genes

If the chromosome of either parent contains a dominant gene which causes a disease and the chromosomes of the other do not (this is the usual situation), the abnormal gene is transmitted to one-half of their children, who will develop the disease and in their time will be capable of transmitting it to half their children. The other children are normal and do not pass on the abnormal gene. If the parents have only one child, it has a fifty-fifty chance of inheriting the abnormal gene.

Diseases produced by dominant genes include:

achrondroplasia

Huntington's chorea

dystrophia myotonica

facio-scapulo-humeral muscular
   dystrophy

peroneal muscular dystrophy

208

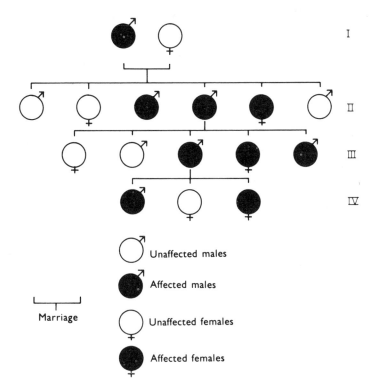

Fig. 66. Pedigree of a typical dominant transmission in four generations (e.g. Huntington's chorea).

◯ Unaffected males

⬤ Affected males

◯ Unaffected females

⬤ Affected females

└─┬─┘ Marriage

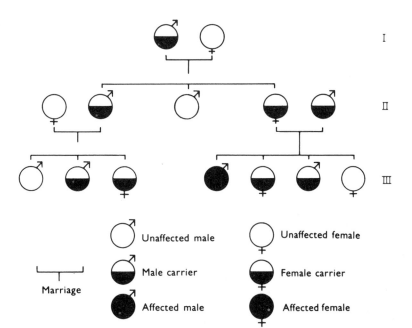

Fig. 67. Pedigree of a typical recessive transmission. The disease appears in the third (III) generation when a female carrier has children by a male carrier (e.g. Phenylketonuria).

◯ Unaffected male   ◯ Unaffected female

◑ Male carrier   ◑ Female carrier

⬤ Affected male   ⬤ Affected female

└─┬─┘ Marriage

The Inheritance of Disease

(b) Recessive genes   These are genes which must be present in the abnormal form in each parent to cause disease in an individual. If only one parent carries a recessive gene, a child will not show the disease but will inherit the actual faulty gene and transmit it to his/her children. If both parents have the same faulty recessive gene, there is a 1 in 4 chance of any of their children developing the disease; this is likely to happen in cousin-marriages.

Diseases produced by recessive genes include:
phenylketonuria
hepato-lenticular degeneration
sickle-cell anaemia
thalassaemia

(c) Sex-linked genes   A number of diseases are the result of a gene that is present on a X chromosome. Sex-linked inherited diseases include:
haemophilia
pseudo-hypertrophic muscular dystrophy

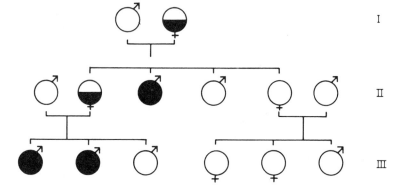

Fig. 68. Pedigree of a typical sex-linked transmission in which half the females transmit the disease and the males develop it (e.g. haemophilia).

12   Auto-immune Diseases; Collagen Diseases

An *auto-immune* disease is one that is believed to be due to the action of certain anti-bodies (called auto-antibodies) against normal components of the same body — a kind of civil war of cells.

Normally, an *immune reaction* in the body is produced as a result of the invasion of the body by micro-organisms (bacteria, viruses, etc.) or the introduction into it of 'foreign' cells from another body (a tissue or organ-graft, an incompatible blood-transfusion). The purpose of an immune-reaction is the defence of the body against infection by micro-organisms or invasion by foreign cells. The body can recognize 'foreign' material introduced into it as not 'belonging' and tries to destroy it. It can recognize micro-organisms and cells introduced into it both from different species or from different individuals of the same species (identical twins are exceptions because basically they, coming from the same cells, are identical in their antigens).

The lympho-reticular system (which includes all reticular cells, lymphocytes and plasma cells, in the spleen, thymus, lymph-nodes, and other lymph-tissue throughout the body) is the system responsible for setting off the immune reaction.

This can be shown diagrammatically:

Micro-organisms ⎫ ⟶ lympho-reticular ⎫ ⟶ Immune
Foreign cells ⎭   system ⎭   reaction.

The immune reaction is a result of various reactions. *Antigens* are substances in the micro-organisms and foreign cells that stimulate the production of *antibodies* in the lympho-reticular cells, as a result of which various changes take place in cells in various tissues and organs.

This can be shown diagrammatically:

Antigens ⟶ antibodies ⟶ immune reaction

This is how normal immunization is established in a body with an attack of an infection or by a course of immunization or vaccination.

Normally, cells in the body tolerate the existence of the other cells — dog does not eat dog; this phenomenon is thought to be due to a build-up of 'immunological tolerance' in early fetal life for antigens experienced at that time do not produce an antibody response.

However, in certain circumstances, cells can be attacked by auto-anti-bodies, the products of cells of the same body — dog here eats dog — and disease results. The following appear to be auto-immune diseases:

haemolytic anaemia

systemic lupus erythematosus and other collagen diseases

rheumatoid arthritis   Sjögren's disease

myasthenia gravis   Hashimoto's disease

ulcerative colitis   pernicious anaemia

sympathetic ophthalmia[8]

    Among other diseases in which auto-immunity is possibly involved are:

diabetes mellitus   disseminated sclerosis

pemphigus   acute peripheral neuritis

    Certain features in common suggest that diseases are auto-immune diseases:

1. An increased serum gamma-globulin (anti-bodies are gamma-globulins); the presence of auto-anti-bodies in the serum.

2. Evidence in a family of the inheritance of one or more auto-immune diseases.

3. The tissues show a similar reaction — the invasion of them by lymphocytes, plasma cells and histiocytes[9].

4. An enlarged thymus gland or a tumour of the thymous gland.

5. Cortico-steroid and cytotoxic[1] drugs produce improvement.

6. Similar auto-immune diseases in animals.

    The mechanisms by which self-recognition fails and these diseases develop are very complicated and not definitely established. The possibilities can be summarized thus:

(a) There has not been in early life the usual build-up of 'immunological tolerance' to a particular antigen.

When that antigen escapes later in life into the circulation, an anti-body is produced in large amounts and causes disease.

(b) Cells can become changed by drugs, irradiation or infection in such a way that they become 'foreign' and are therefore attacked.

(c) Anti-body forming cells may become altered and having thus been altered in this way cannot recognize as 'normal' the tissues in which they are living.

(d) There is a complete break-down of the system of cellular recognition from other causes.

The Collagen Diseases

Collagen diseases are diseases in which inflammatory and degenerative changes of a particular type occur in connective tissue. The causes are unknown; it is thought that they might be *auto-immune diseases* — diseases in which anti-bodies that can destroy connective tissue are produced in the body. In these diseases the fibres of connective tissue show a particular kind of degeneration called fibrinoid necrosis.

    The various collagen diseases have much in common: patients have a temperature, they complain of joint pains and swellings, the ESR is raised, the white cell count of the blood is low or normal, some response to treatment by cortisone is to be

[8] *sympathetic ophthalmia:* inflammation in one eye 2-6 weeks after injury to the other

[9] *histiocytes:* a form of tissue cell

[1] *cytotoxic:* cell-destroying

expected, for most of them (rheumatic fever is the chief exception) the outlook for recovery is poor.

The diseases generally considered to be collagen diseases are:

rheumatic fever   rheumatoid arthritis
systemic lupus erythematosus
polyarteritis nodosa
dermato-myositis   scleroderma

SYSTEMIC LUPUS ERYTHEMATOSUS

Systemic lupus erythematosus (SLE) is a collagen disease most common in women aged 20-50. It can run a benign course for years, with sometimes stationary periods but at any time it can become much worse and kill the patient within a couple of years.

Clinical features

The patient feels ill and complains of joint pains and swellings. He has a raised temperature, a raised ESR and a low or normal white blood cell count.

Lupus erythematosus, which gives its name to the disease, is a rash which appear on the face. It is reddish, hard and raised, and it has a 'butterfly distribution' on the nose and cheeks.

The patient may develop disease in many organs and tissues:
(a) kidneys: degeneration, excretion of proteins in the urine, the nephrotic syndrome, hypertension and uraemia.
(b) lungs: pleurisy and pneumonia.
(c) heart: pericarditis, endocarditis and myocarditis, congestive heart failure.
(d) liver: hepatitis, acute or chronic, liver failure.
(e) blood: iron-deficiency anaemia, haemolytic anaemia,
(f) nervous system: peripheral neuropathy, fits, headache, tremor, mental disorder.
(g) hair: generalized or patchy baldness.

Treatment

The patient is treated with bed-rest, analgesics for arthritis and pain, and with appropriate treatment for any of the conditions that may occur. Chloroquine (an anti-malaria drug) sometimes produces improvement. Prednisolone (a corticosteroid) relieves symptoms and may prolong life.

POLYARTERITIS NODOSA

This collagen disease affects connective tissue in small arteries in all parts of the body. The walls of the arteries degenerate and become weak, and blood is likely to clot in them. The disease usually occurs without any obvious reason, but it has occasionally followed a hyper-sensitivity reaction to a drug. It can occur at any age. It is very serious and 9 out of 10 patients die within 5 years.

Clinical features

The patient feels ill and complains of joint pains and swellings. He has a raised temperature and ESR, but instead of the usual low or normal white blood cell count he may have an increase in the number of eosinophils, sometimes to an extreme degree (normal: 150-300 per mm^3).

A variable number of other conditions occur, according to the particular tissues and organs involved:

(a) lungs: patches of inflammation, going on to abscess formation.

(b) kidneys: renal disease, excretion of proteins, uraemia, hypertension.

(c) alimentary tract: ulceration, colitis,[2] enlargement of liver.

(d) heart: coronary artery disease.

(e) nervous system; peripheral neuritis; fits and other signs of cerebral artery disease.

Treatment   As for systematic lupus erythematosus.

DERMATOMYOSITIS

In this collagen disease the patient develops:

(a) skin rashes of various kinds, usually an erythematous[3] macular[4] rash,

(b) muscular pain, tenderness, degeneration, fibrosis[5],

(c) myocarditis[6], which can be the cause of death.

Usually cortico-steroid treatment is given; but the outlook is poor and patients die of a pulmonary or cardiac complication or sometimes of pre-existing malignant disease.

SCLERODERMA

This collagen disease sometimes appears as a development from dermatomyositis. The patient's skin becomes hard. Sometimes the hardness is only patchy and does not cause complications; but it can occur in a generalized form, beginning in the hands and spreading. Hard and thick at first, the skin wastes later. The fibrosis immobilizes the limbs, and bones and joints degenerate. In one form of the disease, the fibrosis affects internal organs – the heart, kidneys and alimentary tract – and the patient dies of renal failure or heart disease.

Treatment   Steroids are given, but may not check the course of the diseases. Splints are used to try to prevent contractures.

[2] *colitis:* inflammation of the colon

[3] *erythematous:* red

[4] *macular:* spotty

[5] *fibrosis:* abnormal amount of fibrous tissue

[6] *myocarditis:* inflammation of the myocardium

13   Diseases of the Nervous System

The nervous system can suffer the same kinds of illness as other parts of the body. There are many diseases of the nervous system: some, such as vascular conditions, disseminated sclerosis, dementia, are common; others are uncommon and some very rare. The causes of many are unknown.

Diseases of the nervous system can affect the brain, the spinal cord or the cranial and spinal nerves.

Diseases of the brain are likely to lead to a disorder of cerebral functioning, of speech, of movement, or sensation, of co-ordination, of sight, hearing, depending upon the part of the brain affected, the progress of the condition, the type of condition and its effects on other parts of the brain not directly affected by the original disease-process. The functions of certain parts of the brain are known. The motor area of the brain, in which muscle movements are to some extent initiated, is situated in the precentral gyrus of the frontal lobe of the brain; in this region the head is represented in a large part at the lower end; above this the hand is represented; other parts are represented in smaller areas above these. Disease of this gyrus will produce paralysis of appropriate muscle-groups on the opposite side of the body (opposite because in their course in the brain-stem and spinal cord the nerve-fibres cross to the opposite side). Sensation is represented in a similar upside-down manner in the post-central gyrus of the parietal lobe; disease in these areas will cause disorders of sensation on the opposite side of the body. Vision is represented in the occipital lobe and hearing in the temporal lobe. Speech is controlled on the left side of the brain (in parts of the frontal, parietal and temporal lobes) in all right handed people and in most left-handed.

Disease of the so-called 'silent' areas of the brain (i.e. those to which no specific function can be ascribed) are likely to cause disorders of thought, memory, the organization of ideas.

Other parts of the brain have functions which are likely to be upset if they are affected by disease, e.g. disease of the thalamus will cause emotional disturbances and painful sensations; disease of the cerebellum will cause inco-ordinated movements; disease of the hypothalamus will cause disorder of the pituitary gland with which it is closely associated both anatomically and functionally; disease of the brain-stem (pons, medulla oblongata) causes paralysis of various cranial nerves.

Disease of the brain can begin by promoting 'excitatory phenomena', e.g. muscle twitching, epilepsy, abnormal sensation, as a result of the stimulation of groups of nerve-cells. This evidence of irritation may with further progression of the disease be followed by a failure of function — by paralysis and anaesthesia.

Disease of some parts of the brain and of the spinal cord is likely to produce at first irritation and then paralysis of the various tracts of nerve-fibres which pass from brain to spinal cord and vice-versa. If the sensory fibres are affected, abnormal sensation will be followed by anaesthesia of the part affected. If the motor-fibres are affected, the patient will develop an 'upper motor neurone lesion', in which muscles are paralysed but do not become wasted and the tendon-reflexes (e.g. the knee jerk) are exaggerated.

Disease of the cranial or spinal nerves is likely to produce (a) sensory changes, abnormal sensations going on to anaesthesia, and (b) a 'lower motor neurone lesion' in which muscles are paralysed and waste and tendon-reflexes are absent because all connection with the spinal cord is lost.

Vascular Diseases of the Brain

The brain requires a constant and adequate supply of blood. It needs as much blood as the heart. If it does not get this blood-supply mental and physical signs appear of faulty cerebral functioning. If the blood-supply quickly becomes normal, these signs disappear, but if the blood is cut off for more than a few minutes brain cells die.

The blood-supply to the brain is through the two internal carotid arteries and the two vertebral arteries. In the circle of Willis at the base of the brain several communicating arteries connect these four arteries, so that interruption of the supply through any one artery can to some extent be compensated for through the others, but the circle is variable in its connection and in its ability to compensate for the interruption of the blood through any one of its connections.

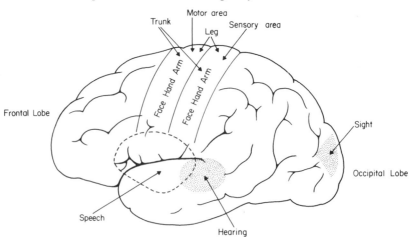

Fig. 69. Functional areas of the cerebral cortex on the left side. The speech centre is on the left side in right-handed people and most left-handed people.

Branches of the internal carotid arteries supply (a) the frontal lobe, the anterior part of the parietal lobe, and much of the temporal lobe, and (b) the white matter within these areas and the basal ganglia. The vertebral arteries and basilar artery (the latter formed by the union of the two vertebrals) supply (a) the medulla oblongata, pons, cerebellum and much of the occipital lobe. The veins of the brain drain into the superior longitudinal sinus and the cavernous sinuses and into the lateral sinus on each side with its continuation the sigmoid sinus, which is continuous with the internal jugular vein.

The type of disturbance caused by interruption of the blood-supply to the brain will depend on (a) the suddenness, (b) the extent, (c) the arteries involved, and (d) the time during which the interference lasts.

The features seen are:

(a) fainting, giddiness, confusion, forgetfulness, insomnia, nausea, vomiting

(b) fits, unconsciousness, coma

(c) paralysis, sensory disturbances, extreme giddiness, blindness.

A temporary interference will cause transient disturbance; the longer the interference lasts the more likely are the symptoms and signs to be severe, lasting or fatal.

Common causes are:

1. Athero-sclerosis of the cerebral arteries.
2. Cerebral thrombosis, embolism and haemorrhage.
3. Venous sinus thrombosis.
4. A failure of the heart to pump adequate amounts of blood to the brain; a sudden fall in blood-pressure; sudden loss of blood; severe anaemia.

DISEASE OF THE INTERNAL CAROTID ARTERY

Athero-sclerosis of this artery (which supplies the frontal lobe and parts of the parietal and temporal lobes) is likely to cause:

(a) at first brief disturbances of cerebral function, with confusion, dysphasia[7], blindness on the same side and paralysis on the opposite side of the body;

(b) subsequently as the damage to the brain becomes permanent, there is likely to be further confusion, dementia and hemiplegia[8].

Special tests

Carotid arteriography: to reveal evidence of obstruction in the artery.

Thermography: finding a cold area on one side of the forehead is a sign of internal carotid artery block on the same side.

DISEASE OF THE VERTEBRAL-BASILAR ARTERIES

Athero-sclerosis of these arteries (which supply the medulla oblongata, pons, cerebellum, midbrain and occipital lobe of the cerebrum) is likely to cause:

(a) giddiness, dysarthria[9], and ataxia by involving the cerebellum;

(b) disturbance of eyesight and blindness by involvement of the occipital lobe;

(c) hemiparesis[1] by involvement of the cortico-spinal (pyramidal) tracts.

Dysfunction of these parts is likely to deteriorate into permanent changes.

Drop-attacks are due to kinking of the vertebral arteries and sudden loss of posture-sense. The patient drops to the ground without warning and without loss of consciousness, cannot rise unaided, but can pull himself up using furniture.

[7] *dysphasia:* impairment of speech due to brain disease
[8] *hemiplegia:* paralysis of one side of the body
[9] *dysarthria:* impairment of articulation
[1] *hemiparesis:* partial paralysis of one side of the body

Diseases of the Nervous System

Once up he can stand and get about. A patient with drop-attacks should not wear tight collars and should avoid making sudden movements of the head.

Special test   *Vertebral arteriography:* to reveal narrowing or blocking of the vertebral arteries.

CEREBRAL EMBOLISM

A cerebral embolism is the blocking of a cerebral artery by an embolus[2]. Commoner causes are:

(a) a detached part of a clot that has formed inside the heart following a coronary thrombosis;[3]
(b) a piece off an atheromatous patch on the aorta or other diseased artery;
(c) a piece of vegetation from a heart valve in rheumatic endocarditis or subacute bacterial endocarditis;
(d) a septic embolus from pulmonary suppuration.

When an embolus becomes stuck in an artery, it blocks the blood-supply to the part of the brain supplied by that artery. The onset is sudden. The features vary with the particular artery and part of the brain involved. The features are similar to those of a very rapid thrombosis. The embolus may in time shrink and allow some blood to get through, or it may lead to thrombosis and a worsening of the patient's condition.

VENOUS SINUS THROMBOSIS

The blood in the venous sinuses inside the skull can become thrombosed as a result of:

(a) general malnutrition in feeble ill-nourished children and in adults seriously ill with a wasting disease, such as cancer;
(b) after childbirth, when an infected clot of blood finds its way from the pelvic veins to the sinuses via the vertebral veins;
(c) infection from middle ear disease, nasal sinus infection, osteo-myelitis of the skull or erysipelas of the scalp.

The general features of thrombosis are an irregular pyrexia, rapid pulse, sweating, rigors, vomiting, headache, meningeal irritation, confusion, and coma leading to death. Other features vary with the particular sinus thrombosed:

Superior longitudinal sinus: fits, hemiplegia, epistaxis.
Cavernous sinus: protrusion of eyes, swelling of eyelids, pain at back of eye, papilloedema,[4] retinal haemorrhages.
Lateral sinus: papilloedema.
Sigmoid sinus: pain, tenderness and swelling over mastoid process; thrombosis extending into internal jugular veins palpable as a cord in the neck.

Treatment   Full doses of penicillin, other antibiotics or sulpha drugs are given. The thrombus is removed surgically.

[2] *embolus:* any abnormal matter that can get stuck in a blood-vessel and block it
[3] *thrombosis:* clotting of blood within the heart or a blood-vessel
[4] *papilloedema:* oedematous swelling of the optic disc, the eminence where the optic nerve fibres appear inside the eye

Complications	Abscesses in adjacent parts of the brain. 'Otitic[5] hydrocephalus' following middle ear disease and faulty reabsorption of cerebro-spinal fluid.
INTRACEREBRAL HAEMORRHAGE	This is usually a disease of the old and a common cause of death. It can occur spontaneously or be caused by sudden exertion. Hypertension and atheroma of the cerebral arteries are contributory factors. The usual site is the centre of a cerebral hemisphere as the result of a rupture of one of the perforating arteries to the interior of the brain. The resulting haemorrhage forces a way into the white matter and basal ganglia, destroying and compressing them, and into the lateral and third ventricles. Occasionally it results from the rupture of a berry aneurysm which happens to be embedded in brain tissue.
Clinical features	The patient may have had a preliminary warning of cerebral arterial disease in the form of headache, giddiness, fainting attacks, peculiar sensations, or may have had a previous attack of cerebral thrombosis. The onset is sudden with severe headache and giddiness, and then a rapid loss of consciousness which deepens into coma. The patient lies breathing stertorously and has a slow pulse, profuse sweating and a flushed face; he may be incontinent of urine and faeces. One side is usually completely paralysed; its limbs are flaccid, the tendon reflexes are absent; and if the two arms are held up and allowed to fall the paralysed arm falls immediately because it is completely devoid of tone. Haemorrhage into the pons causes hyper-pyrexia due to interference with the temperature regulating centre in the brain-stem. Deepening coma leads to death within a few hours or days. Should the patient survive, he is likely to be left with a permanent spastic paralysis and impaired mental faculties; disturbances of speech occur if the haemorrhage has been into the left cerebral hemisphere (in which the speech-centre is situated in all right- and most left-handed people).
Treatment	The patient is put to bed and requires the full nursing care given to an unconscious patient. Removal of the clot of blood is sometimes attempted — when it is fairly superficial, when coma is not very deep or when there are some signs of improvement. Frusemide, a diuretic drug, is used to relieve the associated cerebral oedema.
CEREBRAL ANEURYSMS	Cerebral aneurysms are small thin-walled projections from cerebral arteries. They can be: (a) *berry aneurysms:* small berry-like protrusions, occurring at the junction of two arteries on the circle of Willis or nearby parts of the internal carotid or basilar arteries. (b) *mycotic aneurysms[6]:* the result of the impaction in an artery of an infected embolus during an attack of infective endocarditis.

[5] *otitic:* arising from the ear
[6] *mycotic:* this word means infection by a fungus, but here it means any infection

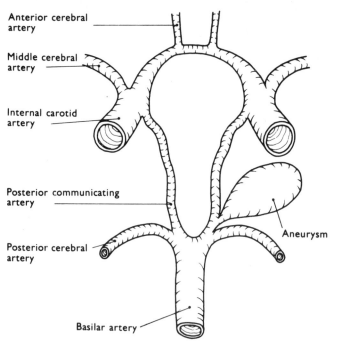

Anterior cerebral artery

Middle cerebral artery

Internal carotid artery

Posterior communicating artery

Posterior cerebral artery

Aneurysm

Basilar artery

Fig. 70. Diagram of the circle of Willis with a berry aneurysm at the junction of the posterior communicating and posterior cerebral arteries.

(c) *atheromatous aneurysms:* due to weakening of the arterial wall

(d) *syphilitic aneurysms:* which are rare.

Clinical features:

The commonest of these aneurysms is the berry aneurysm, which is a deformity often unsuspected until a haemorrhage from it produces an acute emergency and may kill an apparently healthy man or woman in early or mid-adult life.

Aneurysms can produce symptoms and signs:

1. by pressing on cranial nerves in the vicinity, the nerves most commonly affected being II, III, IV, V, and VI.

2. by bleeding into the subarachnoid space.

3. by bleeding into the brain and producing a cerebral haemorrhage. The bleeding may be a slight leak, producing headache, stiffness and pain in the back of the neck, or may be a massive and sometimes fatal haemorrhage.

Special tests

CSF: blood-stained.

Cerebral angiography: likely to reveal the presence, position and size of the aneurysm.

Treatment

Surgical treatment is the only hope for the patient and the only possible way of preventing a second haemorrhage. The patient is usually operated on under hypothermia. The surgeon tries to put a silver clip on the aneurysm or to tie it with thread, and if he cannot do that to put a clip on the main artery supplying it. If he cannot do any of these, he may try to surround the aneurysm with muscle or a rapidly-setting plastic.

SUBARACHNOID HAEMORRHAGE

Haemorrhage into the subarachnoid space around the brain can be due to:-

(a) rupture of a cerebral aneurysm,

220

(b) rupture of a malformation of blood-vessels.

(c) rupture of an atherosclerotic artery.

(d) head injury.

Clinical features The rupture of the aneurysm or vessel is sometimes preceded by small leaks, producing slight headache and stiffness and pain in the back of the neck. When a larger haemorrhage occurs, it produces:

(a) severe headache, running from the back of the head down into the neck and shoulders;

(b) vomiting;

(c) neck rigidity, Kernig's sign[7], signs of pressure on cranial nerves, papilloedema, extensor plantar responses, slow pulse, Cheyne-Stokes breathing[8], slight pyrexia.

(d) death in 30-35 per cent of patients within 3 days and 50 per cent within 6 weeks.

Complications Nearly half the patients who survive this kind of haemorrhage are likely to suffer permanent personality changes, usually apathy, depression, forgetfulness and irresponsibility. Some personalities have been improved, anxious, tense people becoming relaxed. Personality impairment is usually proportional to the amount of brain damage.

Special tests *CSF:* blood-stained and under increased pressure. Xanthocromia (yellow CSF) develops in 6 hours and can persist for 3 weeks.

Cerebral angiography: to reveal the state of the cerebral arteries and to demonstrate an aneurysm.

Treatment The cause is treated surgically if possible. Patients who are seen a few weeks after the haemorrhage and have fully recovered do not require angiography or surgery as the risks of conservative treatment and of surgical treatment are about equal.

Cerebral Tumours

Cerebral tumours are either (a) metastases from tumours that have started elsewhere in the body, especially in the lungs and the stomach, of (b) primary tumours starting in the brain.

Primary tumours are of various kinds, dependent upon the kind of cell that they start in. Some are benign, some malignant. They are classified into:

1. *Meningioma:* believed to start from arachnoid granulations on the surface of the brain; most are non-malignant, hard and smooth, press down into the brain and sometimes erode the skull.

2. *Neurofibroma:* non-malignant, arising from the sheaths of a nerve, especially the eighth (auditory) nerve.

[7] *Kernig's sign:* resistance or pain produced by attempting to extend the leg completely at the knee with the thigh flexed to a right angle

[8] *Cheyne-Stokes breathing:* periods of deep breathing alternating with periods of suspension of breathing

3. *Glioma:* these can be of various kinds, depending on the cell they arise in; they all are malignant, invading brain tissue, but unlike malignant cells in other parts of the body they do not form metastases[9]. Among them are *astrocytomas,* which are of variable malignancy; *ependymomas,* which grow from the linings of the ventricles; *medulloblastomas,* which are malignant and liable to occur in children and start in the region of the fourth ventricle in the hindbrain; *oligodendrogliomas,* which are uncommon.

4. *Pituitary gland tumours:* which cause the clinical features of a space occupying lesion as well as those of pituitary gland dysfunction.

Clinical features

The clinical features of a tumour are:
1. those caused by an increase of intracranial pressure or stretching of pain sensitive tissues inside the skull (large arteries, venous sinuses, sensory nerves).
2. localizing signs which indicate the site of the tumour.

Pressure and stretching features

Headache: is due to stretching the pain-sensitive tissues; it varies from time to time, is not usually throbbing, is at first improved by rest, is made worse by coughing and straining, tends to get worse and more persistent.

Nausea and vomiting: as pressure increases vomiting can occur without nausea.

Mental changes: apathy, loss of memory, forgetfulness, lack of attention, intellectual deterioration.

Sleep: drowsiness, excessive sleep.

Vertigo.

Epilepsy: major or minor or other kind of fit.

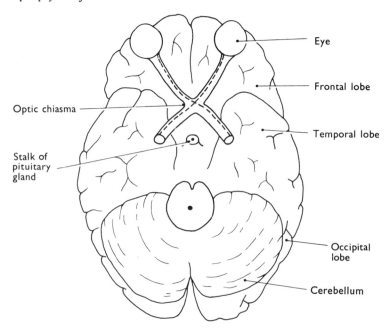

Fig. 71. Inferior surface of the brain to show the proximity of the stalk of the pituitary gland to the optic chiasma.

[9] *metastasis:* a secondary deposit of a tumour in another part of the body

Pulse: slow

Optic disc: papilloedema, due to obstruction of the veins draining the eye.

Localizing signs These vary with the position and size of the tumour and are an indication of destruction or pressure on a particular part of the brain or an interference with its blood-supply. The term 'false localizing sign' is given to a sign produced by pressure and one which does not indicate the position of the tumour.

Papilloedema: can be produced by a tumour in the posterior fossa of the skull — in the region of the third ventricle, the aqueduct, the 4th ventricle and the foramina leading out of it; papilloedema is in these conditions produced by obstruction to the circulation of the cerebro-spinal fluid.

Deafness, facial weakness and ataxia[1] : can be produced by a tumour of the eighth (acoustic) nerve involving the seventh cranial nerve which is next to it.

Visual field defects: can be produced by pressure on the optic chiasma by pituitary tumours, meningiomas, and other tumours arising in that neighbourhood.

Anosmia (loss of smell): produced by pressure on the olfactory tracts.

Special tests 1. *X-ray of skull* to show:- (a) any erosion of the posterior clinoid processes, (b) any expansion of the pituitary fossa, due to a pituitary tumour (c) any erosion of the skull due to a meningioma, (d) any abnormal calcification, as in a slowly growing meningioma, (e) any shift sideways or downwards of a calcified pineal gland due to pressure from a tumour.

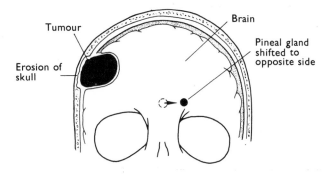

Fig. 72. A cerebral tumour that has (a) eroded the skull and (b) displaced the pineal gland to the opposite side.

2. *X-ray of chest:* for evidence of a cancer of the lung.

3. *Electro-encephalogram:* Tumours may cause abnormal electrical discharges, which are recorded on an EEG.

4. *Cerebral angiography:* a radio-opaque substance is injected into the carotid or vertebral artery to reveal abnormal vascular patterns in the brain, e.g. a cerebral angioma.

5. *Air-encephalography or ventriculography:* The CSF is withdrawn and air introduced into either the subarachnoid space via a lumbar puncture or directly into the ventricles, the skull having been trephined, and X-ray photographs taken. Tumours are likely to cause malformation of the ventricles.

6. *Brain-scanning:* a radio-active substance is injected intravenously, and is taken up and concentrated by tumours, abscesses and vascular lesions. Concentrations of isotopes are detected by a counter outside the skull, and a map is produced which show the concentration and definition of isotopes.

7. *Ultra-soundwaves:* passed through the skull and their bounce-back is recorded; tumours cause an abnormal bounce-back.

[1] *ataxia:* inco-ordination of muscular action, affecting the gait

223   *Diseases of the Nervous System*

Treatment The only hope for a patient with a cerebral tumour is that it can be removed surgically without leaving him with a gross disability. Meningiomas, tumours of the auditory nerve and pituitary tumours are the ones likely to be removable. Pituitary and some other tumours may be treated by deep X-rays, which can give some relief. To reduce intracranial pressure before operation, 150 ml of a 50 per cent solution of magnesium sulphate is given by rectum or 100 ml of sucrose intravenously, Frusemide, a diuretic drug, is given to relieve cerebral oedema.

Infections of the Nervous System
ENCEPHALITIS
MENINGITIS

The nervous system can be infected by (a) bacteria, (b) the *treponema pallida*, which causes syphilis, (c) viruses.

Some of these infections are dealt with elsewhere:
(a) meningococcal meningitis on p. 29.
(b) acute poliomyelitis, a virus infection, on p. 22.

Infections may be mainly meningeal or mainly encephalitic[2], depending on whether they infect mainly the meninges or mainly the brain; in many infections both are involved.

In meningitis[3], the meninges become inflamed, swollen and reddened. There is an effusion of fluid from them, and this fluid may turn into pus. The cerebrospinal fluid is under increased pressure, has an increase in the number of cells and amount of protein in it, shows a reduction in sugar in some, and may show the infecting organism. In encephalitis, there is degeneration and death of brain cells and sometimes the formation of an abscess. Meningitis is likely to cause some degree of encephalitis on the surface of the brain. If the meningitis is not cured during the acute phase, a chronic meningitis may develop, which can involve the cranial nerves and can cause hydrocephalus by blocking the escape-holes through which the CSF passes out of the 4th ventricle into the subarachnoid space.

TUBERCULOUS MENINGITIS

This occurs as a result of a spread from a tuberculous infection elsewhere in the body. It may be part of a *miliary tuberculosis,* in which tuberculosis is spread by the blood-stream to all parts of the body. It is a disease of early childhood, but can occur sometimes in later childhood and early adult life.

Clinical features The onset is slow. The child becomes fretful, peevish, disinclined to play and off his food. He develops a slight irregular temperature. The headache becomes worse; the child takes to his bed, may vomit and have a fit.

On examination he is likely to show neck rigidity, dilated pupils, Kernig's sign and diminished tendon reflexes. He becomes drowsy, confused, resents examination, and lies curled up on his side. If untreated he dies. Miliary tubercles on the retina are sometimes seen as little white spots on ophthalmoscopic examination. The death rate even with treatment is about 30 per cent. Treatment begun late may stop the infection, but the child survives with a badly damaged brain, with blindness, deafness and mental retardation.

[2] *encephalitis:* an infection of the brain
[3] *meningitis:* an infection of the meninges

Special test	*CSF:* under increased pressure: clear or opalescent; increased lymphocytes (to 500 per cu. mm; normal is less than 5); increased protein; decreased glucose and chlorides. Tubercle bacilli may be demonstrated by staining or culture.
Treatment	Combinations of anti-tuberculous drugs are given — streptomycin, isoniazide and PAS (para-amino-salicylic acid) and continued for 12-18 months.

VIRUS MENINGITIS

Infections by viruses include acute poliomyelitis and a number of other infections — mumps, herpes simplex, vaccinia, Coxsackie and ECHO infections.

Clinical features

Those of a meningeal infection — slight fever, headache, vomiting, cranial nerve paralysis, fits, drowsiness, confusion, stupor, coma. Most virus infections of this sort clear up completely.

Special test

CSF: clear or opalescent; increased pressure, increased lymphocytes (from a normal of below 5 to 1,000 per mm^3)

Treatment

There is no specific treatment. Full nursing care will be required until the infection has cleared up.

EPIDEMIC NEUROMYASTHENIA

Other names: Royal Free disease, poliomyelitis-like illness, benign myalgic encephalomyelitis
This is a disease of unknown origin (in spite of intensive investigations), which has occurred in several parts of the world. In Britain epidemics have occurred among the nurses at two London hospitals (Royal Free Hospital and the Hospital for Sick Children).

Clinical features

Clinical features are very varied. The illness usually begins with malaise, a sore throat, and a headache which becomes very severe. The temperature is not raised or raised slightly for a short time. Other symptoms vary considerably.

Common symptoms are:

headache	sore throat
nausea	vomiting
pain in back, neck, limbs, chest, abdomen	
depression	tiredness
giddiness	earache
sore eyes	photophobia
double vision	blurred vision
diarrhoea	bladder disturbance
loss of voice	loss of appetite

On examination the following are likely to be found:
pharyngeal inflammation
enlarged cervical lymph-nodes

neck stiffness

injected conjunctivae

usually no rash

usually no enlargement of the spleen.

The duration of the illness is likely to be 6-12 weeks. Relapses can occur more than once for no obvious reason. Lethargy and depression can continue for a long time, and some patients are not restored to full health for 12 months.

Special tests   Various tests can be performed; their chief value is in excluding other diseases.

Treatment   The patient should stay in bed until she feels well enough to be up. Treatment is otherwise symptomatic. The headache is not relieved by simple analgesics; pentazocine, dihydrocodeine and dextropropoxyphene may relieve it. The patient requires reassurance that she has not got poliomyelitis.

ABSCESS OF THE BRAIN   An abscess of the brain can be due to:

(a) spread of an acute suppurative infection from the middle ear, mastoid antrum, or an accessory nasal sinus;

(b) spread via the blood from an infection elsewhere, e.g. a suppurative chest infection;

(c) a fracture of the skull or an infected wound of the brain.

The abscess may occur in the white matter of the cerebrum or cerebellum. An acute abscess can spread rapidly and provoke a more general encephalitis or a purulent meningitis. Chronic abscesses become enclosed in fibrous tissue and produce the features of a space-occupying lesion of the brain.

Clinical features   Superimposed upon the original infection are:

(a) signs of suppuration: irregular fever, malaise, rigors;

(b) those of increased intra-cranial pressure: drowsiness, confusion, coma, slow pulse and respiration; papilloedema, paralysis of cranial nerves.

(c) localizing signs: *Frontal lobe:* sometimes hemiparesis on opposite side with upper motor neurone lesions (spastic paralysis, increased tendon reflexes, extensor plantar reflex); interference with speech if abscess is on left side of brain. *Temporal lobe:* word-deafness; weakness of lower half of face, interference with vision (due to pressure on some fibres of optic radiation). *Cerebellum:* giddiness, inco-ordination, ataxia, falling to same side as abscess.

Special tests   *CSF:* under increased pressure; slight increase in polymorphs, increase in protein; chloride and sugar normal.

Treatment   Treatment is by the antibiotic and sulpha drug to which the organism is sensitive, with surgical drainage and removal of the abscess.

MENINGO-VASCULAR SYPHILIS   This usually occurs as a "tertiary" or third stage manifestation of syphilis several years after the original infection, but it can occur as an acute illness complicating the primary infection (see p. 48). In the nervous system as elsewhere syphilis

226   *Chapter 13*

attacks the small arteries and causes inflammation of the tissues around the arteries, and can produce gummas, the particular syphilitic lesion with a gelatinous centre enclosed in fibrous tissue.

Clinical features   The usual symptoms and signs are headache, neck stiffness, and paralysis of cranial nerves. Involvement of the optic nerve produces visual defects; paralysis of III, IV and VI cranial nerves produces squint, double vision and ptosis[4]; paralysis of V nerve produces anaesthesia of the face and paralysis of the muscles of mastication; paralysis of VII nerve produces paralysis of the muscles of facial expression; paralysis of VIII nerve produces deafness and giddiness. Mental confusion, irritability, speech disturbances, fits and hemiplegia[5] can occur. A single gumma can mimic a cerebral tumour.

Syphilitic myelitis   This is a form of meningo-vascular syphilis in which the spinal cord is affected. It can occur: (a) in an acute form with a rapid development of paralysis, sensory loss and disturbance of the sphincters; or (b) in a chronic form with spastic paralysis of the legs (due to involvement of the cortico-spinal — i.e. pyramidal — tracts) and wasting of the small muscles of the hand (due to involvement of the spinal nerves in the cervical area, where the disease is most likely to occur).

Special tests   *Blood:* WR usually positive
CSF: pressure raised; cells and protein increased; WR positive.

Treatment   Penicillin is given intramuscularly in doses of 1 million units daily for 12-15 days. A response to treatment is usually obvious within 48-72 hours. Examination of the cell count and protein content of the CSF is a guide to progress. On recovery the patient may be left with some signs of permanent damage to the nervous system.

GENERAL PARALYSIS   *Other names:* general paralysis of the insane, G.P.I., general paresis
This chronic syphilitic infection of the brain and meninges usually occurs 10-15 years after the primary infection. It occurs in less than 5 per cent of people infected with syphilis. Spirochaetes are deposited in nervous tissue during the primary and secondary stages of syphilis, but remain dormant for years before becoming active. In general paralysis, they occur in large numbers in the brain, where they cause degeneration and death of brain cells and thickening of the meninges.

Clinical features   The onset may be slow over several months or rapid over a few days. In the first phase the patient shows evidence of dementia[6]: his personality deteriorates, he becomes irresponsible and acts foolishly. He may complain of vague ill-health

[4] *ptosis:* drooping of upper eyelid
[5] *hemiplegia:* paralysis of one side of the body
[6] *dementia:* deterioration of mental faculties, of memory, reasoning, etc.

Diseases of the Nervous System

or headache. He shows a tremor of fingers and tongue, has slurred speech, and may have a fit. His pupils may show the typical Argyll-Robertson abnormality (reacting to convergence, but not to light) and his tendon-reflexes may be brisk. From this early phase he degenerates into a later phase in which dementia is more pronounced, in which he may express delusions of grandeur (imagining he is extremely wealthy, powerful), or of misery and poverty and disease. He may have more fits. Speech is grossly disordered, writing a meaningless scrawl; walking, standing and balancing are increasingly difficult; a fit may leave him with a permanent paralysis of one side. If untreated he passes into a final phase in which all rational thought is lost; emaciation, physical weakness and total paralysis of the voluntary muscles render him helpless and bedridden, to die of status epilepticus[7] or a respiratory infection or bedsores.

Special tests   *Blood:* WR positive, occasionally negative.
CSF: increased cells, and protein; WR positive; gold curve show the paretic form – of the order of 5554321000.

Treatment   After a day of small doses to detect unusual and dangerous responses, penicillin is given daily in doses of 600,000-1 million units for 12-15 days. Subsequently injections of a long-acting penicillin are given twice a week for 2 months. There should be a rapid improvement; progress is checked by examination of the cells and protein of the CSF; and if there is any subsequent increase in them a further course of penicillin is given.

Early cases should be cured; late cases are likely to show some permanent evidence of damage to the brain.

Tabo-paresis is a combination of general paralysis and tabes dorsalis in the same patient. The disease shows features of both diseases and runs a relatively slow course.

Congenital general paresis can occur in congenital syphilis. It is rare. The patient develops in adolescence signs of progressive dementia with loss of memory, irresponsibility, signs of progressive damage to the brain. Treatment is by penicillin, but the outlook is poor.

TABES DORSALIS   *Other name:* locomotor ataxia
This is a chronic progressive syphilitic disease of the nervous system, in which there is degeneration of the sensory nerve roots and of the posterior columns of the spinal cord. It occurs in less than 5 per cent of patients with untreated or incompletely treated syphilis. It begins between 5 and 40 years after the primary infection.

Clinical features   Pain is experienced by almost all patients. The usual site is the leg, the patient often calling it rheumatic. It varies in intensity from slight to anguishing. 'Lightning pains' are pains which come on in attacks usually in the thigh, leg or foot, now in one place, now in another. 'Girdle pains', encircling the body, can occur. The limbs often feel heavy, weary and numb. 'Visceral crises' are attacks of acute pain with disorder of function of some internal organ, usually the stomach, rectum, bladder and larynx; and when the organ affected is an abdominal one, the severe pain, vomiting and collapse may mimic an abdominal emergency.

[7] *status epilepticus:* epilepsy in which one fit succeeds another without the patient recovering consciousness between them

The muscles of the bladder become weak, and dribbling and incontinence occur.

The gait is characteristic. Because of sensory loss, the patient cannot appreciate the degree of movement in his legs and their relationship with the ground; he picks up his feet too high and slams them down hard, and walks with his feet widely separated. Perforating ulcers on the big toes or the balls of the feet can penetrate the tissues until they reach bone. A Charcot's joint may develop – an arthritis of one of the big joints, which becomes much enlarged, is useless as a joint but quite painless.

Examination of the nervous system reveals many signs of disease: Argyll-Robertson pupils, optic atrophy, paralysis of cranial nerves, loss of pain sensation and of the appreciation of position, positive Romberg sign[8], loss of tendon reflexes. The disease is likely to run a progressive course over many years.

Special tests	*Blood:* WR positive in about 50 per cent of patients.
	CSF: increase in cells and protein; WR positive; gold curve of the 0123454321 pattern. Can be normal in patients who have been treated for syphilis.
Treatment	Penicillin 60,000 units daily for 28 days, followed if necessary by a second course. Pains, abnormal sensation, ataxia and crises are likely to improve, but the damage to the nervous system is likely to persist and may cause permanent disability. Morphine or pethidine may have to be given to relieve pain. Abdominal crises are relieved by adrenaline 0.2-0.5 mg.

Injuries of the Brain

In severe injuries the substance of the brain is torn and haemorrhages occur in it or in the extradural space, or sometimes there are many small haemorrhages in the brain. Cerebral oedema follows, and fibres may lose their myelin sheaths[9].

Concussion is a sudden, immediate disturbance of the functions of the brain, with loss of consciousness and paralysis of voluntary muscles. It can be slight, moderate or severe. In slight concussion consciousness is lost for a few seconds to a few minutes, or sometimes there is incomplete loss of consciousness. When he comes round, the patient is likely to be confused, to be drowsy and to complain of headache. In moderate concussion he is unconscious for several hours; he recovers consciousness slowly; for days afterwards he may be confused, talk at random, misindentify people and misinterpret what is going on around him; occasionally a patient will pass into a state of acute delirium. In severe concussion, the patient is likely to be unconscious for several days, to be severely shocked and to die; if he does not die, he is likely after regaining consciousness to be for days in a state of delirium or pass into a dull, apathetic state.

Retrograde amnesia[1] is common: that is, an amnesia for events immediately before the injury. The motorist remembers driving the car, but not the accident

[8] *positive Romberg sign:* swaying of the body when standing with feet close together and eyes shut; patient may fall if not supported.
[9] *myelin sheath:* the sheath of fatty tissue in which many nerve-fibres are wrapped; loss of it is called demyelination
[1] *amnesia:* loss of memory

that occurred; the footballer remembers starting a game but not the kick that laid him out. With severe concussion the retrograde amnesia may be for weeks, months or years, although islands of memory may stick up out of the sea of forgetfulness. In all but the most demented of patients the retrograde amnesia in time becomes gradually shorter.

During convalescence after concussion the patient is likely to have headaches, to be at times slightly confused, and to have post-traumatic amnesia[7].

Post-traumatic amnesia is the period of time from the injury until the patient is continuously aware of his surroundings. The length of this time is a measure of both the severity of the concussion and of the time the patient is likely to be off work. A patient with a post-traumatic amnesia of under one hour is usually able to return to his work, whatever it is, within 4-6 weeks; with a post-traumatic amnesia of 1-24 hours he is likely to be off work for 6-8 weeks.

Special test   *EEG:* at first all recordable activity may cease. Then abnormal waves appear. The worse the injury the longer the EEG shows abnormal waves, except in a patient whose brain cells have been so extensively destroyed that they do not again show electrical activity.
X-ray of skull: for fracture of skull.

Post-concussional Syndrome is common and likely to become chronic. The people who get it have usually been neurotic or with a strong neurotic predisposition or whose relatives have been neurotic. Symptoms include: throbbing headache, giddiness on change of posture, anxiety, difficulty in concentrating, black-outs, fatigue and intolerance of any noise.

A fugue state, similar to that found in hysteria and in which the patient wanders with impaired consciousness away from home and comes back to full consciousness hours or days or weeks later, may follow brain injury, particularly in a patient with a hysterical or psychopathic personality.

Post-traumatic epilepsy occurs after 2-4 per cent of brain injuries. Fits usually occur within 2 years of the injury, but sometimes much later. The longer the interval between injury and fit the more likely is epilepsy to persist, and fits occurring soon after the injury are the ones most likely to cease. Major fits are usual, but other kinds can occur.

Post-traumatic dementia is most common in old people, athero-sclerotics and patients who have been very severely concussed. Old people hardly ever recover from a severe concussion. The patient does not return to normal but continues to show symptoms, such as poor memory, mental slowness, difficulty in concentrating and studying, moodiness, irresponsibility, lack of control and outbursts of violence. Symptoms of this kind present 18 months after the injury are very likely to persist indefinitely.

Punch-drunkenness is a post-traumatic dementia produced in boxers by injuries to the brain produced by blows to the head or knocking the head against the floor of the ring. Typical features are loss of memory, decline in intelligence, slowness, dullness, fatuousness, slurred speech, ataxia and a coarse tremor of the arms.

[2] *post-traumatic:* after injury

Chapter 13

Chronic sub-dural haematoma is due to bleeding into the subdural space. An apparently trivial injury, such as knocking one's head against the roof above the door in getting into a car, may be sufficient to produce the bleeding. It may not produce symptoms for several weeks or months after the injury. The symptoms are headache, drowsiness, apathy or excitement, confusion, fits and irresponsible behaviour. Very

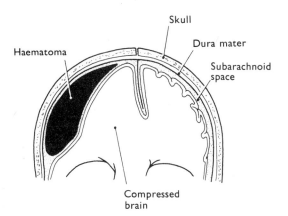

Fig. 73. A subdural haematoma compressing a cerebral hemisphere.

typically the symptoms vary much from day to day; on one day the patient may appear to be perfectly well, on the next very ill. The CSF is likely to be under increased pressure, to be yellow, and to have an increased protein content (normal: 15-45 mg per 100 ml); it can be normal in all respects. Treatment is by surgical removal of the haematoma through burr holes or by open operation.

Psychosis of schizophrenic, paranoid or manic-depressive kind occasionally follows injury to the brain, but rarely if ever is to be attributed to it, for almost all affected in this way have had a psychotic illness previously or have shown a definitely abnormal personality previously.

Treatment   While unconscious the patient will require the full treatment given to an unconscious patient.

As soon as he starts to recover consciousness, psychological treatment must begin. He must be told what has happened to him, the information being if necessary repeated many times over hours or days, for he may have difficulty in appreciating and remembering what he has been told. From the first he must be surrounded by optimism; he must be reassured over and over again that he will recover; and he must hear nothing of symptoms he might have unless he himself complains of them.

As soon as possible he is got out of bed and as soon as possible engaged in exercises, games, interests, occupational and industrial therapy, designed to give him reassurance and to promote a recovery of his former skills and interests. Treatment of an acute neurosis may be necessary. Patients with special disabilities will require re-education and training. A quick payment of any compensation and resumption of work promote recovery.

DISSEMINATED SCLEROSIS

Other name: multiple sclerosis.

This is a common disease of the nervous system. It occurs most commonly in temperate countries and is said not to occur in South Africa and India. It is one of the 'demyelinating diseases', i.e. diseases in which the myelin-sheaths around nerve fibres are affected and disappear. During acute phases of an attack patches of nervous tissue in various parts of the brain and spinal cord become swollen and pink; when the swelling settles down there may be left hard patches of tissue in which nerve-fibres have been replaced by fibrous tissue.

The cause of the disease is unknown. It has been attributed to many things, including viruses and auto-immunity. It is suggested that it is the late result (after a long latent period) of a virus infection acquired in childhood; the virus of measles is a suspect.

Clinical features

The characteristic feature of this disease is that signs of damage to the nervous system are scattered in time and place. First attacks usually occur between 15 and 30 years; subsequent attacks can occur at any time, after intervals of months or years, and in different parts of the central nervous system.

Precipitating factors can be: (a) trauma — injury to a part being followed by sensory symptoms in the part; (b) pregnancy and the puerperium; (c) emotional stress; (d) changes in temperature — a hot bath has been followed by symptoms; (e) exertion and fatigue.

Early features are:
(a) temporary mistiness or loss of vision,
(b) seeing double,
(c) weakness of an arm or leg, dragging a foot on walking,
(d) frequency or urgency of micturition; sometimes retention of urine,
(e) giddiness,
(f) tremor of hands,
(g) tremor of tongue and slurred speech.

Any of these can clear up within a few weeks and leave little or no trace. Physical examination may reveal nothing and at first the diagnosis cannot be definitely made. Later attacks can affect the same or other parts of the central nervous system. In spite of repeated attacks some patients develop little or no disability and can continue to get about their business. Others develop spastic paralysis, painful flexor spasms, slurred speech, severe tremor and inco-ordination, and show a pale optic disc, nystagmus, increased tendon reflexes and some sensory loss. A rise in body-temperature may make some symptoms worse. A few patients become severely paralysed and chair-borne.

Special tests

CSF: may show normal or increased protein, increase of lymphocytes, an abnormal Lange curve, a negative WR.
X-ray of spine: to exclude any abnormality of bone.
Aortogram: to exclude abnormal blood-vessels in spinal canal.

Treatment

There is no specific treatment. Giddiness and tremor are relieved by chlorpromazine. Injections of phenol around the spinal cord may relieve painful spasms, but there is a risk of paralysis. Crutches or wheel-chairs may be needed; the patient may have to live in a ground-floor flat equipped with appropriate gadgets to aid living.

EPILEPSY   The term epilepsy is used to describe sudden losses of consciousness, usually associated with convulsions or convulsive phenomena and due to excessive electrical discharges by brain cells. Epilepsy is not a disease in itself but an expression of something abnormal happening within the brain. The word 'epilepsy' means a seizure, and the words fit, convulsion and seizure all refer to the same thing.

Among the many causes of epilepsy are:
(a) any congenital deformity of the brain;
(b) damage to the brain during birth by shortage of oxygen or by haemorrhage or actual destruction of brain-tissue;
(c) encephalitis, meningitis, syphilis of the brain;
(d) a cerebral tumour, abscess or cyst;
(e) cerebral athero-sclerosis, thrombosis or haemorrhage;
(f) degenerative disease of the brain: any dementia;
(g) chronic alcoholism; lead and carbon monoxide poisoning;
(h) uraemia, hypo-glycaemia, eclampsia;[3]
(i) heart-attacks;
(j) some drugs, e.g. strychnine, camphor, caffeine;
(k) dentition, rickets, acute fevers, gastro-intestinal infections and acute allergic reactions in infants.
(l) watching television from a close distance or adjusting the picture or changing the channel. At least half of these people have normal EEGs. Some people get unusual sensations when exposed to flickering lights and can stop them by covering up one eye.

Idiopathic or cryptogenic epilepsy are the terms used to describe epilepsy when no cause for it can be found.

Epilepsy is a common condition; it has been estimated that 1 person in 200 will have fits at some time in his life. It usually begins in childhood, and about 1 epileptic in 3 has his first fit before the age of 10. Of those infants who have fits when they are teething, etc. (group 'k' above) a few continue to have fits. A fit for the first time in a person over 20 years is strongly suggestive of an organic disease of the brain. If one parent is epileptic, the incidence of epilepsy or psychopathy[4] in their children is about 10-15 per cent and of epilepsy alone about 6 per cent. If both parents are epileptic or one is epileptic and the other has an abnormal EEG the incidence of epilepsy is much higher.

Clinical features   The essential clinical feature of epilepsy is the fit. There are several kinds of fit; some patients have only one kind, others have fits of various kinds.

(a) *Major Fit* (Grand Mal). A major fit can occur without warning or be preceded by an aura. An aura may take the form of moodiness, headache, dizziness, peculiar feelings, peculiar smells or tastes, muscular twitchings; they can come

[3] *eclampsia:* a toxic illness of pregnancy of which fits are a feature
[4] *psychopathy:* aggressive, irresponsible behaviour

Diseases of the Nervous System

days or hours before a fit. The patient may have some warning just before a fit that he is going to have one.

In a major fit the patient loses consciousness and falls down. He may utter a cry. He then passes into the *tonic phase;* this lasts for 30-60 seconds; he has severe muscular rigidity; with extended limbs, clenched jaw, cessation of respiration, deep cyanosis, sometimes a bitten tongue and emptying of the bladder or bowels. He then passes into *clonic phase,* which lasts 1-5 minutes. In it he has alternate muscular contractions and relaxations in which his limbs thrash about and he may sustain a fracture. Breathing is now resumed and is stertorous. He sweats profusely. The tongue may be bitten again. The muscular contractions become weaker as the fit passes and then disappear. Some patients recover quickly; others remain exhausted or in stupor or complain of headache, muscular pains and inability to speak properly. *Post-epileptic automatism* is a condition in which the patient after a fit performs some apparently purposeful but inappropriate action without being aware of what he is doing; the condition is of medico-legal importance for the patient may commit an indecent or violent act in this state.

(b) *Minor Fit* (Petit mal). In this fit the patient loses consciousness momentarily or has a moment of impaired consciousness. He does not convulse, wet himself or fall, unless the fit lasts unusually long. He stops for a moment doing what he is doing, perhaps going pale, staring or dropping anything he is holding, sometimes twitching a little; and then he goes on with what he had been doing, as if nothing had happened. The whole fit is over in a few seconds. Single or multiple attacks occur. Some epileptic children have very many attacks, up to several hundred, in the course of a day. A minor fit can be followed by post-epileptic automatism.

(c) *Jacksonian fit.* This kind of fit can be motor or sensory. A muscular jacksonian fit begins as a muscular contraction in one part of the body — the thumb, the big toe, the corner of the mouth; the contractions may remain in one spot or they may spread to other muscles; consciousness is not always lost, but sometimes a jacksonian fit finishes up as a major fit. Sensory fits begin as abnormal sensations in one part of the body and gradually spread.

(d) *Temporal lobe epilepsy* is produced by disease of one or both temporal lobes of the brain. The patient shows varying degrees of impairment of consciousness, dream states, feelings of unreality, chewing movements, violent behaviour and running about.

(e) *Myoclonic epilepsy[5].* A form of epilepsy in which muscular twitchings occur on their own or sometimes in association with other kinds of epilepsy.

(f) *Status epilepticus:* A condition in which one fit succeeds another without the patient recovering consciousness between them. The number of fits can vary from a few to several thousand. It is said to be precipitated by taking the patient suddenly off a drug, but in the majority of cases no cause can be found. The patient may recover or may die from heart-failure or bronchopneumonia. Serial epilepsy is similar, but the patient recovers consciousness between fits.

Epilepsy runs a very variable course. Some patients have only one fit a year or

[5] *myoclonus:* involuntary muscular contractions

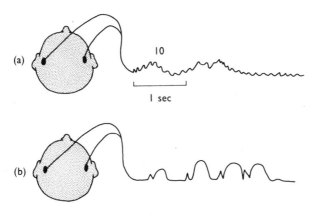

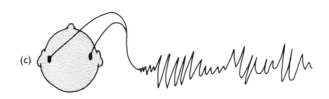

Fig. 74. The electroencephalogram: (a) normal waves, (b) the spike-and-wave seen in minor epilepsy (petit mal) and (c) the larger waves seen during attacks of major epilepsy (grand mal).

even more rarely; others have several a day. A succession of fits may be followed by freedom for weeks or months. Spontaneous cessation can happen or freedom from fits be produced by drugs. A patient occasionally dies in a fit.

Special tests   *EEG* is a recording of the magnified electrical discharges from cells in the brain. Epileptics usually show abnormal waves; especially (a) a violent discharge of abnormally fast or abnormally slow waves, which are characteristic of a major fit, and (b) a pattern of alternating three per second spikes and waves, characteristic of a minor fit. Abnormal waves may be present at times when a patient is not having a fit. Some epileptics have a normal EEG, and some people who have never had a fit have an abnormal one.

Other investigations are directed towards finding a cause for the epilepsy: X-ray of skull, air encephalography, blood tests for syphilis.

Treatment   (a) *Drugs:* The aim of drug treatment is the achievement of the maximum anticonvulsant effect with the minimum of side-effects, the correct dose of a drug for any individual being the one that achieves this for him. Effective control may be achieved by one drug or by several in combination. Except when acute toxic effects are being produced, no drug must be stopped suddenly, because of the danger of increasing the number of fits or of producing status epilepticus; any change should take at least a fortnight, the dose of the old drug being reduced as the dose of the new is increased.

Drugs used for major and jacksonian epilepsy
phenobarbitone: 30-120 mg 2-3 times a day
phenytoin sodium (Epanutin, Dilantin): 50-200 mg daily
primidone (Mysoline): 500 mg-2 g daily
sulthiame (Ospolot): 200-600 mg daily

Diseases of the Nervous System

sodium valproate (Epilim): 1200 mg or more daily
Drugs used for minor epilepsy
ethosuximide (Zarontin): up to 1 g daily
sodium valproate (Epilim): 1200 mg or more daily
Drugs used for temporal lobe epilepsy
carbamazepine (Tegretol): up to 1600 mg daily

(b) *Surgery.* Small lesions of the brain may be localized and removed surgically. Lesions likely to respond to surgery are scars, depressed fractures, bullets, cysts and encapsulated abscesses. Treatment by drugs is continued for at least two years.

(c) *General.* An epileptic child should be encouraged to lead as normal a life as possible. If possible he should attend an ordinary school, but if he has frequent fits he may have to be educated in a special school or at home. On leaving school, the epileptic will require to find suitable work. He should not work with machinery, have to drive a vehicle, work on ladders or high places, not work where there is a danger of his injuring himself or others if he has a fit. Although well controlled epileptics do not have a high accident rate, employers are often unwilling to employ them and other workers to work with them; and it is not at all unusual for an epileptic to hide his disability and hope that he does not have a fit at work.

It is advisable that an epileptic should not sleep alone in case he has a fit at night. As some epileptics are said to have suffocated themselves in a soft pillow, their pillows should be hard. Any sport such as football and boxing in which the patient is likely to get blows to the head should be forbidden. An epileptic should not take alcohol.

(d) If EEG is normal and the patient gets fits only when watching television, there is no need for drug treatment. The patient should watch TV only in a well-lit room, not sit close to the set, not adjust the set or change the channel, and if he has to approach the set cover up one eye.

Treatment during a Fit

(i) *Major Fit.* If possible catch the patient before he falls. Loosen his collar. Remove him from a place of danger. His movement need not be controlled unless he is in danger of knocking himself. Do not attempt to force a gag into his mouth during the tonic phase; you will only break a tooth and if he has cut or bitten himself the damage is already done. During the clonic phase slip something soft, such as the corner of a towel between his teeth. After the fit examine him for any injury. Stay with him until he has completely recovered consciousness.

(ii) *Minor Fit.* No special treatment required. Stay with patient until he has completely recovered consciousness.

(iii) *Status epilepticus.* The patient should be moved to hospital. Diazepam is given intravenously in a dose of 10 mg, followed by 20 mg intravenously if the fits do not stop within a few minutes. Subsequently, if the patient has any fits or twitching, diazepam 5 mg hourly is given in an intravenous saline drip.

NARCOLEPSY

This is a condition in which the patient has attacks of sleep which come on suddenly and last for a short time; the patient may have many in rapid succession; sometimes they are associated with *cataplexy* in which there is a sudden loss of postural tone and the patient falls helpless to the ground. Attacks may begin in childhood or the first half of adult life. There appears to be no connection between them and epilepsy.

No cause is usually found; it can follow brain injury, encephalitis and some tumours of the brain, and complicate some metabolic diseases; but these possible causes account for only a few of the cases. In some patients attacks are precipitated by emotion. A patient can be aroused out of his sleep by calling, touching or sometimes only by shaking. There are usually no signs of physical disease and the EEG shows normal sleep-patterns. In cataplexy the patient is fully conscious but unable to move or speak.

Treatment   Narcolepsy can be prevented by taking amphetamine sulphate 10-50 mg twice daily. There is a danger of addiction to amphetamine developing. No treatment is known to affect cataplexy.

MIGRAINE [6]

This condition is characterized, in the classical form, by attacks of headache, nausea and vomiting, often preceded by visual disturbances. Its causes are not definitely known. The symptoms appear to be the result of abnormalities of blood-vessels inside and outside the skull. Possible abnormalities are: (a) oedema of the arterial walls; (b) contraction of arteries within the skull and dilatation of those outside it. There is a higher incidence of epilepsy in patients with migraine than in the general population, and there is often a history of previous allergic disorder.

A number of people get "migrainous headeaches" of various kinds, but without the full migraine picture.

Classical migraine begins in childhood, and attacks tend to become less common and milder with increasing age. Years of freedom from attacks can be followed by 2-3 years of frequent attacks. Patients with migraine are said often to have an obsessional personality with drives towards exactness and perfection; in some patients attacks occur during a period of relaxation after stress.

Oral contraceptives may (a) appear to precipitate a first attack or make existing migraine worse, or paradoxically (b) reduce the number and severity of attacks.

Clinical features   Attacks often occur unpredictably and may be preceded by feelings of well-being.

Prodromal features can occur and last for 5-45 minutes. They take the form of visual disturbances in which the patient sees flashes of light, dazzling lights or "fortification figures" of pointed, angled patterns like plans of old forts; sometimes there is some loss of sight.

The prodromal features fade with the onset of the headache, which becomes very severe; it may be limited to half the head or involve the whole head, and lasts up to 48 hours. It is associated with nausea, vomiting, pallor and photophobia; and at the end of an attack the patient may pass a lot of urine. The superficial temporal artery may be engorged and visibly pulsating during the attack.

Rarely, aphasia[7] or paralysis of an oculo-motor nerve occurs.

Prevention   Methsergide (Deseril) in doses of 2 mg three or four times a day will prevent attacks in 80 per cent of patients, but they may give up taking it because of its side-effects. Tranquillizers may reduce the number or severity of attacks. Patients learn to avoid alcohol or certain foods (chocolate, fried dishes, etc.) which appear to bring on attacks.

[6] *migraine:* French from Greek: *hemi* – half; *cranium* – skull
[7] *aphasia:* inability to speak, write or understand spoken or written words as a result of disease of the speech centre in the brain

Treatment	The patient will demand to be left alone in a darkened room. There is no one drug which will relieve attacks in all patients. Ergotamine tartrate is the most effective drug and is given by injection in doses of 0.25-0.5 mg or by suppository in a dose of 2 mg. Only very careful patients should take the drug in aerosol form as over-dosage is easy. Chlorpromazine is given by injection to relieve vomiting.
MIGRAINOUS NEURALGIA	This is a paroxysmal headache resembling migraine but occurring more often and lasting for shorter periods. Its cause is unknown. It occurs mostly in middle-aged men − of the ambitious, pushing, conscientious kind.
Clinical features	A severe headache wakens the patient from sleep. The headache starts above the eye and can spread upwards, on the forehead, downwards on the cheek, or backwards into the eye. It lasts for 30-60 minutes. Similar attacks sometimes occur by day, and sometimes more than one a day. In some attacks the eye on the affected side waters and has a constricted pupil and ptosis[8], and the nose on that side is blocked. Attacks occur in clusters, recurring daily for several weeks, with long periods of freedom from attacks between the clusters.
Treatment	As for migraine. Patients must be warned not to take more than 3 doses of ergotamine tartrate a day for it can cause gangrene[9] of the fingers and toes by constricting arterioles.
PARALYSIS AGITANS	*Other name:* Parkinsonism, Parkinson's disease This is a progressive disease of the brain due to degeneration of parts of the basal ganglia[1] and of the cerebral cortex. Its cause is unknown. A similar condition can arise from the use of tranquillizers, from cerebral athero-sclerosis, poisoning by carbon monoxide, and other conditions causing disease of the basal ganglia. It affects about 1 per cent of people over 50. The usual age of onset is between 45 and 65 years of age. It occurs equally in the sexes.

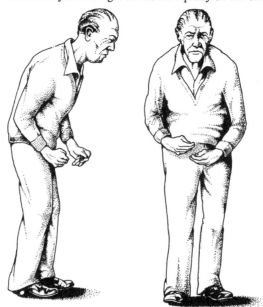

Fig. 75. Paralysis agitans

[8] *ptosis:* drooping of upper eyelid
[9] *gangrene:* death of a tissue due to cutting off its blood-supply
[1] *basal ganglia:* the caudate and lenticular nuclei etc.

Clinical features   The onset is insidious. A tremor usually begins in one limb and may be limited for a time to one side of the body; eventually all the limbs, the head and the trunk show it. The hands are particularly affected, showing the so called 'pill-rolling' movements of fingers and thumb. The tremor is fine or moderate in degree, is present at rest, disappears on voluntary movement, and unless severe stops during sleep.

Rigidity is a feature. Muscular movements are performed slowly, small muscles being more affected than large. Speaking, chewing and swallowing are hampered, and the speech becomes monotonous. The patient's features become mask-like, the eyes unblinking, the ordinary lines washed out. The trunk is held in a stoop. The patient walks in little steps. He is likely to become depressed, peevish, suicidal or psychotic and if the disease is prolonged to develop cerebral deterioration, with loss of memory, lack of concentration and emotional disturbances. Eventually he becomes bed-ridden and dies of an intercurrent infection.

Parkinsonism produced by drugs is usually, but not always, reversible.

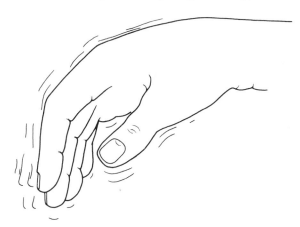

Fig. 76. Tremor of the hand in paralysis agitans.

Treatment   Light massage, passive movements and warm baths are helpful. The patient should be encouraged to take regular exercise for as long as he is able, but not to the point of fatigue.

The following drugs are used:

(a) Levodopa, in doses of 0.25 g twice daily increasing up a total daily dosage of 2.5-5.0 g daily in divided doses, improves all symptoms but does not affect its cause and has to be continued for life. Nausea and tremor are common side-effects which can be reduced by giving carbidopa (MK486).

(b) Amantadine, 200-600 mg daily, for early cases.

(c) Benzhexol hydrochloride (artane, Pipanol), 2-5 mg three times a day; rarely it precipitates a confusional, hallucinatory or depressive state.

(d) Orphenadrine hydrochloride (Disipal), up to 400 mg daily; it can produce euphoria[2] and should be given with meals to prevent gastric irritation.

(e) Procyclidine hydrochloride (Kemadrin) up to 60 mg daily.

(f) Hyoscine hydrobromide, 0.3-0.6 mg daily.

[2] *euphoria:* a feeling of well-being

Several drugs may have to be tried before the one that suits the patient best is found.

Surgical removal or destruction of the affected parts of the brain are sometimes performed.

HUNTINGTON'S
CHOREA[3]

This familial disease is transmitted by a dominant gene and inherited by about half the children of an infected person. Occasionally it will skip a generation or occur without a family history. It affects both sexes and usually begins at 40-60 years. The brain shows degeneration of cortex and basal ganglia.

Clinical features

The disease is characterized by (a) chorea and (b) dementia. Choreic movements may precede the dementia or occur without it. The patient shows irregular involuntary movements, beginning with fidgetiness and advancing to gross, violent movements which interfere with all physical activities and eventually render the patient chair-borne or bed-ridden. Dementia, which can occur without the chorea, begins with loss of memory, apathy and carelessness and progressive to a failure of all mental faculties. In early days suicide may be attempted. The patient can survive for 10-20 years, dying eventually of a pulmonary or other infection.

Treatment

No treatment halts the progress of the dementia. The chorea may to some extent be relieved by trifluoperazine or other tranquillizer. The prevention of bedsores is important because the irregular movements are liable to rub off patches of skin.

CONGENITAL
MALFORMATIONS
OF THE NERVOUS
SYSTEM

About 60 per cent of major congenital deformities affect the nervous system.

Anencephaly[4]: absence of nearly all of the brain; the infant dies shortly after birth.

Microcephaly: an abnormally small brain, with small ill-developed gyri; the child is usually mentally retarded to severe or moderate degree and has a typical 'bird-like' appearance with a tiny head and large nose.

Arnold-Chiari deformity[5]: the cerebellum is enlarged and the medulla oblongata thrust downwards into the foramen magnum; may be associated with meningocoele, hydrocephalus and spina bifida; produces occipital and cervical pain, cerebellar symptoms, and signs of pressure on nerve tracts in the medulla.

Platybasia[6]: a congenital deformity of the base of the skull with pushing upwards and constriction of spinal cord; produces clinical features similar to those of the Arnold-Chiari deformity.

Klippel-Feil syndrome[7]: congenital deformity of cervical part of spinal column producing a short neck, torticollis etc. and sometimes associated with platybasia and syringomyelia (see p. 248).

Spina bifida: a failure of the vertebral arch to close in the course of early development and an associated mal-development of the spinal cord and meninges. It usually occurs in the lumbo-sacral region. It is often associated with other congenital deformities. In severe forms there is a *meningocele,* a protruding meningeal sac containing CSF, or a *myelo-meningocele* the spinal cord and nerve roots being involved in the meningocele. In mild forms there may be only a dimple in the skin over the spot or a pigmented patch or a tuft of thick hair. Involvement of the spinal cord and nerves in the malformation produces difficulty in walking, wasting of legs, deformities of the feet, and sphincter disturbances, especially enuresis.

[3] *G.Huntington* described it in 1872, as the result of observations made by himself, his father and grandfather on families on Long Island, USA

[4] *anencephaly:* Greek: *an* – no; *encephalos* – brain

[5] *Arnold-Chiari:* Arnold described cerebellar condition (1894) and Chiari the medullary condition (1896)

[6] *platybasia:* Greek; *platys* – broad; *basis* – base

[7] *Klippel-Feil:* M. Klippel (1858-1942), A. Feil (1884-   ) French physicians.

Chapter 13

HYDROCEPHALUS

In this condition the ventricles of the brain are dilated and filled by an excessive amount of cerebro-spinal fluid. The causes are:

(a) a congenital malformation preventing the normal circulation of CSF through the ventricles and out into the subarachnoid space;

(b) a meningitis which has blocked the holes in the roof of the 4th ventricle;

(c) a tumour pressing on the intraventricular foramen (between the two lateral ventricles) or the aqueduct between the 3rd and 4th ventricles;

In 10-15 per cent of cases no cause can be found.

It is usually a disease of infancy, but in later life it can be caused by a meningitis or tumour acting in one of the above ways. A hydrocephalus with normal CSF pressure following a subarachnoid haemorrhage or of unknown origin can produce a dementia, incontinence and unsteadiness of gait in an adult.

The ventricles become more and more dilated, the brain becomes thinner and thinner and the cortex may be in the end no more than a thin membrane. The intra-cranial pressure is raised. When present before birth the hydrocephalus may make the baby's head too large to enter the mother's pelvis.

Clinical features

In the infant the head becomes abnormally large in all directions; the fontanelles bulge and the sutures are widely separated. A squint develops. The child fails to thrive.

A spontaneous arrest of the hydrocephalus can occur: the head stops enlarging at an abnormal rate, the child starts to improve mentally and physically, although he may be left with some of the complications detailed below.

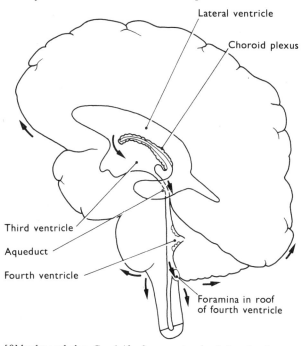

Lateral ventricle

Choroid plexus

Third ventricle

Aqueduct

Fourth ventricle

Foramina in roof of fourth ventricle

Fig. 77. Diagram of the circulation of the cerebro-spinal fluid. Places particularly liable to become blocked, with the formation of a hydroecephalus, are the aqueduct and the foramina in the roof of the fourth ventricle.

[8] *hydrocephalus:* Greek:'*hudor* — water; *kephale* — head

Diseases of the Nervous System

If the hydrocephalus continues, the head goes on enlarging and may be more than 35 cm in diameter. The forehead bulges, the veins on the scalp are distended. The eyes are thrust downwards and the child may learn that to see he has to pull his lower eyelids down. Death is due to wasting, pneumonia, hyper-pyrexia or meningitis.

Complications

Spastic paralysis	Epilepsy	Blindness
Severe wasting	Pressure sores on head	
Mental retardation	Personality problems.	

When the hydrocephalus develops after the cranial sutures have fused, no enlargement of the head is possible and the patient develops the symptoms and signs of increasing intracranial pressure.

Treatment

When hydrocephalus occurs before birth; the head can be tapped *in utero* and the CSF drained off; caesarian section may be necessary.

For hydrocephalus occurring in infancy, conservative treatment is advisable for the hydrocephalus may cease and the results of surgical treatment are unsatisfactory. If the hydrocephalus is increasing rapidly, an attempt is made to drain the CSF out of the brain; the usual method is by a tube leading from the ventricles under the skin of the neck into a jugular vein. A Spitz-Holter[9] valve in the tube allows the CSF to drain into the blood when a certain pressure is reached. The valve is likely to become infected and the tube blocked, and venous thrombosis can occur, and for these reasons the treatment is not often successful. One of these ventriculo-atrial shunting operations can be of great benefit to an adult patient who has developed dementia due to hydrocephalus.

CEREBRAL PALSY

Cerebral palsy is the term used to describe mal-functioning of the cerebral motor functions, present at birth or within the first few years of life, liable to produce paralysis, incordination and involuntary movements, and commonly associated with epilepsy, mental retardation, blindness, deafness and behaviour disorders.

It can be caused by anything which damages the growing brain, before, during, or after birth:
(a) genetic abnormalities affecting the brain,
(b) German measles, kernicterus[1], exposure to radiation, metabolic disturbances in intra-uterine life,
(c) lack of oxygen or brain damage during birth,
(d) encephalitis, meningitis, brain injury after birth.
The brain shows various kinds of degeneration, cysts, and failure of development.

Clinical features

Affected newly-born infants are likely to show breathing or sucking difficulties, to be pale or cyanosed or in some conditions to be severely jaundiced.

According to the parts paralysed the following names are given:

[9] *Spitz-Holter:* names of the engineer who devised the valve for his own baby and the surgeon who operated
[1] *kernicterus:* brain damage produced by severe jaundice in newly-born baby

Diplegia: both arms or both legs affected.

Monoplegia: one limb only affected.

Hemiplegia: arm and leg on the same side affected.

Triplegia: three limbs affected.

Quadriplegia: all limbs affected.

Spasticity is common in affected muscles. Limbs are held in rigid positions; voluntary movements are interfered with; contractures are likely. Legs may be held crossed in the 'scissors' position. If the face is affected, the patient has difficulty in speaking, chewing and swallowing, and saliva dribbles from his mouth. Tendon reflexes are exaggerated.

Involuntary movements may be choreic (jerky) or athetoid (slow, twisting). Any kind of epileptic fit may occur. Mental retardation of varying degree occurs in about 75 per cent, and it is unusual for a patient to have high intelligence. Behaviour disturbances can take the form of restlessness, hyperactivity, inability to concentrate, noisy outbursts and temper-tantrums.

Treatment

This is a long struggle against the effects of a permanently damaged brain. It depends upon the amount of damage and the degree of intelligence of the child. The degree to which the child can be educated will depend upon the extent of spasticity and the degree of intelligence. Education in a special school or training in a day-hospital or training centre, may be required or the child admitted into a hospital for the mentally retarded. Other forms of treatment are by physiotherapy, speech therapy, orthopaedic surgery to lengthen tendons and relieve contractures, and by drugs to control epilepsy or behaviour disorders.

Diseases of the Cranial Nerves and Disorders of the Special Senses
OLFACTORY NERVE (I) AND SMELL

Interference with smell may be due to:

(a) a cold or chronic infection of the nose,

(b) some virus illnesses,

(c) a fracture of the skull involving the anterior cranial fossa,

(d) a meningioma pressing on one or both olfactory tracts,

(e) tabes dorsalis.

OPTIC NERVE (II) AND VISION

Interference with vision may be due to:

(a) errors of refraction, the visual image not falling exactly on the retina,

(b) corneal scarring, following a corneal ulcer,

(c) a cataract, an opacity of the lens,

(d) detachment of the retina from the choroid coat,

(e) glaucoma[2], producing 'tunnel vision', the patient feeling that he is looking down a tunnel, and further impairment of vision leading to blindness,

[2] *glaucoma:* increase of pressure in the eyeball

(f) lesions of the optic nerve, chiasma and tracts as a result of pressure by a berry aneurysm, a pituitary tumour, or a meningioma or other tumour in that region.

(g) pressure on the optic tract and optic radiation or the visual area in the occipital lobe by a space-occupying lesion.

(h) increased intra-cranial pressure producing papilloedema[3].

(i) involvement of the optic nerve in meningitis, syphilis or disseminated sclerosis.

(j) in certain general diseases — severe anaemia, polycythaemia vera[4], diabetes mellitus, athero-sclerosis, hypertension, chronic heart-lung disease, vitamin B deficiency.

(k) poisoning by methyl alcohol, nicotine, quinine.

The term *optic neuritis* is used to describe any degeneration of inflammation of the optic nerve. Optic neuritis may progress to produce *optic atrophy,* in which eyesight is permanently impaired or completely lost.

The treatment of all these conditions is that of the basic cause.

| OCULO-MOTOR (III), TROCHLEAR (IV) AND ABDUCENT NERVES (VI) | These nerves supply the muscles of the eyeball (the 4 recti, 2 oblique). From their points of origin on the surface of the brain to their terminations they are liable to be affected by meningitis, a tumour, a berry aneurysm, disseminated sclerosis, and fracture of the skull. |

OCULO-MOTOR (III), TROCHLEAR (IV) AND ABDUCENT NERVES (VI)

These nerves supply the muscles of the eyeball (the 4 recti, 2 oblique). From their points of origin on the surface of the brain to their terminations they are liable to be affected by meningitis, a tumour, a berry aneurysm, disseminated sclerosis, and fracture of the skull.

The result is likely to be a squint, a ptosis if the III nerve is involved and an irregularity of the pupil.

Abnormalities of the pupil

(a) *Argyll Robertson pupil[5]:* small unequal pupils with irregular outline, do not react to light but do to convergence; almost always due to syphilis.

(b) *Horner's syndrome[6]:* pupil of affected eye is small, does not dilate to darkness; usually associated with enophthalmos[7], ptosis, and reduction in sweating of face on affected side; due to interference with sympathetic nerve pathways in neck or on internal carotid artery.

(c) *Myotonic pupil[8]:* reacts slowly to light and convergence; a harmless condition sometimes associated — in *Adie's[9] syndrome* — with absent tendon reflexes.

(d) *Senile pupil:* in old age pupil can become small, unequal and irregular.

TRIGEMINAL NEURALGIA (V)

Other name: tic douleureux.

Trigeminal neuralgia is characterized by attacks of severe pain in parts of the face supplied by the trigeminal (*V* cranial) nerve. Its cause is unknown; it is sometimes

[3]*papilloedema:* oedematous swelling of the optic disc, the eminence where the optic nerve fibres appear inside the eye

[4]*polycythaemia vera:* disease characterized by an abnormal increase in the number of red blood cells

[5] *D. M. Argyll Robertson* (1837-1909): Scottish ophthalmologist

[6] *J. F. Horner* (1831-86): Swiss eye specialist

[7]*enophthalmos:* recession of the eyeball into the orbit

[8]*myotonic:* Greek: *mus:* — muscle; *tonos* — tone

[9] *W. J. Adie* (1886-1935): British neurologist

associated with disseminated sclerosis. It usually begins at 40-60 years, occasionally earlier.

Clinical features   The pain is severe — shooting, stabbing or like red hot needles or electric shocks. It occurs in sudden spasms lasting for a few seconds; attacks recur rapidly for a few days or a week, with freedom from attacks for weeks, months or years. Attacks occur spontaneously or are precipitated by touching a certain spot (a 'trigger-point'), by eating, talking, yawning, by a loud noise or an acute emotion, or by abnormal dental conditions and the wearing of faulty dentures. The pain starts in one spot and shoots in one or more directions within the area supplied by the trigeminal nerve. Common sites are (a) between mouth and ear and (b) around the eyes and on the side of the nose. The pain is felt deep in the face, gums or side of the tongue. The forehead and back of the head are not involved. The pain sometimes is bilateral, but pain on one side does not shoot into the other. There is no impairment of sensation, and the muscles supplied by the nerve are not affected. The disease is likely to persist, can make old age a misery, and has driven patients to suicide. Spontaneous remission is rare, but long remissions can occur.

Treatment   Medical treatment is by phenytoin or carbamazepine which relieve the pain in many patients. The correction of faulty dental conditions can bring relief. Surgical treatment is by (a) cutting the sensory root of the trigeminal nerve either completely or in part, or (b) injecting the trigeminal nerve-branches with alcohol. Of these, section is preferred. It produces a complete anaesthesia of the parts supplied by the divided fibres; patients get used to the loss of sensation in the face and are completely and permanently relieved of pain. If the sensory fibres to the eye are involved, the cornea will be anaesthetized and as the eye will not blink when a bit of dust falls on it, it has to be protected to prevent ulceration. All that is necessary is to instill twice daily for 3 months a drop of sterile paraffin into the eye. There is no need to cover the eye. The patient should report if the eye becomes red or vision becomes blurred. The surgeon may then sew the eyelids together (tarsorrhaphy) for 3 months.

FACIAL NERVE (VII)   The facial nerve can be pressed on: (a) by an acoustic nerve tumour, involving the auditory nerve, which runs alongside it for part of its course; (b) a fracture of the middle cranial fossa of the skull; (c) in acute and chronic middle ear disease, mastoiditis and operations on the mastoid process; (d) by lymphatic tissue in leukaemia.

Bell's palsy[1]   This is a paralysis of the muscles on one side of the face. Its cause is unknown; it may be due to a virus infection, to spasm of the arterioles supplying the nerve or to compression of the facial nerve by oedema as it passes through the narrow facial canal in the temporal bone. It occurs in both sexes and at all ages, and is occasionally bilateral.

Clinical features   The onset is sudden, the paralysis being at its worst within a few hours. There may be some preliminary pain in the ear, cheek or eye on the same side. The patient

[1] *Sir Charles Bell* (1774-1842): Scottish physician and physiologist

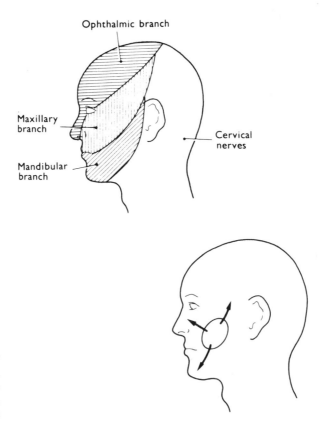

Ophthalmic branch

Maxillary branch

Cervical nerves

Mandibular branch

Fig. 78. Distribution of branches of the trigeminal nerve and a common site and spread of trigeminal neuralgia

finds that one side of his face is paralysed. He cannot speak clearly, he cannot whistle, he has difficulty in eating, he cannot close the eye completely. The mouth is pulled over to the sound side; the paralysed side of the face is flat, the corner of the mouth droops. Between 30 and 50 per cent of patients complain of an unpleasant taste or of impairment of taste (this is due to involvement of taste fibres to the tongue in a branch of the facial nerve).

There may be impairment of taste on the anterior two-thirds of the tongue (which is supplied by the facial nerve) and hyperacusis[2] in the ear on the same side, due to paralysis of a small muscle in the ear.

The paralysis starts to disappear in 2-12 weeks after the onset. Mild cases clear up in 2-3 months, severe cases take up to 12 months; in some a degree of permanent paralysis is left. Complete recovery occurs spontaneously in 60 per cent of cases.

Treatment   The best treatment is prednisolone by mouth in a dose of 20 mg four times a day for 5 days, the dose being gradually reduced during the next 4 days; the best results are achieved when treatment is begun within 2 days of onset. Pain is relieved by analgesics. Stitching the eyelids together for a time may be necessary to protect an exposed eye.

[2] *hyper-acusis:* abnormally acute hearing

ACOUSTIC-VESTIBULAR NERVE (VIII) AND HEARING	*Deafness* may be due to (a) wax in the auditory meatus; (b) acute or chronic otitis media, obstruction to the auditory (eustachian) canal; (c) neuritis of the eighth nerve; (d) otosclerosis; Paget's disease of bone; (e) tumour of the eighth nerve. *Giddiness* and impaired balance may be due to: (a) disease of the internal ear involving the otolith organ or the semi-circular canals, (b) atheroma of the basilar artery, which supplies the brain-stem.

Ménière's disease [3] — This disease is characterized by (a) attacks of vertigo, often with nausea and vomiting and (b) deafness and tinnitus in one or both ears. It begins in late middle age, the cause is unknown; it has been thought to be due to a disturbance of fluid-balance in the internal ear.

Clinical features — Deafness and tinnitus are common early symptoms. The tinnitus is of roaring, singing or hissing sounds. Attacks of acute vertigo then start. Each attack begins very abruptly, sometimes so abruptly that the patient is flung to the ground, and lasts from minutes to hours. During it the patient may vomit profusely, and after it he may stay for some time in a state of collapse. The disease often progresses to permanent deafness.

Treatment — There is no satisfactory treatment. Antihistamine drugs have been recommended for the relief of an attack, and phenobarbitone and other sedatives to relieve anxiety and tension between attacks. Chlorpromazine relieves attacks.

GLOSSO-PHARYNGEAL NERVE (IX) — *Glossopharyngeal neuralgia* consists of attacks of pain, similar to those of trigeminal neuralgia (see p. 242) in the region of the sensory distribution of the glossopharyngeal nerve – the ear, the nasopharynx, the tonsil and the side of the tongue. Its cause is unknown. It usually starts in late middle life. Severe attacks of pain, each lasting for a few seconds, occur in bouts over days or weeks and are followed often by long periods of freedom from attacks. Attacks occur spontaneously or are triggered off by talking, swallowing, yawning, moving the head quickly. There may be somewhere in the distribution of the nerve a 'trigger-spot', stimulation of which shoots off an attack.

Treatment — The only effective treatment is to cut the nerve inside the skull. The subsequent sensory loss and paralysis are so slight as to be practically unnoticeable.

TICS — *Tics* are jerky movements produced irregularly, usually when a person is emotional or anxious. Simple tics occur in children, taking the form of blinking, grimacing, screwing up the eyes, shrugging the shoulders. Occasionally they persist into adult life, occurring when the patient

[3] *Prosper Ménière* (1799-1862): French ear specialist

Diseases of the Nervous System

is under stress. Treatment is by reducing stress, especially when it is the result of parental anxieties and mismanagement.

Torticollis occurs in adult life as a sudden jerking of the head to one side and tilting of it as a result of a sudden contracture of the sternomastoid muscle and of some of the deeper muscles of the neck. The spasm may be painful. The condition is made worse by worry and excitement; rarely it is due to irritation of nerve roots by bony outgrowths. Treatment is by reassurance, by the avoidance so far as possible of anxiety-provoking situations, and by tranquillisers. Complete recovery is unusual.

Hemi-facial spasm is a similar condition in which one half of the face is subjected to violent irregular spasms. Occasionally it follows an attack of Bell's palsy. The other side of the face is sometimes involved later. Treatment is unsatisfactory; psychotherapy and tranquillizers can be given. In severe cases the seventh cranial nerve, which supplies the muscles of the face, is divided as it emerges from the skull just below the ear; but the patient is of course left with a permanent facial paralysis.

DISORDERS OF SPEECH

The term speech in medicine includes speaking, hearing, writing and reading. The motor areas of the brain involved are those that regulate the movements of the lips, tongue, larynx, respiration, hand and arm; the sensory areas are those of vision and hearing and all the associated areas in which the sensory stimuli are sorted out and stored and from which they are recalled into consciousness. The *speech centre*, the master controller of all these functions, is situated in the left cerebral hemisphere for all right-handed people and for most left-handed people. It occupies part of the upper temporal gyrus and parts of the frontal and parietal lobes just above the gyrus. It is usual to ascribe separate functions to different parts of the area; speaking and writing appear to be in front, hearing and reading behind.

The speech area can be affected by diseases of the brain: it can be injured, its blood-supply can be cut off, it can suffer various degenerations, infections can damage it, tumours can grow into it or press upon it. The following terms should be understood:

aphasia: any general inability to speak, to write, to understand spoken or written words as a result of disease of the speech centre.

motor aphasia: the patient is unable to express himself in written or spoken speech while understanding what he hears or reads and not having any paralysis of articulation or writing.

agraphia: the patient is unable to express himself in writing.

word deafness: the patient can hear sounds but cannot understand words.

word blindness: the patient can see but cannot understand printed or written words.

nominal aphasia: the patient can recognize an object and knows its purpose but cannot name it.

agnosia: the patient can recognize an object but cannot understand what it is used for.

motor apraxia: the patient is unable to perform an action he wishes and knows how to perform.

COMPRESSION OF THE SPINAL CORD

The spinal cord can be pressed on by:

(a) a crush-fracture of a vertebral body, a fracture-dislocation of the vertebral column,

(b) a prolapsed intervertebral disc,

(c) a tumour, which can be a tumour such as meningioma or glioma arising as a primary growth, or a secondary carcinoma from a primary growth elsewhere in the body,

(d) bone disease, e.g. Paget's disease, tuberculosis of the spine, cervical spondylosis,

(e) a lymphatic deposit in Hodgkin's disease,

(f) an extra-dural abscess.

Clinical features
1. Rapid compression

With severe sudden damage, e.g. from an injury, to the spinal cord with damage to many tracts or possibly complete section, the patient goes into spinal shock.

Spinal shock is characterized by:

(a) complete paralysis of muscles below the level of the injury,

(b) loss of muscle-tone, the muscles being completely flaccid,

(c) loss of all reflexes,

(d) complete loss of sensation below the level of the lesion,

(e) paralysis of bladder and rectum; as the internal sphincter muscle of the bladder is not involved, retention of urine will develop.

(f) circulatory failure in the parts affected, which become cold and blue; bed-sores may develop,

(g) if the damage is in the upper dorsal region, there will be a fall in blood-pressure due to involvement of the sympathetic tracts.

If the patient survives, the spinal shock will pass off in about 3 weeks. The patient will be left with paralysis and sensory loss, but his muscle-tone will redevelop and there will be a spastic paralysis in place of the previous flaccid one; the tendon-reflexes become exaggerated and the plantar responses extensor. Reflex micturition will develop.

2. Slow compression

(a) *Features due to involvement at the site of the lesion:* Root-or girdle-pain due to

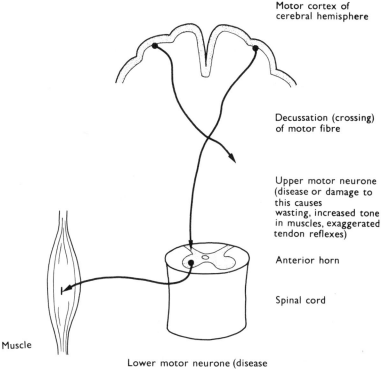

Motor cortex of cerebral hemisphere

Decussation (crossing) of motor fibre

Upper motor neurone (disease or damage to this causes wasting, increased tone in muscles, exaggerated tendon reflexes)

Anterior horn

Spinal cord

Muscle

Lower motor neurone (disease or damage to this causes paralysis, wasting of muscles, loss of tone, loss of reflexes)

Fig. 79. The upper and lower motor neurones.

Diseases of the Nervous System

pressure on dorsal nerve-roots with excessive sensibility to painful stimuli (hyper-algesia) in the part. Pain is increased by sneezing, coughing and straining. Wasting and paralysis of muscle are due to involvement of anterior horn cells in the spinal cord.

(b) *Features due to pressure on tracts in the spinal cord* and so causing symptoms and signs at a lower level.

An *upper motor neurone lesion:* paralysis and spasticity of muscles, increased tendon reflexes, extensor plantar reflex.

Interference with *control of the bladder:* at first precipitant micturition and incontinence, followed by retention, dribbling overflow and sometimes periodic reflex partial emptying.

Special tests
X-ray of spine: for evidence of tuberculosis, recent or old fracture, erosion of bone by a tumour, Paget's disease.

Myelography: the injection of a radio-opaque substance into spinal subarachnoid space, by either the lumbar or the cisternal route, to detect any filling defect.

Lumbar puncture: if the obstruction completely blocks the subarachnoid space, the CSF will show: (a) *Froin's syndrome:* CSF is yellow, coagulates quickly, contains an excessive amount of protein due to increased permeability of the meninges, so that it becomes more like blood-plasma; (b) *Queckenstedt's phenomenon:* when the jugular veins in the neck are compressed, the pressure of the CSF is not raised or raised only slightly.

Treatment
The treatment of spinal compression is surgical. If the cause of the compression cannot be removed, palliative treatment such as for the relief of pain is given.
Care has to be given to the bladder and to the prevention of bed-sores.

SUBACUTE COMBINED DEGENERATION OF THE SPINAL CORD

This is a degeneration of the posterior and lateral columns of the spinal cord occurring in patients with pernicious anaemia (and less commonly with diabetes mellitus, pellagra and sprue). It is due to deficiency in the absorption of vitamin B_{12}. Patches of degeneration occur in the affected parts of the cord and fibres lose their myelin and degenerate. The disease can occur before or after the onset of megaloblastic anaemia.

Clinical features
Numbness, tingling and burning sensations occur in the feet and later in the fingers; later still girdle-pains, encircling the trunk, may be experienced. The legs become weak, and because of this and of ataxia the patient has difficulty in walking. Retention of urine can occur. Eventually the untreated patient develops either a spastic paralysis or, if the spinal nerves degenerate, a flaccid paralysis.

Symptoms of pernicious anaemia are likely to be present: pallor, shortness of breath, dizziness, sore tongue and gastro-intestinal disturbance.

Special test
Blood count: for evidence of megaloblastic anaemia.
Gastric juice: for evidence of achlorhydria [4].

Treatment
The disease is prevented by adequate treatment of pernicious anaemia; but if it occurs a high dose of cyanocobalamin (vitamin B_{12}) is given, such as: 1-4 mg. in divided doses during the first week, followed by 250 mcg once weekly until the

[4] *achlorhydria:* absence of hydrochloric acid

blood-picture is normal or nervous features are fading, and then a maintenance dose of 250 mcg every 3-4 weeks. It is important that treatment should begin at once before damage to the nervous system becomes irreparable.

SYRINGOMYELIA[5]:
SYRINGOBULBIA

In this disease the grey matter of the spinal cord degenerates and cysts are formed and press upon tracts. It is called syringomyelia when it occurs in the spinal cord and syringobulbia when it occurs in the medulla oblongata. It usually begins before the age of 30. Its cause is unknown; it has been thought to result from faulty embryological development, for a patient who develops it is quite likely to show some congenital abnormality, such as a high palate, a pigeon-chest or spina bifida.

Clinical features

In *syringomyelia* the clinical features are the result of:
(a) pressure on and then destruction of anterior horn cells; in consequence the muscles supplied by nerve-fibres from these cells become paralysed and waste; and as the disease usually affects the lower part of the cervical cord and the upper part of the dorsal, it is usually the small muscles of the hand that are affected.
(b) pressure on and degeneration of long motor tracts in the cord, producing a spastic paralysis of the legs;
(c) dissociated sensory loss; by destroying the fibres transmitting sensations of pain and temperature, which cross in the spinal cord
The first thing the patient may notice is that he is painlessly burning a finger with a cigarette or painlessly cutting himself. Other results of the anaesthesia are painless whitlows, necrosis[6] of the phalanges, and Charcot's joints of the spinal column, the shoulder or the elbow. Severe pain is sometimes experienced.
In *syringobulbia* the same sort of clinical features are produced, but in the medulla oblongata the disease affects cranial nerve fibres and their nuclei, the patient is likely to develop sensory loss on the face, giddiness, hoarseness, and wasting of the tongue.
Both forms of the disease run a slowly progressive course with long apparently stationary periods. A sudden enlargement of a cyst can cause a spinal block.

Treatment

The only treatment that is thought to be any good is deep X-ray therapy applied to the affected part of the cord in the hope of arresting degeneration; possibly it may relieve any pain the patient experiences. Surgical decompression of a suddenly enlarging cyst is sometimes performed.

AMYOTROPHIC
LATERAL SCLEROSIS [7]

In this disease (whose cause is unknown) there is rapid degeneration of anterior horn cells of the spinal cord and of the cortico-spinal (pyramidal) tracts. The usual age of onset is 40-50 years; it is said to be sometimes inherited.

Clinical features

It runs a rapid course with:
(a) wasting and weakness of the small muscles of the hand and later of muscles in the arms;
(b) fasciculation[8] in the wasting muscles; (c) difficulties in talking and swallowing, wasting of the tongue and weakness of the palate (due to the disease involving the brain-stem[9]);
(d) spastic paralysis of the legs. Although a patient may survive for 20 years, death usually occurs within 2-5 years of the onset, especially when the brain-stem is involved.

[5] *syringomyelia:* from the Greek: *syrinx* – a pipe; *muelos* – marrow
[6] *necrosis:* death of tissue
[7] *amyotrophic:* characterized by muscular wasting; from Greek: *a* – no; *mus* – muscle; *trophe* – nourishment
[8] *fasciculation:* irregular twitching of muscle fibres
[9] *brain-stem:* medulla oblongata, pons

Diseases of the Nervous System

Treatment	No treatment is known to affect its course.

PERONEAL MUSCULAR ATROPHY

Other name: Charcot[1]-Marie[2]-Tooth's[3] disease

This inherited disease of unknown origin usually begins in childhood and is progressive, with sometimes long stationary periods. The spinal cord is affected: the anterior horn cells and their nerve fibres die and the muscles supplied by them become paralysed and wasted, and the posterior columns (in which some forms of sensation are transmitted to the brain) degenerate.

Clinical features

The patient has difficulty in walking and paraesthesia[4] in the legs. Muscle paralysis and wasting begin in the feet and gradually extend upwards as high as the lower one-third of the thigh; the gait is 'stepping'; foot-drop, claw-foot and talipes equino-varus[5] develop. The hands and forearms are similarly paralysed and wasted. Touch, pain and temperature sensation is impaired and eventually lost in the affected parts.

Treatment

No treatment is known that affects the disease. Pain is relieved by analgesics.

FRIEDREICH'S ATAXIA[6]

Other name: hereditary spinal ataxia

This is usually an inherited disease, with several members of a family being affected by it. It begins usually in adolescence. There is degeneration of the posterior columns, the cortico-spinal (pyramidal) tracts and the spino-cerebellar tracts in the spinal cord.

There are several other hereditary ataxias, resembling Friedreich's ataxia, but differing from it in the tracts involved and accordingly in the predominating clinical features.

Clinical features

The patient walks unsteadily, has weakness in his legs, and cannot control his arm movements properly. He becomes progressively more and more incapacitated by paralysis and ataxia, and usually dies of an infection within 20 years of the onset of his illness.

Complications

Blindness, due to optic atrophy.	Sphincter disturbances.
Fits.	Myocardial degeneration.
Club foot.	Kypho-scoliosis.

Treatment

No treatment is known to affect the disease, and only symptomatic and supportive treatment can be given.

MYASTHENIA GRAVIS [7]

This disease is characterized by rapid or abnormal fatigue of voluntary muscles and recovery with rest. It is believed to be due to a biochemical failure at the neuro-muscular junction, acetyl-choline [8] being too rapidly destroyed. It may be an auto-immune disease. It most commonly begins at 20-30 years of age (when more women than men are affected), but can occur at any age and has been seen as a temporary phenomenon in newly-born babies of myasthenic mothers. In about half the patients the thymus is enlarged or shows a tumour of thymic tissue.

[1] *J. M. Charcot* (1825-93): the most famous French neurologist of his day
[2] *P. Marie* (1853-1940): French neurologist
[3] *H. H. Tooth* (1856-1926): English physician
[4] *paraesthesia:* sensations of tingling, burning, etc.
[5] *talipes equino-varus:* deformity in which foot is plantar-flexed and inverted
[6] *N. Friedreich* (1825-82): German neurologist
[7] *myasthenia:* muscle weakness
[8] *acetyl-choline:* a chemical substance liberated at the endings of nerves in muscle and necessary for stimulation of muscle contractions

Clinical features After using a set of muscles several times the patient finds that he cannot go on using them until he has rested them for a time. The onset of the illness is usually slow, but can be abrupt. The muscles most commonly involved are those involved in vision, speaking, chewing and swallowing. Weakness of the eye muscles causes diplopia[9] and ptosis. The arms and legs can be involved. Patients may have difficulty in shaving or brushing the hair, may have to hold the head with one hand, or have great difficulty in chewing and swallowing a mouthful. Attacks of dyspnoea can occur. In the severe case the patient shows the typical 'myasthenic facies' — with bilateral ptosis, an inability to close the eyes completely, and a half-open mouth.

The course of the disease is variable. Its severity is apt to vary from day to day; there may be remissions for several years; some patients stay at more or less the same level for years; others deteriorate rapidly and die within a few months of the onset. Pregnancy sometimes improves, sometimes worsens the condition. It is likely to be worse immediately after childbirth, during upper respiratory tract infections and during emotional distress. A *myasthenic crisis*, with rapidly developing paralysis can be produced by natural deterioration or precipitated by infection, exercise, childbirth or some drugs (including streptomycin, neomycin, quinine, quinidine, morphine, barbiturates).

Treatment Neostigimine bromide (Prostigmin) prolongs the action of acetyl-choline. It may be given orally in doses of 15 mg when required, which may be many times a day. Pyridostigmine bromide, 60 mg 3-4 times a day has a more prolonged effect. Ambenonium chloride in doses of 10-25 mg has a longer action than pyridostigmine but more troublesome side-effects. In emergencies, neostigmine methylsulphate (also called Prostigmin) is given by injection in doses of 0.5-2.5 mg. In this way the patient can cope with the minor activities of life, but he has still to lead a restricted life with the minimum of muscular activities. Removal of the thymus may produce an improvement. Treatment of a *crisis* is by (a) neostigmine 0.5 mg by subcutaneous or intramuscular injection, (b) artificially assisted respiration with a tracheotomy if necessary.

NEUROPATHY Neuropathy (neuritis) is the term used to describe any degeneration of spinal nerves. Among the many causes are:
1. Bruising, compression, stretching: obstetric injuries, pressure on nerve-roots by disease of the spine, pressure by tools in various occupations; pressure by crutches, cervical rib, narrowing of carpal tunnel; prolapse of an intervertebral disc.
2. As a complication of an infectious disease: diphtheria, tuberculosis, streptococcal infections, tetanus, gonorrhoea, typhoid fever, malaria, leprosy.
3. In some metabolic diseases: vitamin deficiences (beri-beri, pellagra, sprue, chronic alcoholism, food faddism); diabetes mellitus; pernicious anaemia; gout, any severe chronic disease.
4. Poisoning by arsenic, bismuth, lead, mercury, phosphorus, carbon disulphide, etc.
[9] *diplopia:* double vision

Diseases of the Nervous System

5. Vascular disease: athero-sclerosis, poly-arthritis.

6. Some malignant diseases: carcinoma of the lung, multiple myeloma.

Clinical features

There is considerable variation in the nerves affected, the speed of onset, severity and course. In general, a neuritis is likely to show:

(a) *Motor signs:* weakness of muscles, going on to some degree of flaccid paralysis, wasting, loss of tendon reflexes, and in severe chronic neuritis muscular fibrosis and contractures.

(b) *Sensory signs:* pain in the distribution of the affected nerves; pain is variable in intensity, duration and distribution; may be sharp, burning, pricking or deep and severe; there may be hyper-aesthesia, with severe pain being produced by a pinprick or other slight stimulation. Loss of sensation in the area of skin supplied by affected nerve is often small.

(c) *Autonomic nervous system signs:* excessive sweating at first, followed by loss of sweating; the skin becomes dry and shiny, the nails become grooved, there may be osteo-porosis[1].

There can be a general neuritis affecting many nerves, or individual nerves can be affected in particular kinds of neuritis.

1. *Erb[2]-Duchenne[3] paralysis* is due to injury of the upper roots of the brachial plexus (C5 & 6). The arm is held in the 'waiter's tip' position, hanging down close to the trunk with the palm backwards. Sensation is lost on the outer side of the shoulder, upper arm and forearm.

2. *Klumpke's paralysis[4]* is due to injury to the lower roots of the brachial plexus (C8 & T1). There is wasting of the muscles of the forearm and the small muscles of the hand, with sensory loss over the inner side of the forearm and hand.

3. *Cervical rib[5]* (scalenus anterior syndrome). In this condition the brachial plexus or the subclavian artery or both are pressed on by a cervical rib or by the scalenus anterior muscle or are squeezed between clavicle and 1st rib. It occurs mostly in women aged 40-60. The actual cause is obscure: it may be due to a dropping of the shoulder-girdle, or to spasm or over-development of the scalenus anterior muscle.

Clinical features

(a) pain in the back of the shoulder, extending into the neck and down the inner side of the arm, made worse by lifting, carrying and stretching;

(b) hyper-aesthesiae on the inner side of the arm;

(c) weakness and wasting of the interosseous muscles of the hand and of some of the muscles of the forearm.

(d) due to pressure on the subclavian artery:— on the affected side, a slightly lower

[1] *osteo-porosis:* reduction of calcium in bone

[2] *W. H. Erb* (1840-1921), German physician

[3] *G. B. A. Duchenne* ('of Boulogne') (1806-75) French neurologist

[4] *A. D. Klumpke* (1859-1927), French neurologist

[5] *cervical rib:* small rudimentary additional rib attached at one end to 7th cervical vertebra and at the other by bone or a fibrous band to the 1st rib

blood-pressure, weakness or obliteration of the radial pulse; in severe cases gangrene of the finger-tips.

Treatment: Manual work is reduced to a minimum. The arm is carried in a sling. Pillows are arranged at night to throw the shoulder forwards. If these measures fail, the cervical rib is removed or the scalenus anterior muscle divided.

4. *Cervical spondylosis* is a degeneration of the cervical spine with narrowing and protrusion of the intervertebral disc and pressure both on the spinal cord and on the roots of the spinal nerves in their foramina. It is a disease of middle and old age. It produces pain in the distribution of the affected nerves – in the neck, shoulders, arms and hands – hyper-algesia, small areas of cutaneous anaesthesia and slight muscular weakness and wasting.

Treatment is by supporting the head and neck with a plastic or plaster collar. Carrying light weights on the head is likely to decrease the incidence and severity of the disease, and could be used in treatment.

5. *Brachial neuropathy* (plexusitis) is an illness of uncertain cause and mechanics. The brachial plexus becomes tender; pain begins in the shoulder and radiates into the neck and arm; there may be some small areas of anaesthesia; paralysis of the muscles of the shoulder and arm can occur. Recovery is slow and often incomplete. *Treatment* is by rest and supporting the arm in a sling.

6. *Shoulder-Hand Syndrome* is a condition which occurs in some patients who have had a myocardial infarction a few months before. Pain, tenderness and limitation of movement are experienced in one or both shoulders. Later the hands and fingers may swell, become discoloured and develop a deformity like Dupuytren's contracture[6]. It is thought to be due in some way to inactivity, poor circulation and joint damage. About 9 out of 10 patients recover; the remainder develop irreversible changes.

Treatment is by active and passive movements, local heat and analgesics.

7. *Carpal Tunnel Syndrome.* The median nerve passes at the front of the wrist beneath the transverse carpal ligament. The carpal tunnel is the tunnel between the ligament and the bones of the wrist; the tendons of the long flexors of the hand pass through the tunnel. The tunnel can become narrowed by tenosynovitis of these tendons, by osteo-arthritis of the carpus and by thickening of the ligament. The median nerve is compressed, producing paraesthesia, pain and muscle wasting. The syndrome is seen typically in hard-working middle-aged women, and can be bilateral.

In *cubital tunnel syndrome* compression of the ulnar nerve at the elbow produces crippling of the hand.

In *tarsal tunnel syndrome* compression of the nerves to the feet is a cause of "burning feet".

Clinical features   Signs of median nerve compression are:
(a) pain and paraesthesiae in the thumb and index finger, sometimes spreading upwards into the forearm;

[6] *Dupuytren's contracture:* contracture of hand and fingers produced by excessive fibrosis in palm

(b) wasting of the small muscles of the thumb.

Treatment is by supporting the wrist with a splint. If this fails, it may be necessary to divide the carpal ligament. Injection of hydrocortisone into the tunnel may provide relief.

8. *Sciatica* is due to pressure on a lower lumbar or upper sacral nerve-root by prolapse of an intervertebral disc. The sciatic nerve is formed from nerves L 4,5, S 1, 2 & 3. The name was given to this condition when it was thought to be due to a disease of the sciatic nerve itself. Severe pain is felt along the course of the nerve and its branches, from the back and down the buttock, back of the thigh, calf and foot. Sensory loss is usually slight. The knee-jerk is sometimes lost, the ankle-jerk usually. The hamstrings, the gastrocnemius group and the dorsal extensors are weakened. Acute pain is produced by stretching the nerve by flexing the hip with the knee fully extended.

 Treatment is at first by rest, massage, analgesics and local heat. Subsequently the patient's back should be supported with a lumbo-sacral belt. If pain is severe and conservative treatment unsuccessful, it may be necessary to operate and remove the protruded part of the intervertebral disc.

9. *Arsenical neuropathy* is mainly a sensory lesion with pain, paraesthesia, impairment of muscle sense, and tenderness of affected nerves. Ataxia can occur. Other evidence of arsenical poisoning is likely to be present: gastro-intestinal disturbances, hyper-pigmentation of the skin, hyper-keratosis[7] of the skin of the soles and palms.

10. *Lead neuropathy* involves mainly motor nerves. The arms are usually more involved than the legs, and wrist-drop is typical. Sensory symptoms are mild.

11. *Alcoholic neuropathy* is due to vitamin deficiency and not to alcohol itself. It is a mixed motor and sensory neuritis. Usually it begins with pains in the calves and numbness in the feet. Ataxia is common. Muscular weakness is apparent in foot-drop and wasting of arms and legs. Other evidence of alcoholism is usually obvious.

12. *Diabetic neuropathy* is a common complication of diabetes mellitus and can develop when the diabetes is apparently well controlled. Pain, tenderness of the calves, and loss of tendon reflexes occur.

13. *Poly-arteritis nodosa* can produce a *neuropathy* in which cranial and spinal nerves are involved.

Treatment of all kinds of neuropathy

The specific cause of the neuropathy is found and if possible corrected. Rest in bed is usually necessary when the illness is severe. Paralysed muscles must not be allowed to become stretched. For foot-drop a board or box is placed in the bed to keep the feet slightly dorsi-flexed and a cradle to keep the weight of the bed-clothes off the feet. For paralysis of the arm causing wrist-drop a splint is necessary. Other splints are fixed where required. Pain is relieved by analgesics. The services of a physiotherapist will be required for the provision of massage, active and passive

[7] *hyper-keratosis:* hypertrophy of the horny layer of the skin

movements and heat. The patient must take an adequate diet and additional vitamins of the B group should be given where there is evidence of malnutrition.

ACUTE PERIPHERAL NEUROPATHY

This form is of unknown origin; about half the cases follow an infection of the gastro-intestinal or upper respiratory tracts. It has been thought to be an auto-immune disease.

Clinical features

It occurs in several forms, which have been regarded as separate diseases. In one there is a rapidly developing paralysis of the legs, followed by paralysis of arms, trunk and face. Sensory symptoms occur, but are overshadowed by the paralysis. Paralysis of the lips, tongue, pharynx and larynx produce difficulties in speaking, eating and swallowing; respiratory paralysis can be a cause of death. In another form, paralysis is associated with fever, enlarged cervical lymph-nodes and jaundice; in a third form the muscles of the eve are paralysed.

Special test

CSF: may show a great increase in protein up to 2,000 mg per 100 ml (the normal is 15-45 mg), with no increase in the number of cells or only a slight increase.

Treatment

There is no specific treatment. The usual treatment of a neuropathy is carried out. Some patients have responded well to azathioprine. Cortisone is tried. ACTH is given for severe attacks. Artificial feeding, cathererization, naso-pharyngeal suction, and artificial respiration are sometimes needed.

RESTLESS LEGS

Other name: nocturnal myoclonus.
This condition affects both sexes and all age-groups; about 5 per cent of normal people suffer from it. The cause is unknown: it is thought to be due to some disturbance of the nervous or vascular supply of the leg. It can be an early symptom of diabetes mellitus and is also associated with anaemia, uraemia, chronic pulmonary disease, after gastrectomy, and in the later stages of pregnancy.

Clinical features

An intolerable itching and creeping sensation in the legs below the knee and sometimes above it, is relieved only by movement. It tends to occur late in the day, and the patient has to walk about or keep his legs moving; sleep is lost. Many sufferers cannot sit still, and air- and motor-journeys are impossible. The arms are sometimes affected.

Treatment

Diazepam and other anti-convulsants provide relief. Hot baths or cold sponging may be helpful.

14 Mental Illness

There is no absolute distinction between mental and physical illnesses, and the separation of them arose because in some illnesses the patient's behaviour and words became so abnormal that special provisions, in the form of mental hospitals, had to be made either for the patient's own welfare or for the protection of other people. Actually many so-called mental illnesses have definite physical causes: e.g. dementia is due to degeneration of cells in the cerebral cortex, general paralysis to syphilis of the brain. In other mental illnesses the cause appears to be some fault of personality or to be due to some kind of stress arising in the patient's own mind or in the home, the family or the social setting in which he lives or works.

Psychiatry is the branch of medicine that concerns itself with mental illness and mental retardation (see Chapter 16).

Mental illnesses can be classified as:

1. *Neuroses* (psycho-neuroses): anxiety states, hysteria, obsessional-compulsive states.
2. *Psychosomatic diseases.*
3. *Psychopathic states.*
4. *Psychoses:* schizophrenia, affective disorders, dementias, mental illnesses arising from alcoholism, from brain infections or injury (see Chap. 13); etc.

There may in some patients be a considerable overlap of symptoms (a depressed patient may for example, be very anxious), and the division into these four classes is not an absolute one.

Terms

The following terms are used to describe abnormalities of thought, feeling, behaviour, consciousness and speech.

1. Disturbances of thought

Poverty of ideas: the thoughts a patient has are reduced below his normal; he can think of little or nothing.

Thought-blocking: thoughts seem to be prevented from coming into consciousness.

Flight of ideas: thoughts rush abnormally quickly through the patient's mind.

Ideas of depersonalization: ideas that one is not normal, is being altered in subtle ways, that one's limbs do not belong, etc.

Ideas of derealization (unreality): ideas that the world has become unreal, strange, unnatural.

Ideas of reference: patient has ideas that people are referring to him in speech and gesture.

Delusion: a false belief, commonly of some form of persecution, e.g. of being poisoned, followed, secretly x-radiated. *Nihilistic delusion:* that one is dead, turned to dust, has never been born, etc. *Delusion of grandeur:* that one is very wealthy, powerful, titled. *Folie à deux:* delusions or other abnormal ideas shared by two people living together and sharing very much the same life and thought.

Hallucination: a sensory impression without external stimulus to cause it.

Auditory hallucinations: of sounds and voices. *Visual hallucinations:* of shapes, faces or people. *Lilliputian hallucinations:* of tiny people. Hallucinations of smell, taste and touch can also occur.

2. **Disturbances of feeling**	*Euphoria:* a feeling of well-being. *Elation:* a feeling of extreme well-being and happiness. *Depression:* a feeling of intense sadness.
3. **Disturbances of behaviour**	*Stereotypy:* the repetition of the same act over and over again. *Perseveration:* a persistent repetition of words spoken or actions performed in spite of the patient's efforts to say or do something else. *Negativism:* the doing by the patient of the opposite of what he is told to do. *Echolalia:* the repetition in the same words by the patient of anything that is said to him. *Echopraxia:* the repetition by the patient of anything that is done in front of him.
4. **Disturbance of consciousness and memory**	*Disorientation:* a faulty appreciation of time, place or person. *Confusion:* imperfect awareness of what is going on, with muddled thoughts and restlessness. *Delirium:* an acute confusion in which contact with reality is lost partly or completely. *Stupor:* the patient appears oblivious of everything and lies like a log, but may be able to appreciate what is going on and being said around him. *Coma:* patient is unconscious and cannot be roused. *Amnesia:* loss of memory. *Confabulation:* the invention of events to fill up gaps in memory.
. **Disorders of speech**	*Neologism:* a new word invented by the patient. *Word-salad:* a jumbling-up of words *Circumstantiality:* talking in great detail about a topic, wandering round and round it but never leaving it.
ANXIETY STATE	This is a condition in which the patient shows excessive anxiety often associated with over-activity of the autonomic nervous system. By some psychiatrists it is regarded as one of the affective psychoses. Anxiety to some degree is a normal

259 *Mental Illness*

reaction to worry, stress and danger; but in a patient with an anxiety state, his reactions are excessive, prolonged beyond the time of the emergency, or without obvious cause. A family history of anxiety may be obtained, the patient having been brought up by anxiety-ridden parents. An anxiety state can occur in childhood, adolescence, adult life or old age, and in any degree of severity. Anxiety can be a feature of other illnesses, e.g. depression, early schizophrenia, thyrotoxicosis.

Clinical features
An *acute anxiety state* is usually precipitated by acute stress, such as going into battle or having a sudden bereavement, the amount of stress a person can tolerate without breaking down being peculiar to that person. In an extremely acute anxiety state, the patient is terrified, immobilized, unable to do anything; he is drenched in sweat, with a pounding heart, rapid respiration and dilated pupils. From this he can pass into a state of subacute anxiety with headache, fatigue, insomnia, disturbed sleep. A person of previously good personality should recover completely from an acute anxiety state.

In a *chronic anxiety state* the mental and physical symptoms are likely to wax and wane without completely clearing up. Common complaints are of fatigue, palpitations, black-outs, tremor, sweating, diarrhoea or constipation, frequency of micturition, insomnia, fears of dying or going insane, depression, irritability, inability to concentrate, fears of being shut up in a closed room, of open spaces.

An *effort syndrome* (soldier's heart, neuro-circulatory asthenia) is an anxiety state in which the predominating features are fatigue, palpitations, precordial pain and shortness of breath; the patient is usually of asthenic build [8] and an inadequate personality, called upon to engage in hard and potentially dangerous work.

Treatment
Acute Anxiety state. The patient is removed from the stress-provoking situation and sedated by barbiturates or tranquillisers. Convalescence should be short.

Chronic anxiety state. Treatment is more difficult and not very effective. Psychotherapy by simple reassurance and suggestion is given. Sedation at night may be necessary. A tranquillizer, especially chlorpromazine (Largactil), is usually given. Modified insulin treatment is often useful: a course consists of daily treatment 5-6 days a week, for 4-6 weeks of increasing amounts of insulin until mild hypoglycaemia [9] is produced, which is allowed to continue for 2-3 hours and then stopped by giving sugar. A psycho-analyst is likely to advise a course of psychoanalysis.

HYSTERIA
In this condition psychological stress produces disturbances of function, of behaviour or of consciousness. Hysteria takes many forms and mimics many organic diseases. Any one exposed for too long to too severe a strain can produce a hysterical reaction, but signs of hysteria are most likely to occur in a person of hysterical

[8] *asthenic build:* type of physical build characterized by slender trunk, lack of fat, poorly developed muscles
[9] *hypo-glycaemia:* reduced amount of sugar in the blood

personality – one who is immature, dependent upon others and given to self-display, with reactions basically infantile, self-centred and hypersensitive, and liable to become annoyed, moody and querulous if he does not get the attention he demands. He usually comes of a family given to hysterical reactions and with many abnormal members. Hysteria can be brought on by any form of stress, can follow physical illness, and can occur as one of the signs of other diseases – of epilepsy, schizophrenia, depression, anxiety state, disseminated sclerosis, cerebral tumour, cerebral arterio-sclerosis and brain-injury.

Clinical features   These usually take the form of (a) *conversion reactions* with a disturbance of physical functions and (b) *dissociative reactions* with disturbances of consciousness, memory and behaviour. In addition a patient may show *la belle indifférence,* a distinctive lack of concern about his condition, regarding, for example, a paralysed limb as if it was of no importance whatsoever; he can however have outbursts of tantrums.

Conversion reactions   *Muscular paralysis* can occur, usually involving one limb, part of one limb, half the body. The paralysis can be flaccid or spastic. Tendon reflexes and electrical reactions of muscle are normal, and wasting does not occur unless the paralysis lasts a long time. Contractures can be produced. The patient may have a peculiar gait unlike that produced by any physical disease.

Hysterical aphonia is an ability to speak except in a whisper. In *hysterical mutism* the patient can make no sound at all. *Hysterical stammering* can follow an emotional shock.

Hysterical anaesthesia can occur, affect usually a limb or part of a limb, often the part covered by a glove, sock or stocking and with no relationship to the normal distribution of sensory nerves to the skin. Areas of anaesthesia can be readily produced by suggestion. *Paraesthesiae* of various kinds – burning, tingling, itching, etc. – can occur. Anaesthesia and paraesthesia can involve mucous membranes.

Hysterical blindness, sometimes with spasm of the eyelids and photophobia, can come on suddenly and disappear as suddenly, after lasting any period of time from minutes to years.

Hysterical deafness can occur.

Hysterical visceral disturbances can take the form of paroxysms of rapid breathing or of rapid cardiac action, of attacks of diarrhoea, constipation, vomiting, the production of intestinal noises, belching, the expulsion of flatus. Blushing and blanching of the skin can be produced, and dermographia – writing on the skin causing raised lines. Some hysterics appear to be able to raise their temperature by several degrees. A hysterical fit can occur, mimicking a major epileptic fit.

Dissociative reactions   These are conditions occurring in hysterics, psychopaths and early schizophrenics. They are likely to appear when the patient has got himself into trouble and there is no easy way out. The diagnosis from malingering can be difficult.

A *hysterical amnesia* is a loss of memory, complete or incomplete, for people and events in the patient's life. He claims not to know who he is, not to recognize his relatives or associates, not to know what he does. The amnesia can pass into a fugue. A *fugue* is a 'twilight' state, in which the patient wanders about with impaired consciousness, usually not washing or in other ways caring for himself, and unable to state who he is and how he has got to where he is. In a *hysterical trance* the patient lies in a condition resembling sleep, but with anaesthesia to ordinary stimuli and sometimes without tendon reflexes. In *somnambulism* (sleep-walking) the patient, without waking up, gets out of bed and wanders about in the house or in the street. He may put himself back to bed or may wake up where he is, unable to say how he got there. Some quite normal children sleep-walk.

The *Munchausen syndrome* is the name given to the condition shown by some people, often pathological liars, gross hysterics, ex-patients in a mental hospital or ex-prisoners, who get themselves admitted into hospital over and over again, under different names, give a history of medical or surgical *crises* (at which they become adept), and submit to investigations and operations.

Mass hysteria can occur, mainly in institutions for girls or young women or assemblies of them, as an outbreak of disturbed behaviour resulting from a combination of suggestion and shared apprehension.

Treatment The treatment of hysteria is difficult, for the patient has a personality that nothing is likely to change, and symptoms appear and disappear without apparent reason. If an attack is due to known stress, removal from the stress, rest, sedation and psychotherapy can help. Hypnosis has been used to relieve a paralysis or aphonia, but the disappearance of one symptom may be followed by the appearance of another. No one treatment seems to be any better than another, and patients get well or remain ill for inexplicable reasons.

OBSESSIONAL-
COMPULSIVE
STATES

In this condition the patient has to keep on thinking or behaving in a repetitive way. He is often the child of obsessional parents and has always been expected to be neat, clean and tidy. Obsessional-compulsive states are common in childhood, and many children go through periods of having to behave in certain ways. Other people are mildly compulsive — having to make sure that the door is locked, the gas turned off and so on. In an obsessional-compulsive state all this is grossly exaggerated. There are many kinds of obsessional thoughts and compulsive actions, many of them associated with ideas of dirt. The patient may have to wash himself many times a day, with cleansing himself after excretion perhaps being a long anxious ritual; he may have to fold his clothes in certain ways, to keep them in certain places. He may have a fear of uttering four-letter words.

Obsessional ideas can occur in depression or be an early sign of schizophrenia; occasionally a severe obsessional becomes a schizophrenic.

Treatment is difficult to evaluate, for many patients wax and wane without obvious reason. Tranquillizers can help associated anxiety. Psychotherapy of a simple kind or by psychoanalysis may be given.

PSYCHOSOMATIC
DISEASES

The psychosomatic diseases are those 'physical' or organic diseases of which emotional factors are thought to be the predominating cause. It has been estimated that of patients referred to the Medical Out-Patients of a general hospital, one third have an organic disease, one third have a mental illness, and one third have an organic disease largely produced by emotional factors.

Emotional factors play a large part in many conditions and can produce many minor symptoms such as headache, vague pains, nervousness, dizziness, palpitations, rapid or irregular heart-beat, pre-cordial pain or discomfort; dyspepsia, nausea, vomiting, and other disturbances of the gastro-intestinal tract; itching, sweating, paraesthesiae.

In conditions considered to be psychosomatic, the stress produced by emotional disturbance is thought to be the cause of serious organic changes. It is argued that as emotional factors are known to produce such symptoms as those detailed above, so can they produce longer-lasting disturbance and actual chronic physical changes in various tissues of the body.

The patient may show a particular type of personality; the onset should be associated with the onset of an acute emotional emergency; improvement and relapses are likely to be related to changes in emotional life; and psychotherapy should be capable of producing improvement or cure.

Among the diseases thought by some to be essentially psychosomatic are:
peptic ulcer
hyper-thyroidism
essential hypertension
anorexia nervosa.

Anorexia nervosa[1]

This is usually a disease of young women. It occurs rarely in young men. Its precise causes are not clear; it can be precipitated by emotional stresses, often involving the patient's mother, and hence is considered by some to be a psychosomatic disease. She may have a fat mother and has decided not to be like her, she may associate fatness with pregnancy and sex, she may have been over-weight and decided to slim.

Clinical features

The patient develops a great aversion for food. She practically gives up eating and in consequence becomes emaciated, anaemic and constipated. She develops anaemia and a down-like hair grows all over the skin. In spite of emaciation she is over-active and given to long solitary walks.

If the patient does not respond to treatment she is likely to die of starvation or of tuberculosis or some other infection.

Treatment

1. The patient has to be admitted into hospital for the necessary control cannot be exercised at home.
2. All efforts have to be made to get her to eat and precautions have to be taken to ensure that she swallows food and does not throw it away.
3. A course of modified insulin treatment with chloropromazine (Largactil) is given.
4. Electro-convulsive treatment (ECT) is sometimes given.

PSYCHOPATHIC STATES

The term psychopathic state is used to describe some conditions which are not quite neuroses or psychoses, although the person who shows it may at times show

[1] *anorexia:* loss of appetite

features of either. A *psychopath* is a person who behaves irresponsibly, committing anti-social and sometimes aggressive acts regardless of their effects upon others and of any form of punishment he may suffer in consequence. Usually the patient does not alter his behaviour whether he is treated kindly or harshly.

In childhood the potential psychopath may not have been noticed as abnormal, but he may have been regarded as cold and selfish, naughtier than other children, unchecked by discipline, a disturber of other children's play.

The *intelligent psychopath* lives on his wits, usually following no occupation for long, sponging on others, passing dud cheques, stealing. He is often a *pathological liar,* capable of inventing the most wonderful stories about himself and his amorous, financial and military successes, wearing decorations and uniforms he is not entitled to, putting up at the best hotels and leaving them without paying the bill. He can have vivid sexual phantasies and commit sexual crimes. In lower walks of life he lives by stealing or scrounging or on the earnings of prostitutes.

The aggressive psychopath is a moody, irritable and resentful individual, who is liable to attack people without provocation or on the slightest provocation. He is likely to have an abnormal EEG. Treatment by tranquillizers and anti-convulsants may be of some use.

Kleptomania is a morbid impulse to steal. Typically the kleptomanic is a middle-aged woman with no financial need to steal who takes what she can from shops, from the houses of friends, from hotels. The stolen articles may not be used.

SCHIZOPHRENIA [2]

Schizophrenia occurs in many forms; a patient is likely to show a disturbance of normal thinking, a substitution of abnormal thinking for normal thinking, a disturbance of emotion, abnormal behaviour, and withdrawal from the normal world into an abnormal self.

The cause of the disease is unknown, but there is evidence that it is a biochemical disorder of the brain. Heredity is an important factor, and there is a high incidence of the disease and of other mental abnormalities in the families of schizophrenics. It usually begins in early adult life, but it can begin earlier or later. It is most frequent in people living in town-centres and in people from the lowest socio-economic class. Schizophrenics being often rootless, shifting and feckless people, there is a high incidence of the disease among poor migrants.

Between 30 and 50 per cent of schizophrenics show no abnormality or severe personality disorder before the onset of the illness; the others are likely to show a pre-psychotic personality characterized by shyness, timidity, lack of ambition, and self-absorption.

Clinical features

The illness may begin slowly or suddenly.

In the slowly-developing disease the patient withdraws from ordinary affairs. He is likely to develop ideas of de-realization and depersonalization; and from this to develop delusions of persecution — that he is being followed, impersonated, mentioned in newspapers or on the radio, that his thoughts are controlled, that

[2] *schizophrenia:* from Greek: *skhizein* — to split; *phren* — mind

his organs are being tampered with, that he is being poisoned, etc. He is then likely to have hallucinations — usually of abusive voices and less commonly of faces, people, shapes, smells, tastes.

From the beginning he shows emotional changes, losing his natural affections and sometimes developing a viciousness towards his relatives. He can have depressive episodes and attempt suicide.

His behaviour varies from being normal to being very odd, with grimacing, peculiar gestures and apparently purposeless acts.

In the *hebephrenic* and *catatonic* forms of schizophrenia gross disturbances of behaviour occur. The patient can be very excited and violent, or at other times stand motionless or hold himself in peculiar attitudes or show negativism or automatic obedience or pass into stupor. In the *simple form* there is a gradual deterioration into a world of unreality and detachment from ordinary affairs. In the *paranoid form* delusions of persecution are the common feature.

The course of a schizophrenic illness is very variable. An attack can last anything from a few days to a lifetime. Usually, but not always, the more acute the illness the better is the outlook. Recovery from an acute attack is common, but relapse can occur; and the more attacks a patient has the less likely is he to recover. The simple and the paranoid forms usually pursue a steady course. If *chronic schizophrenia* develops the patient lives all day in his abnormal thoughts, behaves oddly, has persecutory or sometimes grandiose delusions, is much hallucinated. He can go on in this state for years, eventually dying of some physical disease.

Treatment
Schizophrenia presents many problems of treatment. There is no specific treatment and as many patients recover from the first attack, it is difficult to assess the value of any particular treatment.

Drug treatment is mainly by tranquillizers, which can in some patients diminish the delusional and hallucinatory experiences and improve behaviour to such an extent that the patient's stay in hospital is shortened, patients who would otherwise have to be in hospital can live in the community, and the lot of the chronic patient is improved. However, these drugs are not a cure; relapse is common if taking them is discontinued. Electro-convulsive treatment (ECT) is used in the treatment of stupor and states of excitement. Many chronic patients are improved by the regular administration of tranquillizers, by employment in crafts and industrial work, by group activities and by the full employment of all the therapeutic facilities of a modern psychiatric hospital.

Infantile Autism
Other name: childhood psychosis
This condition begins during the first two years of life. It can occur in children with any degree of intelligence, from the above normal to the severely retarded. The causes of it are not known. The child becomes self-absorbed, withdrawn, cold, ceasing to show love for his parents, although he may cling to them in an impersonal way. He stops communicating, not speaking, showing echolalia or making up words. He avoids any eye-to-eye gaze. He does not play normally, but engages in apparently

meaningless activity. He may at times show acute anxiety or flashes of normal behaviour. Other features (which can occur in other conditions) are repetitive twisting or flicking movements of the fingers, hands or whole body; hyperactivity; self-injury; feeding difficulties; delayed bladder or bowel control.

Some improve or recover; but others persist in some degree of mental invalidism. Various treatments (psychotherapeutic, educational, drug) are tried, but there is none known that will with certainty improve the condition.

AFFECTIVE STATES

In these mental illnesses there is a marked change in mood towards excessive happiness or excessive sadness. Three conditions are described: (a) manic-depressive psychosis; (b) involutional melancholia; (c) reactive depression.
They may be variations of the same basic condition.

Manic-depressive psychosis

In this condition a person is liable to have recurrent attacks of mania or of depression or of both. The causes are unknown. A family history of the condition is common. First attacks usually occur in early adult life, but they are not unknown in childhood and old age. Having once occurred, recurrence is common. During the intervals, which may last from days to years, the patient is perfectly well, unless he has very frequent or prolonged attacks.

Mania is a state of happiness and excitement. In *hypomania*, the mildest form, the patient is talkative, restless, bubbling over with ideas, rarely finishing anything he starts. His condition may not get any worse and eventually clears up. *Acute mania* is a more severe form. In it the patient is definitely ill. He is extremely excited; very restless, talking non-stop; not sleeping; and wearing everybody out. *Delirious mania* is an even more acute form in which the patient becomes confused, delirious and so physically exhausted that he can die. Attacks are otherwise self-limiting, usually lasting for several weeks and then stopping suddenly.

Treatment is by admission to hospital, sedation, and the provision of adequate nourishment.

Depression can too be of 3 degrees. In *mild depression* (which is often unrecognized for what it is) the patient has feelings of despondency and failure, and complains of headache, tiredness, indigestion. An attack usually clears up in a few weeks or months; it is perhaps only when it has recurred several times that its real nature is recognized. In *acute depression* the patient is obviously ill. He expresses ideas of wickedness, failure and hopelessness, out of which he cannot be argued. Suicide is commonly in his mind and frequently attempted, occasionally the patient murders his family and the family pet. He is retarded — very slowed up in all his mental processes. He is likely to have severe insomnia. Attacks can last from weeks to months. A *depressive stupor* is a depression of such severity that the patient lies like a log, not eating, not speaking, not emptying bladder or bowel.

In about 1 patient in 5 depression becomes chronic, about 1 in 6 commits suicide, and the rest make fairly good recovery from their attacks.

Treatment of depression is by taking adequate precautions against suicide, by psychotherapy, by giving anti-depressant drugs, by maintaining nourishment, by ensuring sleep, and giving electro-convulsive treatment.

Drugs commonly used are:
(a) imipramine: in doses of 75-150 mg daily in divided doses for patients under the age of 60, and in smaller doses for older patients
(b) amitriptyline: in doses of up to 225 mg daily in divided doses for older patients
(c) protriptyline: in doses of 15-60 mg daily in divided doses
(d) doxepin: in doses of 30-50 mg daily in divided doses; it has antidepressive and anti-anxiety properties.

Involutional depression

This form of depression occurs during the 'involutional period' of life — between 45 and 65 years. The patient may or may not have arterio-sclerosis; he may or may not have had an illness, an operation, a bereavement. An attack is characterized by extreme depression, depressive ideas of a very abnormal content — for example, that the patient has no stomach or bowels, that he is already dead, that he will never die. He is agitated and anxious. Suicide is common.

The illness can be a long one and the patient may be left with some degree of mental impairment for the rest of his life.

Treatment is as for depression of the manic-depressive variety.

Reactive depression

This arises as a reaction to some definite event, such as illness, loss of money or job, or bereavement. The patient is likely to be depressed, tired, and unable to concentrate, and to complain of various mild physical disabilities. Treatment is given by improving his circumstances if possible, by giving reassurance, and by tranquillizers and anti-depressant drugs.

DEMENTIA

Dementia is a progressive decline of all mental faculties due to degeneration and death of the cells in the cerebral cortex. It can be:
1. *Senile dementia:* a form of dementia which begins over the age of 65.
2. *Presenile dementia:* certain kinds of dementia (such as Pick's dementia, Alzheimer's dementia) beginning usually in mid-adult life. Jakob-Creutzfeldt's disease (in which presenile dementia is associated with spastic paralysis and parkinsonism) is due to a virus infection.
3. *Athero-sclerotic dementia:* in which the dementia is due to the cutting off of the blood-supply to parts of the brain.
4. *Dementia:* due to other progressive diseases of the brain, such as Huntington's chorea, general paralysis, paralysis agitans, disseminated sclerosis, severe injury of the brain.

Clinical features

All these dementias have many features in common, but some show individual variations. Common features are:
(a) Decline in intelligence; the patient making errors he would not previously have made, not understanding things, and not being able to grasp new situations and problems.
(b) loss of memory: this is usually loss of memory for all events, remote as well as recent, although the patient is characteristically supposed to remember events of childhood when he cannot remember what happened the day before.

Mental Illness

(c) Emotional disturbances: irritability, peevishness, anxiety, agitation, incessant talking.

(d) Insomnia: inverted sleep rhythm (the patient sleeping by day and being awake at night), nocturnal delirium.

(e) Delusional ideas: that he is being neglected, robbed, poisoned.

(f) Previously repressed tendencies asserting themselves: stealing, making homosexual advances, making sexual attacks on children.

(g) Irresponsible behaviour: wandering, getting up at night, trying to light fires, turning on gas taps, not dressing, micturating publicly, assaulting people.

The course of a dementia is downhill. The course is steadily downhill in most dementias: memory becomes completely lost, the mind is blank; excitement is replaced by apathy; physical decline sets in, fractures are common; and a fracture, operation or acute physical illness can precipitate an acute confusional state, in which restlessness, delusions and hallucinations are prominent features. Patients with senile dementia usually die within two years, death being due to an infection, to general weakness, a fracture, or bedsores, which can come on very rapidly. Patients with presenile dementia may live for 5-10 years. In athero-sclerotic dementia, the course of the illness is very irregular, for the patient can suffer attacks of temporary or permanent obstruction of the blood-supply to a part of the brain and then suffer attacks of unconsciousness, paralysis, or speech disorders, from which he may make a partial recovery.

Treatment   The patient should be looked after at home for as long as possible; for many patients admission into a mental hospital is necessary. The patient should be kept ambulant for as long as possible. Attention has to be paid to providing adequate nourishment, to the bowels and bladder, and to preventing bedsores. Insomnia is treated with paraldehyde or chloral hydrate. Restlessness is controlled by tranquillizers.

15   Addictions, Drug-induced Disorders, Poisoning

An addict is a person who takes a substance for the immediate pleasure it gives him, develops a craving for it, acquires a tolerance to it and in consequence has to take more to get the same effect from it, and is liable to become irritable or depressed or to develop severe symptoms when he cannot get it. Addictions to tobacco and alcohol are common forms of addiction. A drug addict is a person who takes excessive amounts of a drug or drugs for prolonged periods, usually without any medical indication, develops a craving and tolerance, and shows symptoms — called symptoms of withdrawal — if he is deprived of it.

ADDICTION TO TOBACCO

Many people are addicted to tobacco, as cigarettes, pipe-tobacco, cigars and snuff. All these forms of tobacco are dangerous; cigarettes are the most dangerous form. Tobacco is:

(a) the most common cause of cancer of the bronchus (lung). The more a person smokes the more likely is he to develop this disease. In England and Wales the number of deaths from cancer of the trachea, bronchus and lung rose from 8,000 in 1946 to 30,160 in 1972;

(b) probably a cause of cancer of the larynx;

(c) an important cause of chronic bronchitis and a factor in the production of respiratory failure;

(d) a cause of angina pectoris;

(e) a factor in the production of thrombo-angiitis obliterans;

(f) a factor preventing the healing of a peptic ulcer;

(g) a possible cause of cancer of the bladder.

Smoking during pregnancy has adverse effects on the developing child, producing retardation of growth, small babies, premature births, and an increased risk of perinatal death from all causes. Infants whose parents smoke have a high incidence of pneumonia and bronchitis due to "passive smoking" (inhaling the smoke produced by somebody else).

Treatment

Treatment is by stopping smoking by an effort of will. There are various aids to this, but in the long run everything depends upon the patient's determination and persistence.

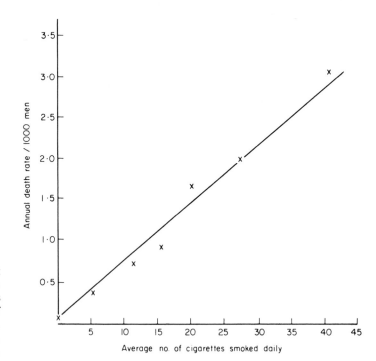

Fig. 80. Graph showing how death-rate from cancer of the lung increases with the number of cigarettes smoked. From Doll, R. & Hill. A.B. (1946) *Brit. med. J.* **i,** 1399.

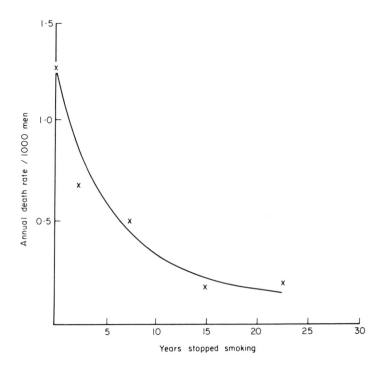

Fig. 81. Graph showing how risk of cancer of lung diminishes when smoking is given up. From Doll, R. & Hill, A.B. (1964) *Brit. med. J.* **i,** 1399.

Chapter 15

| ADDICTION TO ALCOHOL | Alcohol is a depressant of the central nervous system. It produces excitement and elation not by stimulating the brain but by depressing the inhibitory effects of the higher cerebral centres. |

Drinking habits vary widely. Alcoholism is much more common in men than women. It is more common in Switzerland, France, Sweden and the U.S.A. than in Britain. There are thought to be about 400,000 alcoholics in Britain, of whom about 70,000 show mental or physical deterioration. Wherever alcoholism occurs it presents very serious medical and social problems. It is particularly common among workers in the alcohol trade – brewers, publicans, barmen. In recent years in Britain the numbers of young alcoholics (in their 'teens and twenties) and women alcoholics have been increasing.

A person can be considered to be an alcoholic when he cannot control his drinking. Many people drink steadily or heavily but are still able to control their drinking or to stop for a time if they are warned to do so. But the alcoholic has no longer this control, and his life is likely to become one long debauch interrupted by hang-overs. Alcoholism may be an indication of an underlying mental illness – of a manic-depressive psychosis, of anxiety, of epilepsy, of brain damage, of psychopathy; but some people become alcoholics who have not shown any mental disturbance whatsoever.

Alcohol is a common factor in road accidents, both in drivers and pedestrians.

Acute alcoholism: drunkenness

Alcohol is quickly absorbed from the stomach. The rate of absorption is delayed if the concentration is slight, if there is food – particularly fatty food – in the stomach, and if the person has a chronic gastritis. Maximum concentration is reached in 1½-2 hours. A rise of over 0.1 per cent in the blood is likely to produce symptoms, but chronic drinkers may develop a much higher concentration before showing any.

Signs of drunkenness are a blunting of sensory perceptions, inability to think clearly, to concentrate, to appreciate the passage of time; co-ordination and muscular control are affected. The drunk man may be insensitive to pain, behave irrationally and exhibit emotional disturbances and outbursts of rage. He may fall down dead-drunk.

Treatment

Most drunks will 'sleep it off'. If a man becomes unconscious, and his life in danger, the stomach should be washed out with water or sodium bicarbonate solution, 1 teaspoonful to 1 pint of water.

Mania à potu is an attack of extreme violence associated with impaired consciousness produced by only a slight amount of alcohol, such as a single glass of beer or tot of whisky; the person is usually an unstable psychopath or an epileptic.

Dipsomania is an uncontrollable urge to drink excessively in bouts of a few days or weeks in a person who drinks little or nothing at other times.

Chronic alcoholism

Chronic alcoholism can cause:

acute gastritis	cirrhosis of the liver
myocardial degeneration	obesity

271   *Addictions, Drug-Induced Disorders, Poisoning*

polyneuritis   delirium tremens
Korsakov's psychosis   chronic alcoholic deterioration

Acute gastritis

Chronic consumption of alcohol is likely to produce degenerative changes in the mucous membrane of the stomach and a reduction of the secretion of gastric juice. The patient is likely to have loss of appetite, nausea, vomiting and epigastric discomfort.

Cirrhosis of the liver

Cirrhosis of the liver is likely to be associated with malnutrition. The patient will have further gastro-intestinal disturbances and eventually signs of hepatic failure.

Myocardial degeneration

This causes shortage of breath and may go on to produce heart failure.

Obesity

The consumption of alcohol adds to the calorie intake and more fat is laid down.

Polyneuritis

Alcoholic polyneuritis is due to vitamin deficiency and not to alcohol itself. It is a mixed motor and sensory neuritis. Usually it begins with pains in the calves and numbness in the feet. Ataxia is common. Muscular weakness is apparent in foot-drop and wasting of arms and legs. Other evidence of alcoholism is usually apparent.

Delirium tremens

This acute illness is produced by excessive drinking and a failure in consequence of the body to absorb and utilize vitamins of the B group.

It can come at the end of a long debauch or be precipitated by an acute illness, a fracture or another accident sustained by a chronic alcoholic. The patient becomes restless, irritable and sleepless. He has a tremor, ataxia, and slurred speech and he may have a fit. He becomes confused and frightened and misinterprets what he sees, imagining, for example, that patterns on wallpaper are insects or animals. The acute state of the illness lasts for several days and leaves the patient exhausted. Death may occur from heart-failure, pneumonia or a self-inflicted injury. The patient, with his alcoholic habit, is very likely to be obese, and have chronic gastritis, myocardial degeneration or cirrhosis of the liver.

Treatment is by admission into hospital, by giving vitamin B preparations by intravenous or intramuscular injection, and by adequate feeding. Agitation and anxiety is controlled by chlorpromazine. Paraldehyde is given as a hypnotic as it is relatively safe, but prolonged administration must be avoided as an alcoholic can become addicted to it.

An attack of delirium tremens (DTs) should be — but rarely is — a warning to the patient to stop drinking.

Korsakov's psychosis

This can occur in chronic alcoholism, in various kinds of cerebral degeneration and after head injury. It typically consists of a combination of (a) dementia (with loss of memory, judgement, concentration and ability to cope with ordinary affairs) with (b) confabulation — the telling by the patient of fictitious accounts of what

           Chapter 15

he has been doing; a patient, for example, who has spent the day in the ward, may believe that he has spent it in the town. The condition is incurable.

Chronic alcoholism This has developed when drinking has caused the patient's physical and mental health to be impaired, is ruining his working and social life, and cannot be controlled. Mental deterioration shows itself in loss of memory, carelessness, untidiness, disregard of normal social conventions, neglect of work and responsibility, emotional disturbances and empty talk and boasting. By this time the patient is likely to have lost his job. An alcoholic man can become suspicious of his wife, accuse her of having lovers, and attack her. Physically he is likely to show any of the signs of alcoholic deterioration: obesity, myocardial degeneration, neuritis, gastritis, cirrhosis of the liver. He is likely to be drinking methylated spirits as well as what ordinary alcohol he can lay his hands on.

Treatment of Alcoholism To control alcoholism governments have had to introduce measures of control over its consumption — by taxing it heavily to make it expensive and by restricting the places where it can be sold and the hours during which it can be sold.

Young people should be dissuaded from starting to drink and educated in the risks and dangers of drinking.

The treatment of the chronic alcoholic is difficult and usually disappointing. If it is to succeed, the patient has to be mentally strong enough to withstand all inducements to drink, has to change his mode of life, and has to have a family who is willing to become teetotal too. Patients willing to be cured but unable to make the effort by themselves should get in touch with Alcoholics Anonymous (consult Telephone Directory for address of nearest branch), an organization of ex-alcoholics pledged to help alcoholics.

Antabuse (disulfiram) is a drug used in the treatment of alcoholics. By itself it produces no symptoms, but if the patient also takes alcohol within the next 24 hours he is likely to become acutely ill with flushing of the face and neck, nausea and vomiting. The patient takes antabuse in the morning and knows (by a previous test-dose in hospital) that he will become acutely and unpleasantly ill if he takes any alcohol. Most alcoholics, however, stop taking the antabuse after a time and go on drinking.

Aversion therapy is a method of treatment by trying to build up a 'conditioned reflex' against alcohol. In hospital, the patient is given drinks but each is associated with the injection of apomorphine, a very powerful emetic, in the hope that the patient will associate drinking with nausea and vomiting and so develop an aversion to it. The treatment may be effective for a time but relapse is common.

In the treatment of any complication of alcoholism the administration of the vitamin B complex is important.

DRUG ADDICTION AND INTOXICATION A drug addict is a person who takes excessive amounts of a drug for prolonged periods without medical indications, develops a tolerance for it, and shows symptoms of withdrawal if he cannot get it. Any one can become an addict, but most addicts

Addictions, Drug-Induced Disorders, Poisoning

have shown abnormal, psychopathic traits before they become addicts. Any drug with sedative, hypnotic or exhilarating properties can become a drug of addiction.

Barbiturates. Large amounts of barbiturates are prescribed for nervous symptoms and addiction to the drug is probably the commonest of all addictions in the Western World. Large doses produce ataxia, difficulty in speaking, impaired mental function, loss of emotional control, confusion, coma and death. Withdrawal symptoms include anxiety, muscle twitching, irritability, tremor, sweating, nausea, vomiting, palpitations, and insomnia. Sudden withdrawal after the consumption of large amounts can produce a major epileptic fit or delirium. Barbiturate addiction may be combined with alcoholism and heroin addiction. *Treatment* is by slow withdrawal of the drug and simple psychotherapy.

Marihuana (other names: pot, weed, hemp, hashish) has become a common addiction. When smoked it produces variable effects, including exhilaration followed by depression, drowsiness and sleep; inco-ordination, ataxia, flushing of the skin, dilatation of the pupils. Vivid illusions and hallucinations can occur; imagination can be stimulated; time perception is affected, time appearing to pass slowly; schizophrenic like-episodes can occur. Addiction to this drug can be a step towards addiction to 'harder' drugs such as heroin and cocaine.

Amphetamines (Benzedrine, Dexedrine) may be taken by themselves or in combination with barbiturates ('purple hearts', 'black bombers', 'french blues') in order to produce increased energy, euphoria, talkativeness or wakefulness. Some students take them before examinations, some athletes before a race. Dependence on them can occur in people for whom they have been prescribed to reduce depression or suppress appetite. They are sometimes taken in the morning as an antidote to the barbiturate or alcohol of the night before. They are liable to produce irritability, restlessness, over-activity, irresponsible behaviour, insomnia, exhaustion, aplastic anaemia, and short psychotic episodes with delusions and hallucinations. Withdrawal produces anxiety, restlessness and insomnia.

Lysergic Acid Diethylamine (LSD) can produce acute psychotic reactions, anxiety, depression, confusional states, disorientation, hallucinations, self-injury, suicide and anti-social behaviour. It is a dangerous addiction. *Treatment* is by admission to hospital and intra-muscular chlorpromazine (Largactil).

Opium and Morphine addiction is common in the Far East and less common in other parts of the world. The addict who is happy with a small dose is not a problem. Others have to have it in larger and larger amounts and are liable to develop loss of appetite, constipation, anaemia, poor resistance to infections, loss of efficiency, sloth, neglect of appearance, disregard of social conventions, and sudden changes of mood. Withdrawal symptoms include nausea, vomiting, headache, anxiety, depression and muscle cramps. *Treatment* is by slow withdrawal, sedation by other drugs, and psychotherapy. Relapse is common.

Heroin and Cocaine addiction is serious and difficult to treat. The usual story is that the patient has begun with other drugs, starts to take these two by subcutaneous or intramuscular injection, and goes on to giving them to himself intravenously. In Britain addicts rarely take cocaine alone and usually take it with heroin ('H and C'). These drugs are likely to produce elation, restlessness, facile thoughts and glibness; as the effects wear off the patient becomes morose, suspicious and depressed. Addiction can produce delusional and hallucinatory psychoses. Physical deterioration sets in quickly, the addict becoming thin and impotent, having palpitations, and possibly developing heart failure. Sharing syringes among addicts and lack of sterilization is likely to cause infection. An overdose is a common cause of death. Withdrawal symptoms are severe. Addicts to these drugs are usually very unstable, lie to obtain larger amounts of drugs, and frequently relapse after treatment.

DRUG-INDUCED DISORDERS

Other name: iatrogenic[3] diseases.

Many drugs are capable of producing harmful effects. Such effects can be:

1. *A result of over-dosage.* This can be due to (a) the patient is prescribed or given too much; (b) too much is taken by accident or with suicidal intention; (c) the patient is abnormally sensitive to the ordinary therapeutic dose; such sensitivity (which is also called *intolerance*) can be the result of a gene-abnormality; (d) a failure of the body to utilize or excrete the drug so that with further doses the amount accumulates in the blood and tissues.

2. *A side-effect.* A side-effect is an unavoidable effect of a therapeutic dose of a drug, the result of a normal action of the drug on some organ or tissue; thus, chlorpromazine (Largactil) causes dilatation of the peripheral blood-vessels and a fall in BP.

3. *A result of hyper-sensitivity.* As a result of having taken a drug before and developed an antigen-antibody reaction, a patient becomes hyper-sensitive to it and responds with an excessive production of histamine. His reaction can be:

(a) *an immediate reaction:* occurs within a few minutes.

An acute hyper-sensitivity reaction with chest-pain,

dyspnoea, fall in BP, cyanosis;

urticaria, angio-neurotic oedema;

asthma.

   Treatment is by an injection of adrenaline 0.5 ml of 1:1000 solution, and by an anti-histamine drug.

(b) *a late reaction:* occurs in 7-14 days.

skin rashes;

fever, joint-pains, enlarged lymph-nodes;

reduction in number of white blood cells;

haemolytic or aplastic anaemia.

Treatment is by stopping the drug and giving an anti-histamine drug.

4. *The result of idiosyncrasy.* The patient reacts in some abnormal way to a drug (without previously having taken it) as a result of some constitutional defect. An example is prolonged apnoea following the administration of the muscle-relaxant suxamethonium and due to the absence of a particular enzyme.

5. *A secondary effect.* Due to the primary effect of the drug, some other reaction occurs; thus, an antibiotic drug by altering the bacterial content of the bowel can produce vitamin deficiency and a secondary infection by staphylococci and other organisms.

Addictions, Drug-Induced Disorders, Poisoning

6. *By causing an addiction* to the drug.

Among the disorders produced by some commonly-administered drugs are the following:

anti-coagulants: Over-dosage is likely to produce bleeding from the nose and gums; bruising; haematuria; melaena; haemo-thorax; haemo-pericardium; retro-peritoneal haemorrhage; sub-arachnoid haemorrhage.

anti-depressants: Parkinsonism and atropine-like reactions. The monoamine oxidase inhibitors (MAOI) can (a) increase the actions of morphine, pethidine, etc; (b) produce hyper-tensive crises if patient takes alcohol, cheese, 'marmite' or an amphetamine compound, adrenaline, ephedrine.

anti-histamines: Have a hypnotic side-effect.

aspirin: (acetyl-salicylic acid): Can produce gastric irritation, haematemesis, hyper-sensitivity attacks.

barbiturates: Over-dosage produces drowsiness, giddiness, restlessness, confusion, coma, respiratory failure.

chloramphenicol: Can cause (a) aplastic anaemia, purpura, agranulocytosis [4]; (b) growth of fungi on mucous membranes as a secondary effect.

chlorpromazine: (Largactil) Hypotension; anaemia; agranulocytosis; parkinsonism; jaundice; skin rashes.

cortico-steroids: Can cause many complications, including: infection (by the suppression of useful inflammatory reactions); gastro-intestinal bleeding; perforation of stomach and intestine; adrenal failure (likely to cause collapse or death during operation or anaesthetic); nitrogen and potassium loss; sodium and water retention; diabetes; osteo-porosis [5]; obesity; excessive hair-growth; striae [6]; amenorrhoea [7]; psychosis.

cytotoxic drugs: Damage to bone-marrow and reduction in number of blood-cells formed.

digitalis: Coupling of beats; paroxysmal tachycardia; slow pulse; nausea, vomiting, diarrhoea.

diuretics: Excessive excretion of potassium.

phenytoin (Epanutin): Hypersensitivity reactions; hypertrophy of gums; giddiness, ataxia; gastric upsets.

streptomycin: Damage to 8th cranial nerve, producing giddiness.

vitamin D: Over-dosage produces increase of calcium in blood, deposits of calcium in kidneys and arteries with production of renal failure.

POISONING Poisoning is a common medical problem and emergency. Poisoning may be accidental, suicidal or murderous. Drugs are a common method, and carbon monoxide is used less when coal gas is replaced by the non-lethal natural gas.

Questions to be asked are:

1. Has the patient been poisoned or is he suffering from something else?

[3] *iatrogenic:* from Greek: *iatros* – doctor; *gennan* – to produce (i.e. doctor-produced)

[4] *agranulocytosis:* reduction in number of granular white blood cells (polymorphs)

[5] *osteo-porosis:* reduction of calcium in bone

[6] *stria:* white streak or line in skin   [7] *amenorrhoea:* absence of menstruation

2. What type of poisoning is it?

3. If it is a drug, what drug is it and what amount was taken?

4. When was the poison taken?

Principles of treatment
of poisoning
1. *Maintenance of*
respiration

Certain principles of treatment are applicable to many kinds of poisoning.

(i) The patient must have a clear air-way. His mouth should be opened and the air-way explored with a finger. Dentures should be removed.

(ii) The trachea and bronchi are inspected through a bronchoscope and a Magill tube is inserted with or without a cuff.

(iii) If the patient is not breathing, artificial respiration is performed by: (a) mouth-to-mouth method or (b) with the aid of anaesthetic apparatus or artificial respirators.

(iv) Oxygen is supplied via an oxygen mask or by an oxygen tent.

(v) Atropine sulphate 1 mg is given by subcutaneous injection if there is an over-secretion of saliva or mucus.

2. *Removal of poison*

(i) The patient is stopped from taking any more poison, e.g. he is removed from the source of carbon monoxide.

(ii) If poison has been swallowed (a) if he is conscious and the pharyngeal reflex is present, the fauces are stimulated with the finger or he is given salt water to drink (one *dessert-spoonful* of salt to a tumbler of water) to stimulate vomiting; (b) if he is unconscious, gastric lavage is performed; special care is required with old people, young children, people who have had abdominal operations, people who have swallowed a corrosive poison — strong acid or alkali. Washing out the stomach is useless if 4 hours have elapsed since the poison was taken (12 hours for aspirin). During washing a cuffed tube must be in place.

3. *Maintenance of fluid*
and electrolyte balance

(i) A fluid-balance sheet is kept.

(ii) Estimations are made of the blood-urea and of electrolytes, potassium and sodium.

(iii) Forced diuresis by fluids given intravenously is carried out if not contraindicated.

(iv) Dialysis is performed if necessary; it can be done by either intermittent peritoneal dialysis or by haemodialysis.

4. *Maintenance of*
circulation

If the circulation is falling:

(i) The foot of the bed is raised,

(ii) Blood, plasma or dextran is given intravenously,

(iii) Methyl-amphetamine hydrochloride 10 mg is given intravenously or intra-muscularly.

(iv) Venesection is performed if there is acute heart failure,

(v) External cardiac massage is performed if the heart stops.

(vi) Acute pulmonary oedema is treated by bronchial suction, diuretics to remove fluid, digoxin to strengthen the heart-beat.

5. *Prevention of*
infection

Penicillin or another antibiotic is given to prevent or treat infection.

6. *Antidote*	If the poison is known and there is an antidote, the antidote is given, e.g.: morphine poisoning — nalorphine 5-10 mg intravenously pethidine poisoning — nalorphine 5-10 mg intravenously.
7. *Care of bladder*	Catheterization is required if there is retention of urine. The urine is required for examination in the laboratory.
8. *Psychological treatment*	A patient who has attempted suicide is referred to the psychiatrist as soon as he is out of danger.
Acetyl-salicylic acid (aspirin) poisoning	This is a common form of accidental or suicidal poisoning. Young children become pale, drowsy, twitch and overbreathe. Adults show pallor, giddiness, sweating, vomiting and thirst; later they overbreathe, twitch, have a raised temperature and pulse rate. Death can be due to heart failure, respiratory failure, or pulmonary oedema.
Treatment	Treatment is on the usual lines. The stomach should be washed out with water. Fluids are given by mouth if the patient is conscious, which he often is. Intravenous fluids are given to the unconscious patient. Haemodialysis may be necessary.
Barbiturate poisoning	This is the drug most commonly used for poisoning. Some forms act more quickly and some last longer than others, but the basic poisoning is the same.
Clinical features	Patients become confused and drowsy and then pass through stupor into coma. The temperature is low. The pulse rate is increased. Respiration varies, being sometimes rapid and shallow and sometimes slow and stertorous. Skin eruptions can occur. The pupils are small; the tendon reflexes may disappear. Retention of urine is likely. Death is due to cardiac or respiratory failure, to pulmonary oedema, to renal failure, or to bronchopneumonia. Patients who recover are likely to have headache, double vision, nystagmus, and ataxia for some time, and sometimes are mildly excited.
Treatment	This is on the usual lines.
Iron	Young children can poison themselves with iron salts, mistaking sugar-coated tablets for sweets.
Clinical features	The child will be pale and likely to vomit, the vomit sometimes being blood-stained. The pulse and respiratory rates are raised. Drowsiness and stupor are broken by restlessness, twitching and fits. Circulatory, renal or hepatic failure can cause death.
Treatment	The stomach must be washed out with sodium bicarbonate 0.5 per cent solution and

278

some of it is left in the stomach. Desferrioxamine is a chelating agent which can be left in the stomach with the sodium bicarbonate solution and also given by intramuscular or intravenous injection. Treatment for dehydration, electrolyte-disturbance and shock may be required.

Meta fuel   Tablets of meta fuel (metaldehyde) are used by campers as fuel and are scattered on the ground by gardeners to kill slugs. Children can think they are sweets.

Clinical features   Vomiting, diarrhoea, drowsiness, fits, coma and death can occur.

Treatment   Treatment must be given promptly. If the child is conscious, vomiting should be induced by putting a finger into the throat or a drink of strong salt solution given. The stomach of an unconscious child should be washed out and a saline purge given down the tube. Convulsions in coma should be treated by an anesthetist by relaxants and controlled respiration.

Paraffin poisoning   This is the cause of about 10 per cent of children admitted into hospital for poisoning.

Clinical features   If paraffin is swallowed, pallor, nausea, vomiting and diarrhoea are produced. If paraffin fumes are inhaled, pnuemonitis can be produced.

Treatment   For swallowing paraffin, gastric lavage is performed and 100 ml of medicinal liquid paraffin, which dissolves paraffin, is left in the stomach. Oxygen and antibiotics are given for pneumonitis.

Toadstool poisoning   (a) The *Death Cap (Amanita phalloides)* resembles a mushroom; its gills are always white. Its poison is not affected by cooking. Signs of poisoning occur late, after the poison has been absorbed from the alimentary tract: nausea, vomiting, pallor, abdominal pain and diarrhoea are succeeded by collapse, dehydration, and cardiac, respiratory or liver failure. Death can occur 5-10 days after ingestion. If people did not eat a wild "mushroom" that was white underneath, poisoning would not occur.
(b) The *Fly Agaric (Amanita muscaria)* is a red and white toadstool, sometimes eaten by children. It causes gastro-intestinal upset, excitement and hallucinations, but not often death.

Treatment   Treatment of both kinds of poisoning is by (a) washing out the stomach and (b) treating dehydration and electrolyte loss. Atropine sulphate 1 mg hourly can be given for Fly Agaric poisoning, but has no effect on Death Cap poisoning.

Poisonous seeds and berries   Children are likely to eat (a) deadly nightshade berries and berries of similar plants, which contain solanaceous alkaloids and (b) laburnum and lupin seeds.
Deadly nightshade berry poisoning produces fever, flushed skin, rapid pulse, irregular breathing, thirst, dilated pupils and mild excitement. Laburnum seeds etc. produce pallor, dizziness, vomiting, diarrhoea and a slow pulse.

Treatment	There is no specific treatment. The usual treatment for poisoning is given.
Lead poisoning	*Other name:* plumbism Lead poisoning can be due to: (a) Industrial poisoning, the commonest cause. Lead is used in many industrial processes. Workmen can absorb lead through the lungs by inhaling fumes containing lead or by eating with unwashed hands. The risks are known in the various industries concerned and appropriate precautions are taken, e.g. by adequate ventilation, prohibition of eating in the factory, insistence on washing hands. (b) Children licking lead paint. Paint containing lead should not be used indoors or on toys, cot-rails, pen-rails and other furniture for children. (c) Contamination of food and drink by lead-glazed pots or lead pipes.
Clinical features	1. An attack begins with weakness, fatigue, constipation and muscular pains. 2. Abdominal colic occurs, with acute abdominal pain centred around the umbilicus. It is due to spasm of the bowel and can be mistaken for an acute surgical emergency. 3. Confusion, fits, unconsciousness; most likely when a large amount is inhaled quickly. 4. Mental retardation in young children is said to follow lead absorption, but this has been doubted. 5. Patients are likely to show anaemia; to have albuminuria as a result of kidney damage; to have a blue line (due to a deposit of lead sulphide) along the gums where they embrace the teeth, and sometimes a similar line round the anus. Athero-sclerosis is a long-term hazard. The diagnosis may be difficult until the patient's contact with lead is discovered.
Special test	*Blood:* a moderate degree of anaemia is likely, with characteristic basophil (blue-staining) spots in the red blood cells.
Treatment	1. The patient must be removed from any contact with lead. 2. Sodium calcium edetate (Calcium Disodium Versenate) given intravenously in doses of 1-1.5 g daily and penicillamine in doses of 4 g daily by mouth are chelating agents[8] which promote the excretion of lead by the kidneys and rapidly relieve symptoms. 3. Calcium is given by mouth and relieves colic.
Arsenical poisoning	Arsenical poisoning may be the result of (a) industrial processes; arsenic is used in many industrial processes, e.g. the manufacture of glass, enamel, fungicides, alloys; precautions against poisoning are exhaust-ventilation, wearing protective clothing, changing and bathing facilities, regular medical inspection; and (b) accidental or intentional poisoning; arsenic is the classical weapon of the poisoner who can get hold of it.

Clinical features	Acute arsenical poisoning is characterized by acute gastro-enteritis with nausea, vomiting, acute abdominal pain, diarrhoea and collapse going on, with a fatal dose, to coma and death.
	   Arsine (arseniuretted hydrogen) is a gas liberated in some industrial processes. Absorbed, it causes haemoglobinuria, renal damage and jaundice.
	   Chronic arsenical poisoning is the result of the absorption and deposit in the tissues of small amounts of arsenic over a long period. It causes pigmentation of the skin, thickening of the horny layers of the skin, hepatitis, jaundice and polyneuritis, with hyper-aesthesiae, paralysis and muscular wasting.

Treatment	Acute arsenical poisoning is treated by stomach wash-outs, and the treatment of shock. BAL (British Anti-Lewisite) is given in oily solution in order to render the arsenic harmless.

[8] *chelating agent:* drug that combines with a metal to produce a soluble, non-toxic form that can be easily excreted

Chapter 15

Carbon monoxide poisoning

Carbon monoxide poisoning can be accidental or as the result of a suicidal attempt. The commoner sources of carbon monoxide are fumes from cars or other petrol engines, industrial processes and coal gas, where still used for heating or cooking.

Carbon monoxide has a great affinity for haemoglobin, which takes it up instead of oxygen, forming carboxy-haemoglobin. So the tissues are deprived of oxygen. All are seriously affected and in particular the heart and the brain which have a need for a constant high supply of oxygen.

Clinical features

Exposed to carbon monoxide the patient suddenly feels so tired that he cannot move away and has to breathe more in. Patches of erythema appear on the skin and sometimes the patient goes a cherry-red colour from the carboxy-haemoglobin. He loses consciousness quickly and can die if not rescued.

Permanent damage to the tissues can be caused. Shortage of oxygen to the brain quickly causes brain cells to die; disorientation and coma are common; on apparent recovery the patient may develop mental deterioration and fits as a result of damage to the cerebral cortex and rigidity, tremor and athetoid movements as a result of damage to the basal ganglia. Damage to the myocardium can cause a rapid irregular pluse, heart failure and death.

Treatment

The patient is removed from the source of carbon monoxide and if he has stopped breathing, artificial respiration is begun at once. A mixture of oxygen and 5 per cent carbon dioxide is sometimes administered. Such measures are continued while he is being removed to hospital. If possible he is given hyperbaric oxygen with a pressure of oxygen at 2 atmospheres absolute. Hypothermia can be induced to reduce the need for oxygen.

The patient should be kept in bed for several weeks because of possible damage to the myocardium. If he has been unconscious for a long time, the future should be viewed with caution because of the likelihood of cerebral damage. If the poisoning has been a suicidal attempt, the patient should be referred to a psychiatrist.

Addictions, Drug-Induced Disorders, Poisoning

16 Mental Retardation

Other names: mental deficiency, mental subnormality, amentia
Mental retardation is a common condition: about 5 per cent of babies born are likely to be mentally retarded, but with the death of many during the first two years of life and of others later, the incidence in adult life is about 1 per cent.

Among the causes of mental retardation are:

1. *Genetic factors:* genes that cause mental retardation can be inherited; such genes may be dominant or recessive (see Chapter 11). Some patients (e.g. mongols) may show gross chromosomal abnormalities.

2. *Factors in fetal life:* the mother developing German measles (and possibly some other virus infections) during the first 3 months of pregnancy; congenital syphilis; rhesus-incompatability: X-irradiation of the maternal pelvis.

3. *Factors during birth:* during precipitate, prolonged or instrumental delivery, the baby may suffer anoxia or cerebral haemorrhage or injury, with degeneration or death of cerebral cells.

4. *Factors in early life:* encephalitis, meningitis, cerebral tumour or cerebral injury.

DEGREES OF RETARDATION

It is convenient to assess patients with mental retardation as being: severely retarded, moderately retarded or slightly retarded.

Severe retardation

Patients with severe retardation have little intelligence. They show gross physical and mental abnormalities. They are likely to be stunted and mis-shapen and of coarse appearance. The head may be mis-shapen, abnormally large or abnormally small. The ears, palate and teeth are likely to be abnormal. Epilepsy, cerebral palsy, deafness and impaired vision are common among them. The brain is poorly developed and shows gross abnormalities; many patients die within the first two years of life and few live into late adult life.

The patient's mental development is very slow. Many never learn to speak, the best can only mumble a few words. They cannot learn to read, write or do sums. Many of them have to be fed, washed and dressed and are incontinent of urine and faeces throughout life. They can be calm, apathetic or friendly or they may be noisy, excitable, vicious and destructive and eat clothing and swallow rubbish.

Moderate retardation

Moderately retarded patients are likely to show abnormal physical characteristics and disabilities similar to those of the severely retarded, but possibly not to the same degree. Being of greater intelligence, they may be able to speak a few simple sentences, recognize common coins, to print their names, and to be trained in simple tasks. They are not however of sufficient intelligence to earn a living or to live without some degree of supervision and support.

Slight retardation Slightly retarded people do not present as patients unless they are unstable, have other disabilities or commit offences. They are people just below the bottom end of the scale of average intelligence. They are usually of normal appearance and if stable are able to support themselves, by employment in some work that does not demand great intelligence or initiative.

DIAGNOSIS Some severe types of retardation (such as mongolism and microcephaly) can be recognized in a newly born child; babies whose brains have failed to develop or have been damaged during birth are likely to be born blue or white, to have muscular spasticity or flaccidity, to be unable to breathe, cry or suck adequately. Absence of the normal grasp reflex (the hand of the baby closing on a finger slipped into it) or of the startle reflex (the baby's arms being flung apart and then brought together when a loud noise is made or his position abruptly changed) suggests that the baby's brain has suffered anoxia or some injury during birth.

The stages in a child's development which he is expected to reach at a certain age are called his milestones. At 4 weeks he should be noticing his mother; at 6 weeks beginning to smile; at 12 weeks he should be lifting his head; at 9 months he should be sitting up, and at 12 months he should be standing or walking with help and saying 2 or 3 words. Retardation is suspected when a child does not pass his milestone at the expected times, provided that he has no other disability such as deafness, impaired vision, spasticity. A child who cannot hold up his head at 6 months is not developing normally; and a child who at 9 months cannot distinguish his mother, at 12 months is not sitting up, at 18 months is not starting to walk, is almost certainly mentally retarded. The retarded child may not make the usual pleasant sounds of the healthy child, may whimper or cry without obvious cause, or may scream. The very apathetic child who lies motionless and disinterested in his cot is also suspect. Later in childhood, the child going to school is discovered not to be able to cope with academic work such as reading, writing and arithmetic, and may make little or no progress. Psychopathic behaviour may appear.

Special test Intelligence tests measure intelligence — but as almost everybody has had some education, they are not a test of 'pure' intelligence but of intelligence modified by education. There are many kinds of tests and a patient is usually tested by several in order that different facets of his intelligence can be assessed.

A patient's I.Q. (Intelligence Quotient) is often given. This is his score on a particular test and accordingly can vary with different tests. An I.Q. of 90-110 is an indication of average intelligence. More intelligent people score higher. Dull people score less. Severely retarded people have an I.Q. below 30; moderately retarded people an I.Q. of 30-55; slightly retarded an I.Q. of 55-75. An I.Q. is not constant, for a person in poor health, in emotional difficulties or living in a dull, unstimulating environment, is likely to have a low score, which could be raised if the conditions were improved.

CLINICAL TYPES
MONGOLISM

Other name: Down's syndrome
This is a common condition, about 1 baby in every 600 born being a mongol. A

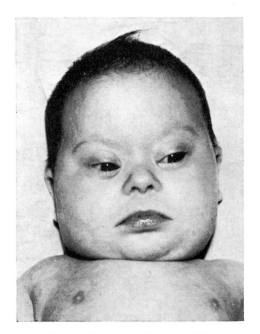

Fig. 82. A young mongol boy (from Jolly H. (1968) Diseases of Children, 2nd ed. Blackwell Scientific Publications).

mongol is usually the child of a middle-aged mother, sometimes of a young mother. A mongol usually has 47 chromosomes in each cell instead of the normal 46 (sometimes the additional one is attached to another) and it is believed that this abnormality is the cause of the condition.

Mongols look very much like one another, although every one does not show all the features of the disease. The condition can be recognized at birth. The mongol has a small round head, a broad flat nose and sparse hair. The eyes slope downwards and inwards; there may be a little fold of skin — the 'epicanthic fold' — at the inner corner of the eye. Nystagmus, a squint, myopia, and small cataracts can develop. The tongue becomes fissured and too large for the mouth and lolls out. The hands are broad and short; a single crease runs across the palm instead of the usual two; the little finger is short and curved towards the others. The neck and trunk are short; the mongol does not grow to average height and in middle age is likely to become fat. The muscles are hypotonic, and this and the laxity of ligaments around

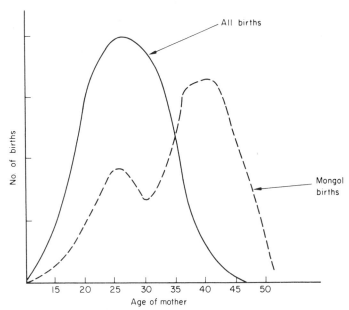

Fig. 83. Graph demonstrating (a) the age of mothers for all births and (b) the age of mothers at the birth of mongols, showing the high incidence of mongol births over the age of 30 years.

joints enable the mongol to put his limbs into unusual positions. The peripheral circulation is poor, and chronic inflammation of the eyelids and nose is likely. Congenital disease of heart and bowel is common. Leukaemia is a complication (possibly as a result of chromosomal abnormality). About half the mongols born die within the first 2 years of life; few survive into old age.

As a baby a mongol is usually placid, apathetic, inactive and a very slow developer. Almost all of them are severely or moderately retarded; and in consequence mongols require care for life. In personality they do not differ from other retarded patients.

PHENYLKETONURIA   This inherited metabolic disease is due to an absence of the enzyme that converts phenylalanine, an amino acid, into tyrosine; the accumulating phenylalanine damages the brain. Some children with this metabolic abnormality are physically and mentally normal.

An affected child may appear normal at birth; if undetected and untreated, the condition produces severe retardation. The child usually has fair hair, a fair skin and blue eyes (as a result of a failure of development of melanin, the skin pigment, due to absence of tyrosine). He is likely to be overactive, have mannerisms, such as twitching the fingers, and an unpleasant personality. He can have an abnormal EEG and fits. A patchy eczema is likely to develop.

Special tests   *Guthrie test:* this is a reliable micro-biological test done on a spot of blood.
Phenistix: stick is pressed into a baby's wet nappy and when positive turns grey or grey green; it is not reliable.

Treatment is by placing the baby on a diet of special foods containing little or no phenylalanine; if the treatment is started in early infancy, there is a likelihood that the child will not develop retardation and the other signs of the disease.

285   *Mental Retardation*

Children in whom the condition has not been diagnosed and treated from infancy may, when placed on the diet, show a rise of intelligence sufficient to enable them to go to a school for the educationally subnormal or possibly a normal school. It is not yet known at what age it is possible to relax dietary restrictions.

TUBEROUS SCLEROSIS

Other names: epiloia, Bourneville's disease
In this condition there is an association of severe retardation (from infancy), with

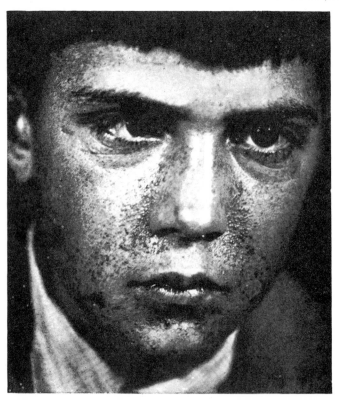

Fig. 84. Tuberous sclerosis, showing the 'butterfly' distribution of the spots on the face (from Ellis and Mitchell, *Disease in Infancy and Childhood* E. & S. Livingstone

epilepsy (from early childhood) with the development (from childhood) of tumours on the face, in the brain and sometimes in the heart and kidneys. The typical rash on the face, which has the name of adenoma sebaceum, begins as small white spots in a 'butterfly distribution' over the nose and cheeks; in later years the spots become darker, larger and more numerous. The skin can show rough patches and disorders of pigmentation. Tumours of fibrous tissue growing in the brain can produce cerebral palsy and hydrocephalus, growing in the heart can produce cardiac abnormalities, and growing in the kidney can produce renal failure. The condition becomes progressively worse and the patient dies young, of an infection or in status epilepticus.

A family incidence is present in about half the cases; it is not unusual for a parent or other relative to have adenoma sebaceum only.

Chapter 16

MICROCEPHALY The head shows characteristic features: a tiny head with receding forehead and a prominent nose and upper jaw. *Complications* are epilepsy and paralysis.

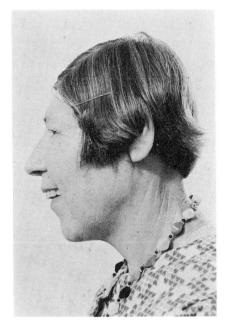

Fig. 85. Microcephaly

NAEVOID AMENTIA
(Sturge-Weber's disease)

This disease shows an angioma within the distribution of a trigeminal nerve, involving face, scalp, skull, meninges; mental retardation is likely to be associated with visual disturbances, epilepsy and hemiplegia.

CYTOMEGALOVIRUS INFECTION

Cytomegalovirus (CMV) is a virus of the herpes group (other members of which cause chickenpox, herpes zoster and herpes simplex) and like other viruses of this group it can lie dormant in the body for years. It is thought to be the most common *infective* cause of mental retardation in Britain today, probably producing about 400 cases a year.

About 1 per cent of women in Britain develop a primary infection (of which symptoms are slight) and others have a reactivation of an earlier infection. About half the babies at risk are infected, and of these 5-15 per cent show the effects of damage to the brain.

Clinical features

Mental retardation, microcephaly and intracerebral calcification can occur in infected babies.

GERMAN MEASLES
(Rubella)

German measles occurring in a pregnant woman during the first 3 months of pregnancy can, in one out of 10 pregnancies at risk, produce mental retardation or other congenital conditions, including microcephaly, cataracts, deafness, deaf-mutism, hare-lip, cleft palate, talipes, and congenital heart disease. If the mother develops German measles after the 3rd month the danger is much less.

GARGOYLISM

Gargoylism is an inborn error of metabolism in which lipids are deposited in the brain and elsewhere. The degree of mental retardation varies. An affected child has an ugly appearance (like a gargoyle on a church), numerous deformities of bone, a large liver and spleen, congenital heart disease, deafness and impaired vision. Death usually occurs in childhood.

Cretinism: see p. 196.
Hydrocephaly: see p. 238.
Toxoplasmosis: see p. 335.

BRAIN DAMAGE   At birth the child's head can be subjected to severe stresses and the brain suffer injury or anoxia. The child is likely to develop mental retardation, spastic paralysis, speech difficulties, choreic[9] or athetoid movements, and epilepsy.

POST-NATAL   After encephalitis or meningitis, a child can be left with some degree of mental retardation,
INFECTIONS   and other signs of brain damage, such as paralysis, epilepsy, ataxia[1], athetoid[2] or choreic movements, emotional instability, psychopathic behaviour.

TREATMENT   Treatment of the mentally retarded is mainly an affair of training retardates to the best of their ability. The care of the retarded is more a social and educational matter than a medical and nursing one.

Home Care. It is generally recommended that a retarded person is looked after at home and in the community for as long as possible. Parents will need psychological help in their emotional difficulties, advice on training and prospects for their child, and material assistance such as better housing, laundry facilities and financial help.

Community Services. In Britain the local authority of the area in which the patient lives will provide many facilities:
a day hospital for severely retarded, handicapped, incontinent children to go to by day.
a training centre for children who cannot be educated at school.
a school for the educationally subnormal.
a hostel and adult training centre or sheltered workshop for older patients.

Hospital Care. Retarded children and adults can be admitted into a hospital for the retarded when facilities for looking after them at home or in the community are not adequate or the patient's behaviour is such that he cannot stay at home or in a hostel. In the hospital he will, in addition to ordinary medical and nursing care, receive appropriate training in school, adult training centre, industrial sheltered workshop, etc. The hospital will be provided with facilities for recreation, sport, and will aim at providing as full a life as possible for its patients.

[9] *choreic:* jerky
[1] *ataxia:* incoordinated muscular actions
[2] *athetoid:* slow, twisting

Diseases of the Skin

The skin is liable to be affected by the same kinds of disease that affect other organs — by congenital deformities, injuries, infections, allergic reactions, metabolic disorders, new growths and degenerations. By virtue of its position on the outside of the body it is particularly liable to injury, infection and extremes of heat and cold. An allergic reaction — in the form called dermatitis (eczema) — is particularly common. Other antigen-antibody reactions of the skin are used in special tests, such as the Heaf, Tine and Mantoux tests for tuberculosis.

Itching, produced either by local disease in the skin or by some general condition such as jaundice, is a common symptom; itching leads to scratching, a scratch to infection; and when this happens extensively, the original condition may be hidden behind infected scratches.

The skin is an organ much used for self display and adornment — as by the use of cosmetics (themselves often capable of producing allergic reactions) and tattooing. It is also an organ by which emotions are expressed; blushing is a result of a loss of tone in the blood-vessels of the skin, pallor of an increase in tone. Sweating and erection of the hairs can be other signs of emotion. Moreover, a patient can see for himself the state of disease in his own skin; he may be tempted to treat it and overtreat it himself; and he can see for himself the effect of any treatment prescribed. For some skin diseases treatment is not very effective, and to a prolonged, extensive and apparently incurable condition the patient may develop severe psychological reactions.

The following terms are used in dermatology:
bulla: a large vesicle.
crust: dried mass of cells, exudate and micro-organisms.
eczematization: development of eczema-like lesions.
erythema: redness of skin.
excoriation: abrasion or scratch.
lichenification: thickening and roughness of skin due to rubbing and scratching.
macule: a flat spot.
nodule: a large papule in deep layers of skin.
papule: a raised spot, up to 1 cm in diameter.
plaque: a firm, raised patch.

pustule: a papule containing pus.

scale: a dry or greasy mass of dead tissue from horny layer.

slough: a patch of dead cells and dried secretions.

ulcer: an area of loss of substance of the skin.

vesicle: a papule containing clear fluid.

weal: a blister.

Eczema [3]

Other name: Dermatitis[4].

This, by far the commonest of all skin lesions, can be due to:

(1) heredity and type of skin

(2) external, traumatic, infective and psychological factors.

Whatever the cause, it can occur in acute, subacute and chronic forms, characterized by redness, oedema, papules which scale, vesicles which weep, itching which causes scratching which leads to lichenification.

1. ATOPIC ECZEMA[5]

Other names: Besnier's prurigo, allergic eczema

In this kind of dermatitis there is a family history of allergy (asthma, hay-fever, rhinitis, urticaria) and the patient is likely to show similar allergic reactions. It occurs at 3 epochs of life:

(a) Infantile eczema

This begins at about 3 months and with improvements and recurrences lasts for 2-4 years. The usual sites are the face (except immediately around eyes, nose, mouth), the forearms, legs and flexures. Vesicles appear and weep over the reddened, itching, slightly oedematous skin, and the infant scratches himself furiously.

(b) Childhood eczema

This can be a first attack, a recurrence of infantile eczema or a continuation of it. Papules and lichenification occur usually on flexor surfaces. It tends to clear up at 10-12 years.

(c) Adult eczema

The patient usually has had previous attacks in infancy or childhood. Papular and lichenified areas appear in the flexures and on the face, neck, wrists, hands and feet. The tendency is for it to become chronic with periods of freedom now and again.

Complications

Scratching can lead to secondary infection.

Children with eczema should not be vaccinated against smallpox because a very severe reaction can flare up and can cause death. They must not come into contact with recently vaccinated people. Vaccination in adult life is not undertaken lightly.

Treatment

1. Considerable psychological help is required throughout a long, trying illness with the likelihood of many recurrences.

[3] *eczema:* from Greek: *ek zein* — to boil out

[4] *dermatitis:* inflammation of skin; from Greek: *derma* — skin

[5] *atopic:* natural, inherited hypersensitivity

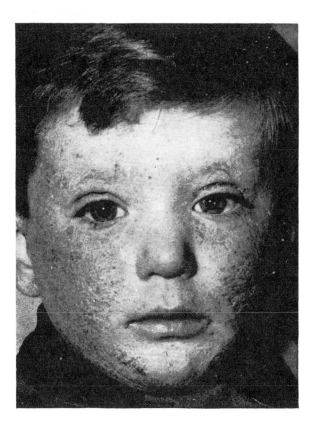

Fig. 86. Infantile eczema.

2. Sudden changes of temperature have to be avoided; washing with soap and detergents are avoided. Woollen underclothes are not worn. The finger-nails should be kept short, smooth and clean.

3. For weeping lesions, lotions are used, e.g. calamine lotion, aluminium acetate lotion (Burow's solution), or potassium permanganate 1/8000-1/16000 solution.

4. For dry lesions, ichthammol in zinc ointment, tar ointment or a steroid cream is used.

5. Itching if relieved by a sedative or anti-histamine by mouth.

6. Removal from home to a relative's home or to hospital can work wonders.

7. Some patients improve if they live in a different climate.

2. POMPHOLYX In this dermatitis the hands (on the palms and sides of the fingers) and feet (on the soles) are affected with very itchy, burning, deep-seated vesicles; the nails can become deformed. It can be associated with emotional storms, contact dermatitis, excessive sweating, ringworm of the feet. Recurrences can occur months or years later.

Treatment is by removal of any known cause, permanganate baths and zinc or steroid creams.

**3. NUMMULAR[6]
DERMATITIS**

In this variety coin-shaped lesions occur on the hands, forearms, thighs and calves of young and middle-aged people, develop weeping vesicles and crusts, and itch. The cause is unknown, the course variable.

Treatment is by coal tar and occlusive bandages.

DERMATITIS DUE TO EXTERNAL (TRAUMATIC) FACTORS

Other names: contact dermatitis, occupational dermatitis

A very large number of substances are capable of producing redness, oedema, vesicles and itching. A *primary irritant* is any substance — such as an acid or alkali — which will produce a reaction in the skin of anyone if it is in strong concentration and left in contact with the skin for long enough; dermatitis is prevented by wearing special gloves or protective clothing, by barrier creams and by washing. A *sensitizer* is any substance that produces a dermatitis not at the first exposure but after a number of exposures, a number that can vary from a few to several hundreds; they cannot easily be prevented and complete avoidance of contact is the only way to prevent recurrence.

The number of substances that in solid, liquid or gaseous form can produce dermatitis is legion. They can be classified as:

(a) *Occupational:* paints, varnishes, resins, plastics, oils, petrol products, insecticides, dyes, cement, etc.

(b) *Household:* detergents, soaps, polishes, rubber gloves, etc.

(c) *Clothing:* nickel in suspenders, zips, watch-buckles; dyes in nylon, furs, etc.; wet napkins in infants; etc.

(d) *Cosmetics:* lip-stick, nail-varnish, hair-lacquers and dyes, deodorants, orris-root powder, lanolin (which is a base of many cosmetics and therapeutic applications), etc.

(e) *Plants:* primula, chrysanthemums, daffodils, narcissi, tulips, celery, parsnips, etc.

(f) *Drugs:* chlorpromazine, penicillin, sulphonamide, anti-histamines etc. applied to the skin. Nurses and doctors who become sensitive can develop an itchy skin or other reaction on entering a ward or room in which traces of the drug are present in the air.

The site of the eruption is often an indication of a likely cause; a dermatitis of the thigh in a woman may be due to nickel in her suspender or dye in her nylon stocking or nail-varnish she has used to stop a ladder. A search for the possible offender is a detailed enquiry into everything the patient is in contact with at work and at play.

Special test

Patch test: some of suspected substance is applied to skin in middle of back, covered with cellophane stuck on with adhesive plaster, and left for 48 hours (or shorter if itching is severe). An inflammatory reaction is positive. The test is not done during an acute attack.

Prevention

In industries where the risks are known it is advisable to test workers' reactions before they start, but this is not always practicable (e.g. with shifting, casual labourers). Gloves or other protective clothing may have to be worn in certain industries and dust extracted from workrooms. Desensitization measures do not usually work.

[6] *nummular:* coin-shaped

| *Treatment* | 1. Patient is removed from source of dermatitis.
2. Bland lotions are applied, e.g. saline, potassium permanganate 1/8,000 solution etc.
3. Steroids can be applied. |

| **OTHER CAUSES OF DERMATITIS** | Exposure to sunlight: hypersensitivity to sunlight can occur.
Exposure to heat or cold.
Exposure to ionizing radiations – radium and X-rays.
Dermatitis artefacta: self-imposed lesions produced by chemical or physical means usually by a young, female, hysterical psychopath. |

Infections of the Skin

Healthy intact skin is able to resist invasion by micro-organisms; but infection can follow any abrasion, cut, scratch or fissure, being aided by excessive sweating, by seborrhoea with its excessive production of sebum, by diabetes and any chronic disease.

IMPETIGO[7] CONTAGIOSA[8]

This staphylococcal infection of the skin affects usually children and adolescents. It can be a complication of a purulent discharge from nose or ear, or of scabies or pediculosis. People who are carriers of pathogenic staphylococci on the skin or around one of the body-orifices or in the scalp may reinfect themselves. The disease is very contagious; small epidemics can occur in families and small communities; epidemics of wound-infection in hospital can be due to impetigo or a boil on a nurse, doctor or other member of the staff.

Clinical features

The usual sites are the face, the limbs and the chest. The patient develops papules, which quickly turn to vesicles, which quickly turn to pustules. The pustules then crust over with a yellow or greenish crust. Fissures develop at the corners of the mouth and nose. With treatment an attack should clear up in a few days; untreated, it persists for weeks.

Treatment

1. Any known cause is treated.
2. A course of penicillin or other antibiotic of the penicillin series is given.
3. Local treatment is by: (a) removal of crusts with 1/10000 potassium permanganate solution; followed by (b) 4-hourly application of one of the following antibiotics: neomycin, framycetin or fucidin.

ECTHYMA[9]

This chronic streptococcal infection with crusting, ulceration and scarring, is a disease of tramps, filthy people and neglected children. Treatment is by (a) treating the usually present parasitical infection, (b) washing, (c) cetrimide 1 per cent to aid the cleansing, (d) the application of an appropriate antibiotic cream, and (e) training in hygiene and improvement of nutrition.

[7] *impetigo:* from Latin: *impetere* – to attack
[8] *contagiosa:* contagious, i.e. infectious by touch
[9] *ecthyma:* from Greek: *ekthuma* – pustule

FOLLICULITIS OF THE BEARD AREA	*Other name:* sycosis barbae[1] This is a staphylococcal infection of hair-follicles in the beard-area, due usually to infection from the nose or to cuts from shaving; it can occur in other hairy places.
Clinical features	Small papules and pustules with a hair sticking out of each appear as a generalized outbreak or in small groups. With treatment the condition clears up in a few days, but relapse is common.
Treatment	1. The sensitivity of the organism should be found before treatment is started. An appropriate antibiotic cream (usually a tetracycline or neomycin with bacitracin) is applied and treatment continued for at least a fortnight after apparent cure. 2. If the patient is a nasal carrier, the inside of the nostrils is treated simultaneously with the antibiotic cream.

BOILS AND CARBUNCLES	These are essentially the same, both being staphylococcal infections beginning in hair-follicles: boils remain local infection around the follicle; carbuncles are more extensive lesions with destruction of skin and subcutaneous tissues, a general reaction and scar-formation, all following a breakdown of the tissue's resistance to infection.
	    Boils can follow any break in the surface of the skin — a scratch, a cut, parasitic infection or skin disease. Some patients, carriers of staphylococci in their noses or on the perineum, keep on infecting themselves. Diabetics and patients with chronic renal and other diseases are particularly liable to develop boils.
	    Furunculosis[2] means multiple boils.

Clinical features	A boil begins as a painful spot, which enlarges, hardens and eventually softens with the discharge first of pus and later of the 'core' of the boil. Eventually a small scar is left. A carbuncle forms a large brawny inflamed patch, discharging in several places. The patient is ill and runs a temperature. In time a slough separates off; scarring is likely to be extensive. For a weak, ill, aged, ill-nourished or chronic alcoholic patient, a carbuncle can be fatal.
Complications	A boil on the face can cause a spread of infection via communicating veins in or near the orbit to veins inside the skull, with the production of meningitis, cavernous sinus thrombosis or cerebral abscess.
Special tests	*Urine:* should be examined for sugar and albumin, especially when a crop of boils or a carbuncle develops unexpectedly.
Treatment	1. A single small boil usually clears up with local treatment e.g. the application of industrial spirit 75 per cent to keep the skin dry and control infection, by dry heat, by hypertonic saline.

[1] *sycosis:* from Greek: *sukosis* – fig-shaped ulcer
[2] *furunculosis:* from Latin: *furunculus* – a boil

2. For multiple boils and carbuncles, neomycin ointment is applied and penicillin or other antibiotic given by injection.

3. Carrier sites in nose and on perineum are treated with neomycin cream for 2-3 months, or with other appropriate antibiotics.

4. Fresh air, good food and a holiday help. Hexachlorophane soap is used.

5. Raw areas after a carbuncle may require a skin-graft.

AXILLARY ABSCESS

This is an abscess of the apocrine glands, large sebaceous glands in the axilla. They are liable to become infected by shaving, by the use of hair-removers, by irritation from rubber in dress-protectors, and the infection is therefore usually one of women. Oblong tender swellings form and go on to suppurate, pus being discharged from several holes; the whole is likely to become a chronic infection with recurrences and scarring.

Treatment is by antibiotic creams or industrial spirit 75 per cent. In chronic cases, persisting in spite of treatment, surgical removal and grafting of the whole area can be performed.

Tuberculosis of the Skin
LUPUS VULGARIS[3]

This tuberculous infection of the skin can result from (a) direct inoculation of a scratch by infected dust, (b) spread from a tuberculous focus elsewhere, (c) miliary tuberculosis. It usually occurs in children under 10. It is rare in countries where tuberculosis has been controlled.

Clinical features

An 'apple-jelly' nodule appears – a smooth semi-transparent yellowish nodule usually on the face, sometimes on the neck, limbs, hands or peri-anal region. When the face is affected there are likely to be other similar lesions in the mucous membrane of mouth, nose, pharynx and larynx. Untreated, the lesion is likely to spread slowly for years and ulcerate, destroying soft tissues and cartilage (disfiguring nose and ears) but not bone. There may be evidence of tuberculosis elsewhere. With treatment the lesions should clear up in less than 6 months.

Treatment

1. Isoniazid 300-400 mg. daily for 12-18 months, i.e. for about 6-12 months after apparent recovery, in combination with PAS; streptomycin is sometimes given.
2. Improvement of general health by better food, better living conditions, and ultra-violet light.

TUBERCULIDES

These are reactions due to a hyper-sensitivity of the skin to the tuberculin produced by tubercle bacilli elsewhere in the body. Among them are:

(a) *erythema induratum* (Bazin's disease): painful, tender dusky, indurated areas eventually going on to ulceration of the legs of young women with poor peripheral circulation.
(b) *erythema nodosum:* sometimes due to tuberculosis.
(c) *papulo-necrotic tuberculides:* papules break down, ulcerate and scar, occurring on the limbs often in crops.

MOLLUSCUM CONTAGIOSUM[4]

This virus infection spread by direct contact and liable to occur anywhere on the skin, causes the appearance of small, umbilicated[5], pearly grey yellow or pink nodules, singly or in small crops. Secondary infection can occur. There is no impairment in general health.

Treatment is by dipping a pointed orange stick in carbolic acid, inserting it in to the centre of each nodule and twiddling it round. The patient should report 3 weeks later for the treatment of any nodules that may have escaped attention the first time. The treatment is painful.

[3] *lupus:* from Latin: *lupus:* wolf, *vulgaris* -- common
[4] *molluscum:* Latin for soft tumour
[5] *umbilicated:* with a depressed centre like the umbilicus

Diseases of the Skin

INFECTIVE WARTS	*Other names:* Juvenile warts, verruca[6] vulgaris

INFECTIVE WARTS

Other names: Juvenile warts, verruca[6] vulgaris
This is a virus infection of the skin usually occurring in childhood or early adult life. Infection is commonly via swimming pools or the changing-rooms of gyms. Warts occur on the hands, knees, face, scalp, soles (where they are very painful), under the nails (which they deform) and on the external genitalia; they have differing appearances on the various sites. They are infectious and a person may keep on infecting himself. They tend to disappear spontaneously within 6 months.

    Treatment is by (a) waiting for them to disappear, (b) applying carbon dioxide snow or liquid nitrogen, (c) removal with a cautery or curette, (d) applying salycylic acid, formalin or podophyllin to plantar warts, (e) strapping with Elastoplast.

SENILE WARTS

Other names: seborrheic warts, basal cell papillomata
These are rough brown excrecences, possibly due to a virus, likely to appear on the face, scalp or trunk of people over 40. They can be scraped off, leaving a raw surface behind. They are not malignant.
Treatment is by curettage.

FUNGUS INFECTIONS

Fungi are a low form of plant life, some types of which can grow on the skin and hair in long branching chains. Fungus infections are usually described, not by the name of the particular kind of fungus, but by the part affected; several places may be affected by the same fungus at the same time.

RINGWORM OF SCALP

Other name: tinea capitis[7]
This is an affection of children only, for at puberty the hairs develop a resistance to this kind of infection. It is usually spread by direct contact between children or indirectly by sharing caps, hair-nets; there is a rare form that is caught from infected kittens and puppies.

Clinical features

Circular patches of short, broken or bent hairs appear on the scalp, which is covered with dirty scales and sometimes pustules. Unlike alopecia areata there are no completely bald patches.

Special test

Wood's light: affected hairs show a bright green fluorescence under ultra-violet rays passed through a nickel-glass filter.

Treatment

1. All child-contacts are examined, preferably with Wood's light, and all treated.
2. Griseofulvin is given in up to 500 mg in a single dose after a meal containing a large amount of fat. Treatment is given daily for 4-6 weeks. By the end of this time all newly grown hair is healthy. A close hair-cut is done and the hair shampood.

RINGWORM OF THE BEARD

Other name: tinea barbae
This fungus is acquired by farm workers and grooms from infected cattle and

[6] *verruca:* Latin: wart
[7] *tinea:* Latin: moth. *capitis* – of the head

horses or occasionally from cats and dogs. Papules and pustules develop in the beard area, which becomes inflamed and swollen.

Treatment is by tolnaftate cream and a course of griseofulvin.

RINGWORM OF THE FEET

Other names: tinea pedis, athlete's foot

This fungus is spread by wearing infected socks, walking with bare feet, and sports' dressing-rooms and swimming baths are common sources. Vesicles appear on the soles; in the clefts between fifth and fourth toes and between fourth and third, infected skin is likely to itch and be thick, sodden and fissured. Skin in other parts of the body can become infected.

Treatment (a) *If inflammation is present:* by soaks or compresses of potassium permanganate solution, followed by an ointment or cream containing a cortico-steriod and hydroxyquinolone. (b) *If inflammation is not present:* Whitfield's oint-ment (benzoic acid compound ointment) applied locally and griseofulvin 500 mg taken once daily by mouth for 6 weeks.

RINGWORM OF NAILS

Any of the nails of the hands or feet can be affected, but usually not all of them. The nails become thickened, rough, friable and grey or brown.

Treatment is by a course of griseofulvin, 0.5 g daily for at least 6 months. If only one nail is affected, it is removed under griseofulvin cover.

RINGWORM OF AXILLAE AND THIGHS

Other name: dhobie itch [8] (in East)

Red itching areas appear in the axillae and genito-crural folds and sometimes else-where.

Treatment is by a fungicidal[9] cream.

TINEA CIRCINATA

This is 'ring worm' — the fungus, of human or animal source, producing a ring of itching reddened tissue with scales and vesicles encircling an area of healthy skin. It can occur in children with ringworm of the scalp or in adult contacts.

Treatment is by a fungicidal cream.

PSORIASIS[1]

This common disease is characterized by raised reddish patches of skin with sharp edges and silvery scaling. Its causes are obscure; the basic lesion appears to be a biochemical abnormality in the formation of epidermal cells. There may be a family history. It usually begins at 10-16 years, sometimes earlier or later.

Clinical features

The thickened reddish patches are typical. Psoriasis does not usually itch and there-fore is not scratched and secondarily infected; it is not infectious. The following types have been described:

[8] *dhobie:* Indian washerwoman (the supposed source of infection)
[9] *fungicidal:* fungus-killing
[1] *psoriasis:* from Greek: *psora* — itch (often a mis-nomer)

Diseases of the Skin

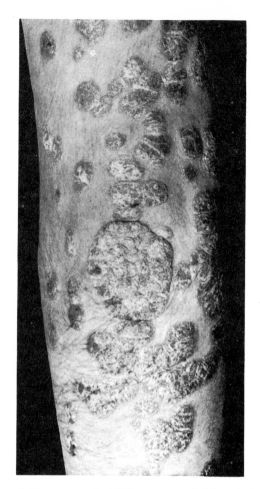

Fig. 87. Psoriasis.

1. *Guttate psoriasis[2]* occurs in childhood; the first attack may have been pre-ceeded 2-3 weeks earlier by a viral infection (chickenpox, mumps, etc.) or an acute streptococcal infection of the throat. Spots of psoriasis appear all over the skin, and, although some persist, usually clear up in about 3 months. More psoriasis is to be expected later in life.

2. *Extensor psoriasis* occurs predominantly on extensor surfaces:— elbow, back of forearm, knee, scalp, lumbo-sacral region; in various shapes: circular, nummular (coin-shaped), circinate (ring-shaped) or geographic (like irregular maps). Beginning in childhood or early adult life, it increases or decreases without obvious reason, and to a greater or less degree is likely to persist for life.

3. *Flexural psoriasis* appears as smooth, shiny, salmon-pink patches in the axillae, under the breasts, in the genito-crural folds and the inter-natal cleft. It is particularly likely to occur in diabetics and old or fat people.

4. *Generalized psoriasis* is a spread from a localized to a widespread distribution, a change sometimes seeming to be due to stress, anxiety, an infection or over-

[2] *guttate:* drop-like

Chapter 17

treatment. The various kinds of psoriasis appear all over the skin, the parts least affected being the hands and feet. Arthritis — usually of small joints — can occur. The condition persisting, the patient is likely to develop a depression — the 'leper complex' of being unclean and shunned. Severe attacks can cause death.

5. *Psoriasis of nails* causes them to be pitted, thickened, opaque and discoloured.

6. *Psoriasis of palms and soles* appears as scaly patches and pustules containing creamy or yellow pus and is very resistant to treatment.

Complication
: *Steatorrhoea* (an excess of fat in faeces) can be caused by disturbance of small intestine structure and function, the amount of disturbance being related to the extent of skin involvement.

Treatment
: 1. During an acute attack the patient may have to go to bed, but at other times he should be encouraged to lead an active life with fresh air and sunshine.

2. He may require psychological help to get him through his periods of depression.

3. Among the ointments applied locally are: oily calamine lotion with or without ichthammol; coal tar with or without salicyclic acid; betamethasone 17-valerate beneath occlusive polythene sheeting for 3-day periods; dithranol ointment; hydrocortisone cream. Care has to be taken not to over-treat.

4. A daily bath is taken with liquor picis carbonis (tar) 60 ml added to the water.

5. Course of ultra-violet light may be combined with local treatment.

6. Azathioprine 100 mg daily, increasing to 200 mg daily.

7. Regular chiropody when nails are affected; the nails should be kept short and debris removed.

LICHEN PLANUS
: This is a disease of unknown origin.

Clinical features
: Violet, flat shiny papules appear all over the skin (sparing usually the face) and itch intensely. On the mucous membranes of mouth, throat, vulva, vagina, and rectum appear white papules or sometimes white streaks and patterns. The skin papules can coalesce to form plaques. On the scalp scarring can cause a patchy baldness. Itching can disturb sleep and affect the general health. Pigmentation can persist after the papules have vanished. The nails may become atrophic and deformed.

The illness runs a quite unpredictable course. Mild attacks can go on for months, new spots appearing as the old vanish. On the legs papules become warty and persist when all others have gone. Apparent complete recovery may be followed by relapse months or years later.

Complication
: Epithelioma is a rare complication of lichen planus of the mouth and vulva.

Treatment
: 1. Any drug suspected of being the cause is discontinued.

2. A severely affected patient is admitted into hospital for a course of 3-4 weeks suppressive treatment by prednisone.

3. Fluocinolone cream or betamethasone 17-valerate cream is applied under an occlusive polythene film.

4. Attempts are made to relieve any stress situations.

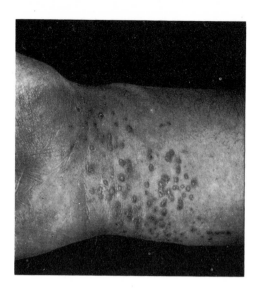

Fig. 88. Lichen planus.

PITYRIASIS ROSEA[3] This is a scaly eruption of unknown origin, sometimes following an infection and possibly then an indication of sensitivity to a virus. It usually affects children and young adults.

Clinical features A week or two after an upper respiratory tract infection – or sometimes without such a history – the patient develops on his trunk a 'herald patch' – an oval or round, rosy patch, which scales. Then, a week or two later, the general eruption appears – of macules, plaques or papules Macules appear on the trunk first and then on the neck and arms; the face and legs are usually not involved. The macules are pink spots, which can spread to form plaques edged with tiny scales, and eventually, after lasting for 4-10 weeks, disappear altogether. Second attacks are uncommon.

Special test WR: the eruption resembles the skin rash of secondary syphilis, and in doubtful cases the WR is tested.

Treatment No special treatment is required except the application of calamine lotion and assurance that all will be well.

PRURITUS[4] Pruritus is itching. The commonest causes are:
1. Scabies
2. Pediculosis
3. Diabetes mellitus, gout, renal failure, cirrhosis of liver, leukaemia, lymphadenoma, carcinomatosis, obstructive jaundice.
4. Old age, with atrophy of the skin.
5. Emotional factors.

Clinical features The patient complains of itching, which is usually made worse by heat and is at its worst at night. Scratching can lead to eczema, urticaria, lichenification and secondary infection.

[3] *pityriasis:* from Greek: *pituron* – bran (i.e. scales)
[4] *pruritus:* from Latin: *prurira* – to itch

Scabies — the 'itch' — is the commonest cause of itching and careful examination for it should be made of every itching patient. Pediculosis causes itching of the trunk. In any case of unexplained itching the urine is examined for sugar.

Treatment
1. The cause should be treated.
2. The patient is kept as fully occupied as possible so that he has less time to worry and scratch.
3. Woollen underclothes should not be worn.
4. Local applications of lead and glycerin lotion or lead and calamine lotion are applied.
5. Phenobarbitone or other barbiturate is given in small doses.
6. Methyl testosterone 5-10 mg. three times daily relieves senile pruritus.

PRURITUS ANI
Itching around the anus is caused by:

haemorrhoids	anal fissure
lack of cleanliness	threadworms
fungus infections	pubic louse infestation
proctitis[5] with discharge	emotional disturbances

intolerance of drugs (a) applied locally, or (b) taken internally, e.g. phenol-
phthalein   leakage of liquid paraffin

Clinical features
In some patients the anal region appears normal; in others there are scratches and lichenification. Emotional disturbances (often in the male associated with passive homosexuality) may be a factor in the appearance and maintenance of the itching. Some patients show excessive peri-anal sweating.

Special tests
If threadworms are suspected but not seen, Scotch tape applied to the perianal region may come off with some of the eggs attached.

Treatment
1. Strict personal cleanliness is insisted on. The part should be dried by dabbing rather than rubbing.
2. The cause is treated. Aperients should not be taken.
3. Hydrocortisone ointment is applied locally.

PRURITUS VULVAE
Itching of the vulva is likely to be due to:
1. Lack of cleanliness
2. Trichomonas and other infections of the vagina and cervix.
3. Threadworms (in children); pubic louse infestation.
4. Sensitivity to contraceptives, soap or powder; excessive use of antiseptics.
5. Diabetes mellitus, glycosuria, urinary incontinence.
6. Skin diseases: infective dermatitis, lichen planus, psoriasis, lichen sclerosus et atrophicus.
7. Atrophic vulvo-vaginitis.

[5] *proctitis:* inflammation of rectum or anus

Diseases of the Skin

8. Nutritional deficiencies.

9. Emotional disturbances.

Clinical features There may be no signs except scratches and secondary infection.

Treatment 1. Treatment is essentially that of the cause.

2. Secondary infection is cured by an appropriate local application, e.g. neomycin with hydrocortisone.

PRURIGO[6] This term describes a number of conditions in which itching and scratching cause patches of lichenification. It is thought of as primarily a psycho-somatic disease in which the patient's tensions and anger, prevented from other outlets, are directed against his own skin.

Clinical features Beginning as red or reddish-brown spots, diamond-shaped patches of lichenification appear. Scratching causes bleeding and secondary infections with boils and impetigo. On the scalp excoriations become scabbed over; on the palms over-growth of the horny layer is likely. In the inter-natal cleft and genito-crural folds the skin becomes white, moist and fissured.

Prurigo may last indefinitely or clear up completely.

Treatment 1. Relief of tension by psychotherapy and sedation by tranquillisers or barbiturates.

2. Sedation at night.

3. Local applications of hydrocortisone, betamethasone 17-valerate cream, or tar as ether-soluble tar paste (ESTP).

ROSACEA[7] This is usually a disease of middle-aged women, but men and young women are sometimes affected. Psychological factors are incriminated; it is predominantly a disease of obsessional women striving at perfection, the blood-vessels of the face dilating in response to frustration, shame, anger. It has been attributed to diet, drugs, hormonal imbalance, acne vulgaris, an unstable vaso-motor system, etc.

Clinical features The patient's face becomes warm and red in the middle of the forehead and on the nose and cheeks. The symptoms are likely to be made worse by embarrassment, worry, exposure to extremes of temperature, and at the pre-menstrual period. Flatulence and indigestion are usually complained of. After a time the redness becomes permanent; red papules appear in the affected regions and becoming infected form crusts and scars. Heavy infestation with *Demodex folliculorum*[8] produces enlargement of the hair follicles.

Complications Conjunctivitis, blepharitis[9] ;

Corneal ulceration, impairment of vision.

Treatment 1. Stress should be treated and anxiety-producing situations avoided.

2. The general health is improved by an adequate diet; hot drinks are not taken; plenty of time is allowed for meals.

[6] *prurigo:* from Latin – itching

[7] *rosacea:* from Latin: *rosa* – a rose

[8] *Demodex folliculorum:* a parasite found in hair-follicles and sebaceous glands

[9] *blepharitis:* inflammation of the edges of the eyelids

3. The face is washed with toilet soap. Cleansing creams are not used.
4. Oxytetracyline or buffered tetracycline 250 mg. daily given for a few months is sometimes effective (the reason for this is unknown).
5. 2 per cent precipitated sulphur is applied as an ointment to treat the *Demodex folliculorum* infestation. Betnovate lotion can be used.

RHINOPHYMA[1]

This is a form of rosacea that is liable to affect the nose in middle-aged men. The veins of the nose dilate; the nose becomes grossly enlarged, irregular in shape and flushed, with very dilated follicular openings. Treatment is by plastic surgery.

URTICARIA[2]

This is an allergic reaction of the skin marked by the development of papules and weals in the skin and subcutaneous tissues as a result of the dilatation of small blood-vessels and the transudation of fluid from them. Causes are:
1. Nettle-stings, insect-bites (mosquitoes, fleas, bed-bugs), contact with 'hairy caterpillar' or jelly-fish.
2. Scabies.
3. Anxiety and stress.
4. Some foods (e.g. strawberries, shell-fish), some drugs (e.g. penicillin, barbiturates, aspirin), in sensitive people. Penicillin can get into milk if a cow is being treated with it.
5. Foci of infection, intestinal parasites.
6. Friction of skin.

Clinical features

Pink papules appear, itch intensely and disappear completely. Swellings appear in the skin and subcutaneous tissues, especially round the eyes and mouth. Single or recurrent attacks can occur. Spontaneous recovery is common.
   Papular urticaria (lichen urticatus) is a form of urticaria in young children in which very itchy red papules appear on the limbs and trunk, form vesicles and crust. Usually it is a hypersensitivity reaction to bites by fleas and other insects.
   Giant urticaria (angio-neurotic oedema) is a form of urticaria with huge non-itching swellings usually on the hands and feet.

Complications

Suffocation may be caused by a weal in the back of the tongue, pharynx or larynx.

Treatment

1. The cause is found and dealt with.
2. Antihistamine drugs are given by mouth, with the usual precautions against driving, cycling and taking alcohol.
3. If all else fails with children with papular urticaria, admission to hospital promptly cures the attack.

ERYTHEMA MULTIFORME[3]

This occurs in young adults. Usually no cause can be found; sometimes it seems to be a reaction to a drug or infection.

[1] *rhinophyma:* from Greek: *rhis* — nose; *phuma* — growth
[2] *urticaria:* from Latin: *urtica* — a nettle
[3] *multiforme:* having many shapes

Diseases of the Skin

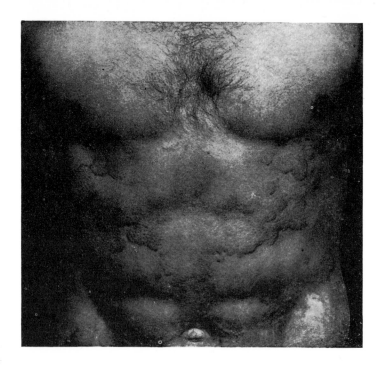

Fig. 89. Urticaria

Clinical features   An attack begins with slight fever and malaise. Then areas of skin, usually on the limbs or face and of all shapes and sizes, become raised and red. Papules, vesicles, bullae, and haemorrhagic lesions can appear, and ulceration of the lips and mucous membrane of the mouth. An attack usually clears up completely within 2-6 weeks. Recurrences can occur.

Complication   In a severe form of the disease (the Stevens-Johnson syndrome) with extensive lesions on the skin and mucous membranes and greater general disturbance, conjunctivitis and corneal ulcers can appear and vision become impaired. The patient may have a high fever, bronchitis or renal disease. Death can occur.

Treatment   The patient should go to bed for a few days. Calamine lotion is applied. Anti-histamine drugs are sometimes given. A patient with the Stevens-Johnson syndrome is a medical emergency for admission to hospital and a course of prednisone to prevent eye complications.

SEBORRHEIC DERMATITIS

This chronic inflammatory disease of the hairy parts follows an excessive secretion of sebum from the sebaceous glands. Possible factors in its causation are excessive intake of fats and carbohydrates, obesity, applications to the skin, and some drugs.

Clinical features   The condition can be considered as occurring in 3 phases:

Phase 1. This is the stage of seborrhoea. Dandruff (scurf) appears on the scalp and sometimes on the other hairy parts as fine, dry, grey scales. There is no reddening.

Phase 2. The scaling becomes worse, the scales are coarse. The nostrils, chest and back are likely to be particularly affected.

Phase 3. Inflammatory changes take place. The skin becomes red, pustules appear, a sero-purulent discharge is present. Staphylococci, streptococci and other organisms infect the areas. More extensive lesions can now appear:

Scalp: extensive, greasy, itching scaling; can extend below the hair-line on to the forehead; hairs fall out.

Ears: pinna inflamed (otitis externa); scaling and inflammation of meatus can cause pain and deafness; painful fissures below and behind the ears (can become secondarily infected, with production of erysipelas).

Eyes: blepharitis[4]; styes; loss of eyelashes; conjunctivitis.

Nose: nostrils and naso-labial folds particularly affected.

Mouth: fissures at angles.

Trunk: likely to be affected especially in obese people, under breasts, under any pendulous fold of fat, in umbilicus, in genito-crural and inter-natal folds; in coronal sulcus of penis.

Toes: infection between toes.

When no definite cause can be found and treated, the condition is likely to become chronic.

Treatment	1. Any cause is treated; fat and carbohydrate consumption is reduced.

1. Any cause is treated; fat and carbohydrate consumption is reduced.
2. The scalp and other hairy parts are shampooed with cetrimide 1 per cent.
3. Any of the following are applied locally; salicylic acid and mercuric chloride lotion, sulphur and calamine lotion, coal tar preparations; hydrocortisone cream combined with an antibiotic to inflammatory areas.
4. Dusting powders of boric acid or zinc and salicylic acid are applied to skin-folds, which can be separated by gauze.

ACNE VULGARIS [5]

In acne there is at puberty an over-activity of the sebaceous glands (which open into the hair-follicles), as a result of an excess in the male of testosterone and in the female of progesterone; and the excessive secretion becomes blocked in the hair-follicle by a thickening of tissue around the opening of the follicle on to the skin. Oxidation occurs in the outer part of the sebum and a blackhead (comedo) is formed. Inflammation and pus develops around the follicle. This can go on to scar-formation; in some people and some places — especially the back of the neck and in front of the sternum — the scarring can be keloidal [6]. Men are usually more severely affected than women. In many people it is very mild.

Acne usually begins at 12-14 years and subsides before 30. Sometimes it persists throughout adult life.

Clinical features

People with acne have usually a greasy, muddy complexion and may be excessively hairy.

Blackheads are seen on the face, neck and upper half of the trunk and to a lesser

[4] *blepharitis:* inflammation of the margin of the eyelid
[5] *acne:* from Greek: *akme* — a point. *vulgaris:* common
[6] *keloid:* excessive fibrous tissue forming a large thick scar

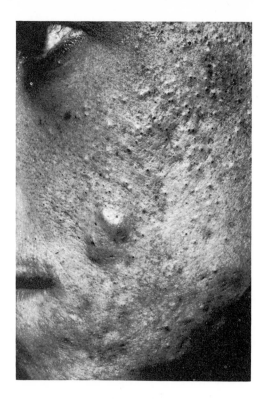

Fig. 90. Acne vulgaris.

extent elsewhere. They are little grey specks at the openings of the hair follicle. If they become inflamed, a little papule forms, topped by the blackhead. A papule can become a pustule; a pustule can form a cyst or a scar. All kinds of lesions can be present at the same time. Keloidal scarring can be very disfiguring.

Treatment 1. Affected parts are washed several times a day with Cetavlon. Blackheads must not be squeezed but can be removed with a 'blackhead remover' (available at large chemists).
2. The patient should be out of doors in all weathers as much as possible.
3. Moderate or severe acne is treated with long-term antibiotics, usually tetracycline or clindamycin.
4. Ultra-violet light treatment produces temporary improvement.

DERMATITIS HERPETIFORMIS This is a disease of unknown origin, occurring occasionally in childhood, more commonly in mid-adult life, and characterized by vesicles and bullae. Intestinal malabsorption and abnormalities of the mucous membrane of the jejunum occur in two-thirds of people affected.

Clinical features The patient develops an eruption of papules, vesicle and small bullae on a normal or reddened skin. Any part of the skin can be affected, in particular the buttocks, genitalia, elbows and upper back. Affected parts itch intensely. The general health is not impaired. The condition can wax and wane over years before eventually disappearing.

306   *Chapter 17*

Treatment	Dapsone (an antibacterial drug used for leprosy) is the best treatment given in doses of up to 100 mg daily for long periods. As it can cause anaemia, blood counts are done and the Hb estimated periodically, and ferrous sulphate and vitamin B given. Malabsorption is treated; a gluten-free diet improves the intestinal condition.
MORPHOEA	This is a disease of unknown origin, more common in women than men. Round or oval plaques develop in the skin, which around them can be violet or pink. The plaques, white and firm at first, eventually become brown and soft. There may be slight itching. *Lichen sclerosus et atrophicus* is a similar condition, especially liable to affect the vulva and perianal region. There is no effective treatment except hydrocortisone ointment or cream to relieve the itching.
PEMPHIGUS	This skin disease can be fatal. Its cause is unknown, it is especially liable to affect Jews and it usually occurs in people of 55-65.
Clinical features	On skin that looks perfectly healthy bullae, large and small, well up, rupture and spread and do not heal. Over the pressure areas deep ulcers can form. In time the whole skin can be affected; secondary infection follows; smelly warty outgrowths appear in the flexures, the mucous membrane of the mouth and other orifices is shed; swallowing is difficult or impossible; fluid, salt and serum protein loss is severe, and eventually the patient dies, usually within two years of the onset. Treatment by cortico-steroids may produce remissions and prolong life. *Senile dermatitis herpetiformis* is a rather similar affliction of old age, but the lesions itch and the skin around them is reddened.
Treatment	1. This being an extremely serious disease, the patient should be admitted into hospital. 2. Prednisone is given in doses of 60-150 mg daily until a remission is produced and then in smaller doses and with corticotrophin by intra-muscular injection. 3. Antibiotic ointments are applied to the lesions and later tulle gras.

Tumours of the Skin
RODENT ULCER

Other name: basal cell carcinoma

This is a malignant tumour occurring in late adult life, usually on the face near the ear, nose or eye but occasionally elsewhere. In a common type a rodent ulcer begins as a pearly nodule, which enlarges slowly over the years, has small visible blood-vessels coursing over it, and ulcerates. Some ulcerate deeply, some extend in the skin without ulceration. Secondary growths are very rare.

Treatment is by excision, X-radiation or radium; the results are very satisfactory. Plastic surgery may be required if there has been much tissue-destruction.

SQUAMOUS CELL CARCINOMA

This is a rapidly growing cancer of the skin. The tumour is firm, nodular and liable to ulcerate or to form cauliflower-like projections. Common sites are the face, ears, and back of the hands. Local lymphatic nodes can be invaded.

Treatment is by X-radiation or excision; block-dissection of lymph nodes is sometimes necessary.

[7] *stenosis:* narrowing
[8] *leuocoplakia:* grey-white thickened patches, often pre-cancerous

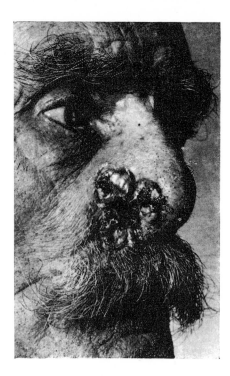

Fig. 91. Rodent ulcer.

MELANOMA

Benign melanomas are moles, pigmented raised patches, sometimes hairy. They are likely to become slowly bigger, they may become malignant. Treatment is by excision, usually for cosmetic reasons.

A *malignant melanoma* can arise in (a) a lentigo, which is a non-hairy mole, a dark brown macule that does not darken on exposure to sunlight (unlike a freckle, which does and is harmless) or in (b) a melanoma. When one of these becomes malignant, it enlarges, darkens, bleeds, ulcerates, scabs over and is painful. A malignant melanoma is the most malignant of all tumours of the body, for it invades local lymph nodes very quickly, rushes into other lymph nodes, and has secondaries in liver, lungs, brain and other organs in less than no time. *Treatment* is by excision with block dissection of glands, but this is often too late.

FIBROMATA MOLLE[9]

These are soft harmless tags or pedunculated tumours of normal connective tissue. They can be removed with a diathermy or more simply, if pedunculated[1], by tying a piece of cotton round the stalk and so cutting off the blood-supply.

NEURO-FIBROMATOSIS

Other name: Von Recklinghausen's disease[2]

In this condition multiple lesions develop on the skin; yellowish-brown macules called *café-au-lait* spots, flat skin-coloured or brownish tumours, pedunculated tumours. Nodules of fibrous

[9] *fibroma:* tumour of fibrous tissue. *molle:* soft
[1] *pedunculated:* having a stalk
[2] *F. D. von Recklinghausen* (1833-1910) German pathologist

tissue develop on nerves, on internal organs, under the periosteum; and these, unlike the tumours of the skin, can become malignant.

Treatment is by surgical removal when necessary.

HAEMANGIOMA

A haemangioma (naevus) is an overgrowth of blood-vessels.

1. *Spider naevus* (stellate haemangioma [3]) consists of a central vein with capillaries radiating out of it; usual sites are the face and hands. They occur in healthy people, pregnancy, chronic liver disease and any condition in which the oestrogen level in the blood is high.

2. *Strawberry mark* (haemangioma simplex) is a bright red naevus, which appears shortly after birth, anywhere on the skin, enlarges for about 9 months, then starts to disappear but does not go completely for several years. Treatment is by leaving it to run its natural course, for any treatment leaves a scar behind, which a natural recovery does not; a rapidly growing naevus in an awkward site, such as around the mouth, might have to be excised or have radiotherapy.

3. *Port·wine stain* (naevus flammeus) is a purple patch of skin due to dilated vessels, likely to persist for life. Nothing very much can be done except to hide the lesion with a suitably tinted cosmetic preparation.

XANTHOMA[4]

Xanthomata are yellow or orange papules or plaques containing cholesterol and likely to occur in middle-aged women with a high blood-cholesterol (normal: 100-300 mg per 100 ml). Treatment is by excision or the application of tri-chlor-acetic acid, and a low fat diet.

TOXIC ERYTHEMA

This is a scarlet or blotchy eruption, associated with mild malaise and slight pyrexia, produced as a result of hypersensitivity to a food, to a drug or to pressure. It can occur in the late stages of pregnancy. The usual sites are the face, trunk and upper parts of the limbs. An attack clears up in a few days. No treatment is required except the application of calamine lotion.

REACTIONS TO DRUGS

In some hyper-sensitive people drugs can produce skin rashes. Many diseases can be mimicked and various lesions produced — erythema, pigmentation, acne, papules, vesicles, pustules, bullae, purpura, scaling, etc. Rashes are usually bright, widespread and symmetrical, and usually present some differences from the condition they most closely resemble. Most of them clear up within a few days of stopping the drug, but at any later time a very small dose of it will provoke an attack.

EXFOLIATIVE DERMATITIS

Other name: erythrodermia

This persistent redness of the skin, which can go on to extensive peeling, is commonly the result of (a) over-treatment of eczema, psoriasis or other chronic skin disease (b) a toxic reaction to a drug, e.g. arsenic, bismuth, gold, mercury. In severe cases, the peeling is very severe and continuous; heat-loss is a complication, and death can follow broncho-pneumonia, nephritis or hepatitis. It often persists for years in a subacute state.

Treatment is by: (a) stopping the cause; (b) applying oily calamine lotion or zinc cream, (c) avoiding exposure and heat-loss, (d) in severe cases giving a course of prednisone, beginning with 30 mg daily, (e) giving a course of dimercaprol if a heavy metal is the cause.

ERYTHEMA NODOSUM

This is a condition in which tender, red or blue-brown nodules appear on the shins or forearms of young people. They subside spontaneously within a few weeks; rest in bed and aspirin are all that is necessary.

An attack is an indication of the hypersensitivity of the blood-vessels of the skin to (a)

[3] *stellate:* star-shaped

[4] *xanthoma:* from Greek: *xanthos* – yellow; *oma* – tumour

Diseases of the Skin

tuberculosis, (b) sarcoid, (c) a streptococcal or other infection — an attack may follow an upper respiratory tract infection, (d) in U.S.A. coccidioidomycosis[5]. An attack should suggest above all things that the patient has somewhere a primary tuberculous focus; it should be sought diligently and the patient, if it is not found, kept under observation and the search renewed.

SUNBURN

Sunburn is due to exposure to ultra-violet light and not to heat, and can be caused by 'cold light' off snow and the sea.

Clinical features

An affected part develops an erythema, which itches, becomes oedematous, and can go on to form vesicles and ulcers. The patient can run a temperature, feel ill, have nausea, vomit.

Complications

Sepsis, following rupture of bullae.
Dehydration, vascular failure, death from very extensive burns.

Prevention

It is prevented by (a) graduated exposure to sun, both of area of skin exposed and length of exposure, (b) use of 'sun-tan' creams that specifically absorb ultra-violet light.

Treatment

Any sunburn should be treated as seriously as a burn of similar degree from any other cause. Liquid paraffin or calamine lotion is applied. Blisters are left intact or opened aseptically. Antibiotics are given by injection or mouth for any infection. Dehydration and vascular failure are treated in the usual ways.

PRICKLY HEAT

This is a common condition in very hot tropical countries where people are likely to sweat heavily and continuously. Newcomers are more likely to be affected than natives or old-stagers; young children and fat people can get it badly. White-skinned people only are affected.

Clinical features

A rash appears in the folds and moist areas, and can become generalized. Reddish papules appear, surrounded by areas of erythema, and vesicles develop in them. Itching is severe, scratching leads to secondary infection, purulent eczematous areas can appear. New crops of papules appear as the old disappear and in this way the condition is likely to persist for months, becoming worse with any exacerbation of the heat; itching being severe, sleep is lost and tempers become frayed.

Treatment

Clothing is changed frequently. Frequent cool baths are followed by careful drying and the application of dusting powder or calamine lotion. Regulated sun-bathing can be helpful. Severely affected infants have to be taken to cooler climates. In some people large doses of Vitamin C seem to prevent it.

TROPICAL ULCERS

These occur on the feet and legs of ill-nourished labourers in the hot wet parts of Africa and the Far East. Arising in a minor injury, the ulcer causes gangrene of the tissues, invading if untreated the subcutaneous tissues, muscles and eventually bone. In spite of the depth and extent of the ulceration, the patient's general health is little affected.

Prevention is by careful treatment of minor injuries and improvement in nutrition.

Treatment is by removal of sloughs, application of antiseptics, occlusive dressings, antibiotics by mouth or injection, and surgical removal of resistant ulcers.

[5] *coccidioidomycosis:* a fungus infection, mimicking tuberculosis, occurring in hot dry parts of America

DISTURBANCES OF PIGMENTATION	The amount of pigment in the skin can be increased or decreased.

Hyper-pigmentation can be:

(a) pigmented naevi;

(b) freckles: a summer eruption of pigmented patches, most common in blondes;

(c) chloasma[6]: brown patches on the face of the pregnant, due to a pituitary hormone;

(d) a result of Addison's disease, thyrotoxicosis, chronic liver disease, etc.

Hypo-pigmentation can be:

(a) albinism[7]: a congenital absence of pigment from the skin (which is pale), the hair (which is white) and the eyes (which are pink); patients have to avoid sunlight, which distresses them and can eventually produce malignant changes in the skin; (b) leprosy;

(c) vitiligo[8]: patchy disappearance of pigment from the skin and sometimes from the hair; sometimes with hyper-pigmentation in other areas of skin; of unknown origin; usually persistent.

ICHTHYOSIS[9]

This is a congenital scaling of the skin, which can vary in degree from very slight braniness to fish-like scaling. It can occur in conjunction with spasticity and mental retardation (Sjögren-Larsson syndrome). Keratosis of the palms and soles is a congenital thickening of the skin in those parts, possibly related to ichthyosis. Greasy applications to the skin can be helpful; soaps and detergents are avoided as much as possible. Frequent baths should be taken.

Diseases of the Hair
ALOPECIA (BALDNESS)
Congenital alopecia

This is rare, can be associated with other congenital abnormalities, and is more common in males. A later growth of hair sometimes occurs but cannot be counted on.

Common (acquired) baldness

This is more common in men than women. The cause is usually unknown; possible factors are genetic or hormonal, dandruff and the use of hair-brushes with bristles of nylon ending in a point. Hair can fall off the crown or sides of head or in both places together. There is no effective treatment. Alopecia can also occur in lupus erythematosus, hypothyroidism, hyperthyroidism and iron deficiency anaemia, and be produced by antibiotics and anti-coagulants.

Alopecia areata

The causes are unknown. It can occur in families; the onset is usually between 10 and 35 years. Both sexes are affected. Hair falls out suddenly in round or oval patches of variable size. Hairs that are left have the shape of an exclamation mark! Loose hairs can be easily pulled out. Regrowth of hair can occur. Recurrences are likely; sometimes they are seasonal.

Alopecia totalis is loss of hair from the whole scalp.

Alopecia universalis is complete loss of hair from scalp and body.

Treatment

1. Injection of steroid preparations into the patch can stimulate re-growth, but is not recommended in childhood.

2. A wig can be worn.

[6] *chloasma:* from Greek: *khoazein* – to be green
[7] *albinism:* from Latin: *albus* – white
[8] *vitiligo:* Latin: *vitiligo* – a rash
[9] *ichthyosis:* from Greek: *ichthus* – fish

Diseases of the Skin

HIRSUTIES   *Other name:* hypertrichosis

This is excessive growth of hair. It can be:

1. Congenital: either general or local.

2. Acquired: (a) on face in women at the menopause or later, (b) temporarily during pregnancy, (c) in Cushing's syndrome, adreno-genital syndrome, acromegaly, thyrotoxicosis, etc.

Treatment is (a) treatment of the cause, (b) diathermy of individual hair-follicles, (c) application of waxes, shaving, use of pumice stone, (d) excision of small areas.

Diseases of Bones, Joints and Muscle

Bone is living tissue and its health depends upon an adequate supply of calcium and of vitamin D. In some conditions calcium is removed from the bone, and bones then become weakened, liable to bend or collapse, and liable to develop pathological fractures; the removal of calcium from bone causes an increase of calcium in the blood and can lead to the development of stones in the kidneys. Much less common are conditions in which there is an increase of calcium in bone.

GENERALIZED OSTEOPOROSIS

This is a condition in which there is a reduction in bone-mass without any change in the chemical composition of bone. It is seen most commonly in elderly women and less commonly in elderly men. It can also occur in acromegaly, hyperthyroidism, Cushing's syndrome and the intestinal malabsorption syndrome, when a person is immobilized for long periods, and when a person is undergoing treatment by cortico-steroids.

Degeneration of collagen tissue in bone appears to be the basic change. The high occurrence in old men and women suggests that there is then a calcium deficiency in the diet.

Clinical features

These are usually due to degeneration of the vertebrae and long bones.

Vertebral degeneration produces pain in the back, made worse by lifting and stooping, attacks of acute back pain when a vertebral body collapses, and girdle pains; the patient becomes shorter because of this degeneration and collapse and develops lordosis or kyphosis.

Fractures are likely to occur in the long bones, particularly in the neck of the femur, and especially in elderly women.

Special tests

X-ray: for lack of density in bone, collapse of vertebral bodies and fractures.

Treatment

1. The patient is kept mobile except when pain is very severe.
2. A high protein diet is given with additional calcium, 1.0 g three times a day.
3. Hormonal treatment is given: oestrogens to women, androgens to men; they are not very effective.
4. Analgesics are given to relieve pain.
5. Fractures are treated appropriately.

OSTEITIS DEFORMANS	*Other name:* Paget's disease of bone

OSTEITIS DEFORMANS

Other name: Paget's disease of bone

This is a disease of unknown cause. It is peculiar that simultaneously it affects some bones extensively, others slightly, and some not at all; occasionally only one bone such as a single vertebra or one of the long bones is involved. It begins in late middle life, more commonly in men than women. Bones commonly affected are the sacrum, pelvis, vertebrae, skull, ribs and long bones of the limbs; the hands and feet are usually not affected. The bony changes are a degeneration of bone-matter with excessive repair, the two changes producing weak, deformed bones.

Clinical features

These vary with the bones involved. In some patients no clinical features are produced, the disease being discovered on X-ray examination or autopsy.

The patient complains of headache when the skull is involved and of backache when the spine is involved. Affected bones are painful, thickened and deformed, and the soft tissues over them are swollen, red and hot. The head becomes enlarged; the long bones of the leg become bowed and the patient's height shortened; involvement of the pelvis and femora produces a wide posture and difficulty in walking. Involvement of the spine produces backache and girdle-pains. The illness runs a long, painful disabling course.

Complications

Pathological fractures   Sarcoma of bone (rare)

Deafness (from pressure on auditory nerves)

Blindness (from pressure on optic nerves)

Compression of spinal cord (from collapse of vertebral bodies)

Heart failure (affected parts being very vascular, they act as *arterio-venous shunts,* causing back-pressure on heart, increased pulse-rate, dilatation of heart)

Special tests

X-ray: shows typical bony changes.

Blood: serum alkaline phosphatase is raised (normal: 3-13 King Armstrong units/100 ml)

Treatment

Mithramycin and actinomycin (antibiotics with anti-malignancy actions) may be given, but they are so toxic that their use is restricted to elderly patients with severe bone-pain or severe disabling complications. The patient should be kept mobile as long as possible.

OSTEO-GENESIS IMPERFECTA

Other name: fragilitas ossium

This is a congenital inherited disease of bone and fibrous tissue. Severely affected infants die *in utero* or shortly after birth. Survivors have:

(a) very fragile bones which break easily, (b) abnormally thin long bones, (c) deformities of the skull with frontal, parietal and occipital bossing, (d) blue sclerae of the eye, (e) poorly developed muscles; excessive movements at joints, (f) spontaneous haemorrhages, (g) otosclerosis and deafness in later life

Treatment

No treatment is possible except that of the fractures when they occur.

ACHRONDROPLASIA

This is an inherited form of dwarfism due to a disturbance of bone formation in cartilage. Severely affected infants die *in utero* or early childhood. Survivors show a particular kind of dwarfism.

The arms and legs are abnormally short and this shortness causes the dwarfism. The legs are usually bowed. The length of the trunk is normal. The head is large with frontal bosses. The vertebrae are abnormal, causing lordosis and prominent buttocks. Prolapse of the intervertebral discs leads to compression of the spinal cord and nerve-roots.

Treatment   No treatment is possible. Achondroplastic dwarfs sometimes earn a living as clowns and tumblers in circuses.

OSTEOPETROSIS   *Other names:* marble bone disease, Albers-Schönberg's disease[1]
This is a rare disease in which there is an increase in the density of bones. It occurs in: (a) fetal life: affected children have hydrocephalus and die shortly after birth;
(b) childhood: affected children show mental retardation, compression of cranial nerves, anaemia (because of involvement of bone-marrow), and pathological fractures; they die young;
(c) adult life: the disease is less severe and may be diagnosed only when a pathological fracture[2] occurs; fractures heal badly and produce deformities. The juvenile and adult forms show a familial incidence in about half the cases.

Special test   *X-ray:* bones show the typical increased density and loss of normal structure.

Treatment   There is no effective treatment. Especial care to avoid deformity has to be taken in treating fractures.

Diseases of Joints

Arthritis is an inflammation or degeneration of joints. In osteo-arthritis only one joint is usually affected, but in most other conditions of which arthritis is a feature several joints are affected at the same time. Arthritis shows itself in the joint becoming swollen, painful and tender and by some loss of function; there can be an effusion into the joint; the cartilage is affected by degeneration in some kinds of arthritis.

Arthritis as a complication of a fever is not now often seen when appropriate chemotherapy or antibiotic treatment is given; it can occur as a complication of septicaemia, meningo-coccal infection, tuberculosis, gonorrhoea, bacillary dysentery, certain virus infections (especially German measles), syphilis and yaws. It is a prominent feature of gout and Reiter's disease.

RHEUMATOID
ARTHRITIS   This is a very crippling arthritis of small joints. Its cause is unknown; it has been attributed to an error of metabolism, to infection, to an auto-immune reaction, and to severe mental stress. It occurs commonly in temperate climates and not in very cold or very hot countries. There may be a familial incidence; about three times as many women as men are affected. The age of onset is usually in the first half of adult life.

Clinical features   The disease begins with a period of malaise, slight pyrexia, fatigue, stiffness, pain

[1] *Albers-Schönberg, H. E.,* German radiologist (1865-1921)
[2] *pathological fracture:* one occurring in diseased bone as a result of a stress or injury that would not produce a fracture in healthy bone; can be a *spontaneous fracture,* occurring without any apparent stress

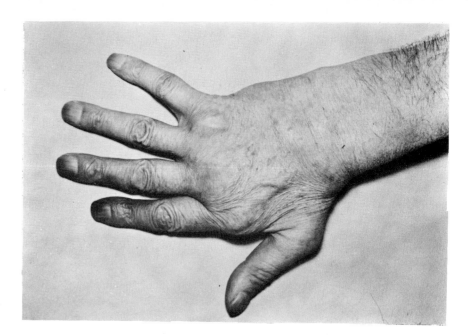

Fig. 92. The hand in rheumatoid arthritis with swollen phalangeal joints and wrist.

in the joints, sweating and loss of weight. Sometimes there is a much more acute onset.

The arthritis affects many joints, beginning with interphalangeal joints as a rule and then spreading to the other joints of the arm and leg. Any joint in the body can be affected eventually. When many joints are involved the patient becomes severely crippled and unable to do anything for himself. Small joints may become dislocated; there is ulnar deviation of the hands. The joints of the cervical spine are commonly involved with the production of instability of the head, paraesthesiae and pressure on the spinal cord.

The patient is likely to develop severe muscular wasting. The bursae are often swollen and subcutaneous nodules appear around the joints. The peripheries have a poor blood supply and become cold and blue. Pleurisy, anaemia, pulmonary fibrosis, enlarged lymph-nodes, malabsorption and neuropathy can occur.

The progress of the disease is uncertain and it is not possible at the onset to predict the outcome. With modern treatment about 20 per cent of patients recover completely, up to 10 per cent are severely and hopelessly crippled, and the rest show various degrees of chronic arthritis. When the disease begins over the age of 60, it can be a self-limiting disease with complete recovery for 25 per cent.

A number of varieties of the disease are known. *Still's disease* is a form of the disease that occurs in children and is associated with enlarged spleen and lymph-nodes, and sometimes with cataract and calcification of the cornea. *Felty's syndrome* is a form in adults who in addition to the usual features have an enlarged spleen and lymph-nodes and pigmentation of the skin, and can develop cirrhosis of the liver. *Sjögren's syndrome* is a form in which there is also deficient salivary and lacrimal secretion, causing a dry mouth and dry eyes.

Chapter 18

Treatment 1. General measures	During the acute stage of the illness the patient stays in bed. Affected joints are splinted with light removable splints of plaster of Paris or plastic. The splints are removed twice a day so that the joint can if possible be put through the full range of its movements. A collar is worn for cervical spine arthritis. Large muscle-groups are exercised several times a day to prevent muscle wasting and stiffness. An ordinary diet can be taken supplemented with iron, calcium and vitamins B and C. Sedatives and hypnotics are given to provide rest and sleep.
2. Drugs	(a) *Gold* is given in weekly injections of sodium aurothiomalate (Myocrisin) 10-50 mg. intramuscularly. Toxic effects are blood disease and renal damage. (b) *Cortico-steroids* are given with gold for short periods. Withdrawal of the drug can be followed by a relapse. Hydrocortisone in a single dose of 50-100 mg can be injected into a joint, usually after the aspiration of fluid. (c) *Acetyl-salicylic acid* (aspirin) is given in the maximum doses the patient can tolerate. But aspirin can produce bleeding from the gastric mucosa. (d) *Penicillamine* is given as D-penicillamine or D-penicillamine hydrochloride by mouth in increasing doses up to a total daily dose of 1-1.5 g. The treatment is continued for 12 months according to the therapeutic effect and the patient's tolerance of the drug. Its mode of action is not known. (e) *Iron* is injected intramuscularly or intravenously for anaemia; a *blood transfusion* is often beneficial both to relieve the anaemia and for its general effects.
3. Physiotherapy	From the beginning the patient should be under the care of a physiotherapist who will carry out appropriate passive movements, supervise active movements and give faradism. Orthopaedic surgery may be needed to correct deformities. Removal of the diseased synovial membrane of an affected joint is sometimes performed.
OSTEO-ARTHRITIS	This arthritis is a degeneration of the articular cartilage and weight-bearing surface of a large joint. Usually only one joint is affected — the hip, the knee or the shoulder. Causes are obesity; injury such as a fracture involving the joint; repeated small injuries to a joint as can occur in certain occupations; old age; syringomyelia.
Clinical features	The patient complains of stiffness and pain in the joint, and later of limitation of movement. Crepitus[3] can be felt in the joint; sometimes there is an effusion of fluid into it; muscles around it may waste. A progressive deterioration of the condition is likely.
Treatment	1. Obesity is reduced. 2. Trauma-producing occupations have to be given up. 3. The following drugs are used to relieve pain and inflammation: acetyl-salicylic acid, phenylbutazone, chloroquine and ibufenac. 4. Physiotherapy provides heat to the joint by short-wave therapy and muscle-strengthening to give stability to the joint. 5. Orthopaedic operations include arthrodesis[4] and replacement of a joint by an artificial joint made of vanadium.

[3] *crepitus:* the grating sensation felt and heard when two injured or degenerated bony surfaces are rubbed together
[4] *arthrodesis:* fusion of a joint by removing the articular surfaces and fixing the ends together

Diseases of Bones, Joints and Muscle

ANKYLOSING SPONDYLITIS

This is a form of arthritis that usually affects young men. Its cause is unknown. There may be a familial incidence.

Clinical features

The onset is insidious. The patient complains of low back pain or 'fibrositis'. He develops a gradually worsening stiffness of the spine and can finish up with a 'poker-spine' with the vertebrae fused together. Joints of the limbs may be affected before those of the spine. Tenderness over bony points occurs.

General symptoms and signs include slight pyrexia, sweating, lack of energy, loss of weight. The aortic and mitral valves can develop stenosis or incompetence. Abdominal herniae are common.

Special tests

X-ray: typical changes can usually be seen in the sacro-iliac, vertebral or any other affected joint.
Blood: ESR is raised; anaemia is likely.

Treatment

1. Physiotherapy is given to check deformity and relieve pain.
2. Acetyl-salicylic acid (aspirin) relieves pain and inflammation.
3. Phenylbutazone or oxyphenbutazone is given in doses of up to 300 mg daily.
4. Corticosteroids are given for acute attacks.
5. Radiotherapy relieves symptoms early in the disease.

Diseases of Muscle
PSEUDO-HYPERTROPHIC MUSCULAR DYSTROPHY

Other name: Duchenne's disease [5]
This is one of the kinds of myopathy or muscular dystrophy. Its cause is unknown. It is an inherited disease, inheritance being either sex-linked or recessive (see Chapter 11). It is most common in boys, but can occur in a milder form in girls and in adolescence or early adult life. There is a very characteristic enlargement of the muscles for some years before they waste, but the enlargement is thought to be due to overdevelopment of still unaffected muscle-fibres.

Clinical features

The history begins in infancy or early childhood. The boy may have been late to walk and always walked badly, or he may have walked all right to begin with and then become clumsy. He stands with feet apart, walks with a waddle, does not romp and move easily like other children, has particularly difficulty in climbing stairs, and when he falls, which is often, he picks himself up by holding on to the furniture or by 'climbing up himself' — turning over on his front, getting on to knees and hands, and then putting his hands on his knees and thighs and pushing. Affected muscles are usually those of the calves (which look like rugby-footballs), buttocks, back, thighs and upper arms. Wasting eventually occurs in them or may appear, without any hypertrophy, in other muscles. Fracture from falls can be a complication. Eventually the weakness and the contractures that develop cause the child to be chairborne, and with increasing helplessness life is usually terminated by a respiratory illness before the patient reaches 20. In girls and adults the progress of the disease is less rapid and the crippling can be much less.

[5] *C. B. A. Duchenne* (1806-1875), French neurologist

Treatment	There is no known treatment. Physiotherapy may prevent the development of contractures. It is advisable not to keep the patient in bed for any infection or other condition because even a few days in bed can put him off his feet and precipitate him into a wheel-chair life. Education of the patient may have to be at home or in a school for the physically handicapped; but if the patient cannot be looked after at home and when home conditions are poor, admission into a residential school becomes advisable. Morale has to be kept as high as possible in what usually is a crippling and before long fatal disease.
LIMB-GIRDLE DYSTROPHIES	These are inherited dystrophies in which the muscles usually affected first are those in the shoulder-region (the scapulo-humeral type) or in the pelvic region. The cause is unknown. The onset is usually at 10-30 years, atrophy is present from the first, and the course is only slowly progressive. There is no effective treatment.
FACIO-SCAPULO-IUMERAL DYSTROPHY	This is a form of dystrophy of unknown origin, affecting both sexes, occurring in adult life and affecting in particular the muscles of facial expression and of the shoulders. The patient has a 'myopathic face' – expressionless with a pouting half-open mouth; typically he cannot whistle. The course is slowly progressive; there is no effective treatment.
DYSTROPHIA MYOTONICA	This is an inherited disease of unknown origin, beginning usually at 20-35 years. It can begin in childhood. The typical features are:

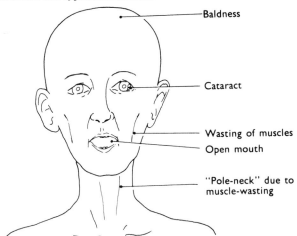

Fig. 93. The face in dystrophia myotonica.

(a) wasting of the muscles of the face and of mastication (producing a flat expressionless face with a pouting half-open mouth), of the sternomastoids (producing a 'pole neck') and of other muscles;

(b) myotonia – an inability to relax muscle after contraction, e.g. the patient cannot let go after shaking hands and has difficulty in swallowing;

(c) other degenerations – cataract[6], baldness, atrophy of testes, wasting;

(d) mental changes in some patients: suspicions, ideas of reference, delusions of persecution.

Treatment	The myotonia is treated by quinine bisulphate or procaine amide.

[6] *cataract:* degeneration and opacity in the lens of the eye

Diseases of Bones, Joints and Muscle

19   Diseases due to Physical Factors

A number of disorders are produced by physical factors — by motion, altitude, extremes of heat and cold, and ionizing radiations.

TRAVEL SICKNESS

Other name: motion sickness

This is vomiting produced by travel by car, train, ship or aeroplane. It is particularly liable to occur in people with a history of migraine or of 'biliousness' in childhood. The cause appears to be an over-stimulation of the vestibular apparatus in the inner ear. The sufferer feels sick and faint and goes on to vomit profusely. He may recover in a few hours or be prostrated for days. *Prevention* is by taking drugs of the anti-histamine or hyoscine groups. Glucose drinks may be given during an attack.

ALTITUDE SICKNESS

This is due to oxygen-want produced by a diminution of the partial pressure of oxygen in the atmosphere, a result of low barometric pressure at heights. The effects vary with the rate of ascent. A healthy mountaineer, climbing slowly, develops 'mountain-sickness' at about 12,000 feet. He has headache, nausea, vomiting and emotional disturbances. After a few days at a height he becomes acclimatized as a result of changes in his blood and respiratory system; the number of RBCs increases and more oxygen is taken up, respiration is deeper. An aviator, climbing in an aeroplane without oxygen, develops symptoms at about the same height but develops them much more acutely. His judgement becomes grossly impaired and if he continues to climb he becomes unconscious, paralysed and likely to die.

CHILBLAINS

Chilblains are the result of peripheral arteriolar spasm and venous stagnation in response to cold. They are most common in girls and young women. The toes, fingers, nose and ears can be affected, becoming swollen and blueish-red, burn or itch intensely and can ulcerate. They are liable to return every winter.

Prevention

1. Wearing warm clothes.
2. Avoiding cold, draughts, standing on cold floors.
3. Taking more exercise.
4. Having an electric blanket instead of a hot-water bottle.

320   *Chapter 19*

5. Having a course of ultra-violet light treatment to the whole body in September-October of every year.

6. Applying toilet lanoline daily as a heat-insulator.

FROSTBITE Frostbite is due to freezing of the soft tissues and a stopping of the circulation in affected parts. The frost-bitten person notices first severe burning and then numb-

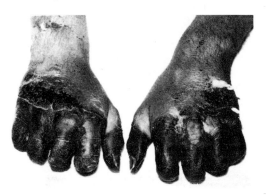

Fig. 94. Frost-bitten hands.

ness of the part, which becomes white and can go on to become gangrenous.

Treatment is by rapid warming. The part must not be rubbed.

HYPOTHERMIA Old people may develop hypothermia during cold weather when they live in a cold house, cannot afford to buy fuel, live alone and cannot look after themselves, and have insufficient food and clothing. Old people with apparently adequate clothing can still develop hypothermia because in old age the temperature-regulating mechanism (in the hypothalamus of the brain) becomes inefficient. Myxoedema is another cause of hypothermia.

Clinical features The patient, after a period of confusion and drowsiness, passes into coma. The body is cold to the touch and the rectal temperature below 32°C (90°F). The pulse is slow, the BP low, respiration slow and shallow. Death is common, in spite of treatment.

Treatment Treatment is by gradual warming with warm blankets or a warm bath, by the maintenance of the air-way, and the administration of intravenous fluids.

HEAT Excessive heat can cause illness in several ways.

Heat-stroke is due to a rise in temperature above about 41°C (106°F) and can be produced by malaria, the heat of a desert or the heat of an engine-room. The patient collapses with a high oral and rectal temperature, a hot dry skin, confusion, restlessness, twitchings, fits and coma. *Treatment* is by immediate cooling with preferably a cold spray combined with fanning.

321   *Diseases due to Physical Factors*

Heat exhaustion occurs when a person is exposed to heat without means of obtaining water, as can occur when a man is adrift on a raft in the tropics. He develops thirst, dehydration, loss of weight, a rapid pulse, anuria, restlessness and coma. *Treatment* is by a high fluid intake by mouth or intravenously in cool surroundings.

Salt depletion occurs when people exposed to heat, sweat profusely and lose salt which they cannot replace, as can occur when a man is working under very hot conditions. He develops fatigue, weakness, giddiness, muscular cramps, vomiting and cardio-vascular collapse. It is very likely to occur in a man who has not become acclimatized to the working conditions.

Prevention is by taking salt drinks while working. *Treatment* is the administration of salt solution by mouth if the patient can retain it or as isotonic saline intravenously.

CAISSON DISEASE

Other name: decompression sickness
This is due to too rapid decompression of a diver or a man who has been working in a caisson, a compressed air chamber in which the pressure has to be higher than the atmosphere in order to keep out water. When a man is exposed to such pressure, his tissues take up an excessive amount of nitrogen from the air; and if on returning to the surface he is decompressed too rapidly, bubbles of nitrogen form in his tissues.

Clinical features

Workmen have their names for the symptoms (a) the 'staggers' – for the giddiness and headache; (b) the 'bends' – for the abdominal pain, nausea and vomiting. If bubbles form in the nervous system, hemiplegia, paraplegia, coma and death can occur.

Prevention

This is by not allowing too long a period at work and taking an appropriate time over the decompression technique in which the workman is gradually restored to a normal atmospheric pressure and gets rid of the nitrogen through his lungs.

Treatment is by putting the man back under pressure again (when the bubble will be reabsorbed) and then decompressing him very slowly.

IONIZING RADIATIONS

Man has always been subjected to some radio-activity, for radiations are given off by soil and rocks and some reaches the earth from outer space; but the amounts received in this way are small.

New sources of radiation are (a) X-rays used in diagnosis and treatment, (b) radium, radon, cobalt-60, etc. (c) radio-active isotopes used in diagnosis and treatment, (d) luminous dials on watches, (e) X-rays used in industry, (f) atomic power-stations, (g) atomic and hydrogen bombs.

Clinical features

The features produced by overdose of ionizing radiations depend upon the dose of radiation received.

With small doses there is in time a reduction in the number of white cells and then of all the cells in the blood; diarrhoea and a falling out of hair can occur. With larger doses attacks of nausea, vomiting and diarrhoea are followed by fatigue, breathlessness, aplastic anaemia, agranulocytosis, purpura, intestinal ulceration, infections, and often death.

With very large doses severe vomiting and diarrhoea are followed by circulatory collapse and death within a short time. The amount of radiation received is measured on a photographic film such as is worn by the staff of X-ray departments. The rate at which it is received is measured by a Geiger counter or a scintillation counter.

Prevention   It is very important that a nurse should obey absolutely all safety regulations where ionizing radiations are being used. Special regulations are in force where X-rays, isotopes, and atomic material are used. It is advisable not to wear a watch with a luminous dial and not to have one's feet examined by X-ray machines in shoe-shops.

Diseases due to Physical Factors

20   Parasites

Parasites are creatures that live in or on the bodies of other creatures and get their nourishment from them.

In tropical countries parasites are a common cause of serious illness, but in temperate climates and where there are high standards of hygiene, they are less of a menace. With the movement of people from one country to another, however, tropical parasites can be brought into countries they are not usually found in.

I. External Parasites
1. FLEAS

Fleas are small insects, with flat bodies and long legs for jumping. They are not 'selective parasites': they do not mind what species of animal they live on and will transfer themselves from one to another.

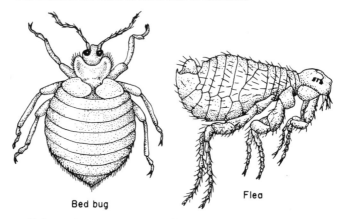

Fig. 95. Bedbug and flea (greatly magnified).

Bed bug   Flea

Pulex irritans, the common human flea, lives on men, dogs, rats, mice and cattle. It feeds on the blood of the animal by biting it, but it can go for 3-4 months without a meal. A bite causes itching, a papule, and in some people an urticarial reaction. It lays its eggs in the cracks of furniture and floors. Each egg becomes a larva and each larva becomes a pupa (chrysalis), which can pass a year in that state if conditions are unsuitable for it to develop into a flea. Bubonic plague and anthrax can be spread by this flea.

Rat fleas will in some circumstances transmit themselves from rats to man. They are transmitters on their bodies of the organisms that cause bubonic plague and flea-borne typhus.

Fleas are killed by insecticides, such as DDT. The main preventive measure is the destruction of rats.

2. LICE

Lice are small flat insects. They can walk over the skin, holding on to hairs with tiny claws at the ends of their legs. They live by sucking blood. They are 'selective parasites': they can live on only one species of animal; human lice live only on

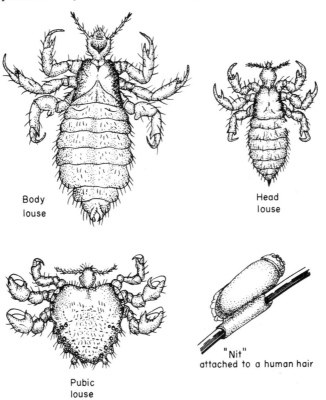

Body
louse

Head
louse

"Nit"
attached to a human hair

Pubic
louse

Fig. 96. Three varieties of louse and a nit (greatly magnified).

human beings. There are three kinds of them: head louse, body louse, and pubic louse. There are small differences between them.

The *head louse* lives in the scalp and beard. Being greyish-white and about 2-3 mm long it can be seen with the naked eye in dark hair, but not very easily in fair hair. It lives for about 4-6 weeks. The female louse lays several hundred eggs, which have the popular name of 'nits'. The greyish-white nits are attached on the hair close to the skin; they can be distinguished from tiny pieces of scurf by not coming off when the hair is run lightly through the fingers.

Recently infected people complain of irritation in the scalp, but people who have been infected for years may feel nothing. Itching leads to scratching and scratching to secondary infections of the skin.

Lice are passed from person to person by direct contact or by sharing a pillow or headwear. They are an infection of the unwashed.

The *body louse* is slightly larger than the head louse and lays its eggs not on hair but in the creases of clothes and bedclothes. It causes papules, itching and secondary infection of scratches. Old vagrants with a chronic resident population of lice upon them can develop a generalized pigmentation rather like that seen in Addison's disease.

Body lice can spread the organism that causes typhus fever.

The *pubic or crab louse* is the smallest of these human fleas. It lives in the pubic hair and elsewhere in very hairy people. Its eggs are attached to the pubic hairs close to the skin. It is spread by sexual intercourse.

Prevention is by cleanliness of body and clothing and avoiding contact with people likely to be infected. *Treatment* is by killing the lice with insecticides. A 2 per cent solution of DDT or of gamma benzene hexachloride is rubbed into the infected areas twice, with a week between applications; the insecticide will be effective long enough to kill any new lice that hatch out. All infected members of a family should be treated at the same time. Underclothes are disinfected by thorough washing and ironing. Bedclothes are autoclaved. Melathion (an organo-phosphorus insecticide) in 0.5 per cent solution is used to treat head lice.

3. BEDBUGS

A bedbug, an insect which lives in cracks in walls and furniture and under wall-paper, is an inhabitant of slums. It is a parasite on man only when at night it comes out for a feed of blood. Usually it does this every 2-3 nights, but it can survive for a year without a meal. It hibernates in cold weather. Its bites cause irritation, scratching and secondary infection; it does not transmit any disease. It is destroyed by insecticides such as DDT. Furniture should not be moved from an infected house to another without being disinfected.

4. SCABIES MITE

Scabies is an infection of the skin by a small insect called a mite.

The female mite is responsible for the features of the infection, the male dying after fertilizing her. An infected person usually has about a dozen females on him.

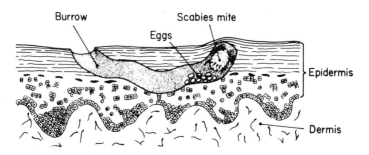

Fig. 97. Scabies mite laying eggs in burrow.

The mite is just large enough to be seen with the naked eye. After fertilization the female burrows into the epidermis at the rate of about 5 mm a day to make a burrow about 1 cm long and lays up to 50 eggs behind it as it burrows. The eggs hatch out into larvae, which make new burrows and turn into mites.

Chapter 20

Infection is by close direct contact with an infected person or occasionally by contact with his clothing or bedclothing. Epidemics can occur.

Clinical features An intensive itching is *the* symptom. This gives the disease the popular name of 'the itch' and anyone developing an itch should be inspected closely for burrows. Burrows appear as thin, grey lines with a tiny speck — the female mite — at one end. The most common sites of infection are: clefts of the fingers, ulnar side of hand and front of wrist, inner side of elbow, anterior axillary fold, abdomen, the external genitalia in men, and in women under the breasts. The female mite can be picked out of her burrow with the point of a needle.

The itching area is scratched and scratching leads to secondary infection, urticaria and eczema. *Norwegian (crusted) scabies* is a rare but very infectious form in which the encrusted skin swarms with mites; it is particularly liable to cause epidemics in small residential communities.

Treatment Any of the following preparations can be used:
(a) gamma benzene hexachloride cream or lotion (Lorexane) 1 per cent,
(b) monosulphiram (Tetmosol), 25 per cent solution, diluted with three parts of water immediately before use,
(c) crotamiton lotion or ointment (Eurax),
(d) benzyl benzoate solution 25 per cent; this has a slight smell and can cause a mild dermatitis.
Day 1. The patient has a hot bath, scrubbing infected areas with a nail-brush. He is then painted from the neck downwards with the solution, no part below the chin being omitted. He goes to bed in his ordinary night clothes and bedclothes.
Day 2. Without having a bath, he is painted all over a second time.
Day 3. He has a bath.

Intimate contacts of the patient should be similarly treated at the same time. Tetmesol soap helps to prevent the spread of infection in a closed community (e.g. a ward or hostel). Failure usually means that this routine has not been scrupulously followed. It is not necessary to disinfect outer-clothing and bedclothing. Underwear is thoroughly washed and ironed. Itching is relieved by hydrocortisone or calamine ointment.

II. Intestinal Parasites
1. THREADWORMS (pinworms).

Threadworms are thin white worms 0.5-1 cm long and look like pieces of cotton. They are a very common infection of man, who is their only host. They are most common in children but can occur in adults. They inhabit the large intestine, especially the caecum.

After fertilization the female worms wriggle along the large intestine and out through the anus to lay their eggs outside the body, in the peri-anal region or on the buttocks. Anal irritation can occur. The eggs stick where they are laid, and if the part is unwashed they can on a warm wet site survive for several weeks. An already infected person reinfects himself by transferring the eggs from the peri-anal region to the mouth with his fingers or on to his food, and the larvae which form from the eggs can also crawl back through the anus. Other people infect

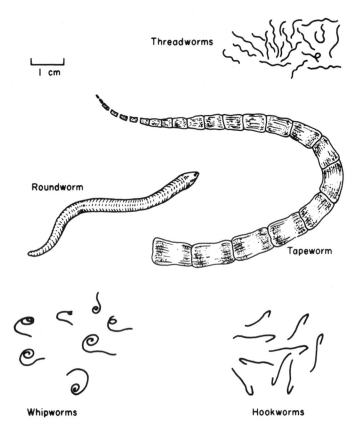

1 cm

Roundworm

Tapeworm

Fig. 98. Threadworm roundworm, tapeworm, whipworm and hookworm.

Whipworms

Hookworms

themselves by contaminating their fingers, by swallowing eggs that have been shaken off underclothes or bedclothes, or from lavatory seats. Several members of a family are usually infected.

Threadworms appear, uncommonly, to be a cause of acute appendicitis, the appendix being sometimes found at operation to be swarming with them.

Threadworms can be seen in the faeces. The eggs can be seen on microscopic examination of a piece of sticky cellulose tape that has been pressed on to the peri-anal region.

Prevention is by washing the hands after defaecation or wiping a child, by washing the hands before meals, by adequate washing of underclothes and bedclothes, and by keeping lavatory seats clean.

Treatment   All members of a family should be treated at the same time as probably more than one is infected.

Viprynium in doses of 5 mg per kilo of body-weight (up to 12 years) is given as a single dose. The faeces are stained red.

Piperazine is given in doses of 1-2 g daily in divided doses for an adult; for children under 6 in doses of 250 mg-1 g daily, and over 6 in doses of 500 mg-1.0 g Treatment is given for a week, then stopped for a week, and then given for a week.

Hydrocortisone ointment can be used for peri-anal irritation.

2. TAPEWORMS

Tapeworms have to live in two 'hosts' if they are to complete their life-cycle. Man can be infected by:

beef tapeworm	pork tapeworm
fish tapeworm	hydatid tapeworm.

(a) Beef tapeworm (taenia saginata).

This is the only common tapeworm in Britain. The fully developed worm is white and flat, lives in the intestine for years, and can grow to a length of 12 metres (40 feet). There is usually only one present at any one time, but sometimes several are present. It consists of a head, a neck and a chain of hundreds of short segments up to 1 cm broad. The pin-head sized head is attached by suckers to the mucous membrane of the duodenum or jejunum; the neck is the part from which the segments grow. As each segment grows it pushes away the one formed previously, and in this way the chain grows in length. Each segment produces and fertilizes thousands of eggs, becomes detached, is discharged in the faeces or wriggles out through the anus, and deposits the eggs in the peri-anal area or on the clothes.

To complete the cycle the eggs have to be eaten by cattle, which can happen when cattle graze on fields that have been contaminated with infected human sewage. Having been ingested by cattle, the eggs become larvae in the intestine and the larvae pass through the wall of the intestine and into the blood stream to become deposited in muscle. There each larva turns into a cyst containing the head. Such beef is called 'measly beef'. If beef with cysts in it is eaten in a raw or only slightly cooked state, the cyst-wall degenerates in the human intestine and the head attaches itself to the mucous membrane and starts to grow into a new worm.

Clinical features

The appearance of segments in the stools is usually the only sign. Some patients complain of abdominal discomfort, colic or diarrhoea.

Prevention

1. Human excreta should not be used untreated as manure where cattle graze.
2. In slaughter-houses beef is thoroughly inspected for cysts.
3. Beef is not eaten raw or only lightly cooked.

Treatment

There are several drugs capable of killing beef tapeworm. *Niclosamide* is given in doses of 1 g followed by 1 g one hour later and a purge after the second dose. *Mepacrine hydrochloride* is given in doses of 100 mg at intervals of 5 minutes until 10 doses have been given or through a duodenal tube that has been in place since the night before. A saline purge is given 30 minutes later. *Male fern extract* draught is given in a single dose of 6 ml, the patient having had nothing but liquids for 48 hours; a saline purge (not castor oil) is given 2 hours later. The other treatments are less toxic.

(b) Pork tapeworm (taenia solium).

This worm grows to a length of 5 metres. It is slightly different in structure from the beef tapeworm and its other host has to be a pig. 'Measly pork' is pork containing the cysts of the worm. Prevention is by proper disposal of human sewage, meat inspection, and not eating raw or imperfectly cooked pork. Treatment is by extract of male fern or niclosamide.

Cysticercosis is the occurrence of cysts in tissues. This can happen in humans as a result of invasion of the body by the larvae of the worm, which sometimes happens. The larvae being distributed by the blood-stream, cysts are formed in many tissues and organs, such as subcutaneous tissue, muscle, eye, brain, lungs and heart. Cysts in the brain can cause epilepsy. When the larvae eventually die, the cyst sometimes becomes calcified and visible on an X-ray. There is no specific treatment except by surgical removal of the cysts where possible. Epilepsy is treated by anti-convulsants.

(c) Fish tapeworm

Found in freshwater fish in countries bordering the Baltic Sea and in Iceland, and in men who eat them uncooked. They can cause macrocytic type anaemia because they interfere with the absorption of vitamin B_{12}.

(d) Hydatid[8] tapeworm (taenia echinococcus).

Only 0.5 cm long, it lives in the intestine of dogs, cats and other animals, and is a common infection of sheep-dogs in Australia, New Zealand, South Africa, the Middle East and parts of Europe. Man is infected by eating contaminated food or fondling infected dogs.

It differs from the other tapeworms in that it does not exist in man as a worm but only as eggs and larvae. After they have been swallowed, the eggs turn into larvae and the larvae penetrate the wall of the small intestine, get into the blood, and are distributed all over the body. Where they lodge hydatid cysts[9] form. A cyst has a capsule and contains fluid with the heads of new worms inside it or smaller 'daughter' cysts with heads inside them. Cysts can grow very large. In the liver they cause hepatic enlargement and jaundice; in the lungs, cough and haemo-ptysis; in the brain, epilepsy. The walls of cysts eventually calcify.

Special tests

Skin: Casoni's test by intra-dermal injection of an antigen prepared from cyst-fluid shows a positive reaction in about 80 per cent of cases; false positive reactions can occur.
Radio-active scanning techniques: for liver cysts.
Blood: often shows eosinophilia[1].
X-ray: reveals a cyst in a bone and any calcified cysts.

Prevention

In countries where the disease is common, a dog is not a pet allowed in the house; it is kept away from food and kitchens, is not fondled, and is de-wormed and treated with DDT.

Treatment

Drugs have no effect. Some cysts can be removed surgically. No cyst-fluid must escape into the tissues for it can cause dangerous anaphylactic[2] reactions.

3. ROUNDWORMS

Roundworms are about 15-25 cm long and are like pale versions of the common earthworm. Infection of man by them is a sign of faecal contamination of his environment.

Man becomes infected by swallowing fertilized eggs from the faeces of another human being, on lettuce or uncooked vegetables. The eggs survive for a long time outside the body, resisting heat, drying and antiseptics. Inside the intestine the eggs develop into larvae. The larvae then follow a peculiar course to finish up where

[8] *hydatid:* from the Greek *hudation,* a drop of water
[9] *cyst:* a little sac containing fluid
[1] *eosinophilia:* increase in number of eosinophil cells in blood
[2] *anaphylactic:* hyper-sensitive to a protein as a result of a previous dose

they started. Piercing the intestinal wall, they get into the veins and so into the pulmonary circulation. Then they pass out of the capillaries and into the alveoli of the lungs, are coughed up in the sputum and re-swallowed. Back in the small intestine they change into the adult worms, which live there freely. A heavily infected person can be a host to several hundred worms at the same time. Worms and fertilized eggs are passed out in the faeces.

Clinical features

A worm in the faeces is often the sole sign of infection. Some people get diarrhoea and abdominal pain. Severely infected children do not thrive and have chronic abdominal disturbance. Some worms, managing to get up the common bile duct, cause biliary obstruction and jaundice.

Treatment

Piperazine phosphate in a single dose of 4 g for an adult or older child and 3 g for a young child paralyses the worms and a saline purge then drives them out. Bephenium hydroxy-naphthoate is also effective in a single dose of 5 g without previous preparation.

Toxocara is a roundworm of cats and dogs; children can become infected by eating contaminated food or soil. The worm wanders round the human body, causing fever, malaise, and an enlarged liver; the eye can become infected. Treatment is by diethylcarbamazine.

4. HOOKWORMS
(two kinds: *Ancylostoma duodenale, Necator americanus*).

Hookworms are mainly an infection of tropical and subtropical countries and evidence of lack of adequate sanitation.

The worms, about 1 cm long have hooks with which they attach themselves to the mucous membrane of the small intestine. The eggs are passed in the faeces and in moist warm soil they hatch into larvae. Larvae infect others by piercing the skin, and the infection is likely to occur in those who walk bare-foot or handle faecally contaminated soil. The larvae get into the bloodstream and in the lungs pass out of the capillaries into the alveoli and thence crawl up the bronchi and trachea and down the oesophagus. In the intestine worms then develop from the larvae.

Clinical features

Many infected people show little or only slight evidence of infection. Others are in chronic ill-health from bleeding in the intestine, diarrhoea and loss of weight, and can eventually die. This is particularly liable to occur in people who are ill-nourished and whose diet lacks protein and iron. Itching at the site of penetration of the skin occurs. The diagnosis is made by the discovery of the characteristic eggs in the faeces.

Treatment

Tetrachlorethylene is given in a dose of 4.0 ml, the patient having fasted from the night before, and a saline purge is given 2 hours later. Or bephenium is given in a single dose fo 2.5-5 g. Iron or a blood-transfusion may be necessary to treat the anaemia. Protein deficiency should be corrected.

5. WHIPWORMS
(*Trichuris trichura*)

This is a common tropical infection of the intestine. The worms are 3-5 cm long, with one end curled up like a whip. Man is the only host. The characteristic eggs are found in the faeces. Some patients have diarrhoea, but the infection is relatively harmless. There is no satisfactory treatment.

6. TRICHINELLA SPIRALIS

These tiny worms infect pigs and rats; man can acquire them by eating raw or imperfectly cooked pork, ham or pork sausages. Several people may be infected simultaneously by the same food. It is common in Europe and North America; epidemics have occurred in England, The muscle of infected pigs can contain enormous numbers of larvae enclosed in cysts. When eaten, the larvae penetrate the wall of the small intestine, are distributed round the body in the blood, and settle in muscle, where they form cysts which eventually become calcified.

Clinical features
Slight infections cause no symptoms. Heavy infections begin with nausea, vomiting, diarrhoea and abdominal pain; as the larvae pass into the body acute reactions develop, with fever, rapid pulse, stiffness of muscles, and oedema of the face, eyelids and conjunctivae. Involvement of the myocardium can produce cardiac failure; involvement of the diaphragm can cause dyspnoea; involvement of the nervous system can cause paralysis, confusion and coma. Very heavy infections can kill.

Special tests
Blood: eosinophilia is common.
Muscle biopsy: to reveal cysts.
X-ray of muscles: to show calcified cysts.

Prevention
1. Proper disposal of garbage; extermination of rats.
2. Thorough meat inspection in slaughter-houses.
3. Thorough cooking of all pork meats.

Treatment
There is no certain cure. Thiabendazole in doses of 50 mg per kilo body-weight for two days is thought to kill the larvae. Anthelmintics and saline purges can be used for recent infections while the parasites are still in the intestine. Severe reactions may be reduced by cortico-steroids.

III. Other Parasites
AMOEBIC DYSENTERY

This is an infection by an amoeba (a uni-cellular organism) called *Entamoeba histolytica.* It is common in the tropics. The amoeba, which is about 5 times the size of a red blood cell, has an active phase in which it can move about, is killed by gastric juice and cannot survive for long outside the body, but it can pass into an inactive phase in which it forms a cyst. This cyst can resist measures which would kill the amoeba in the active phase and is the means by which infection is transmitted from person to person. It is a disease of faecal contamination, spread by infected water, food and flies. Carriers are a source of infection: they can be convalescents temporarily harbouring the organisms in the intestine after an attack or symptomless carriers more or less permanently infected.

Infection causes inflammation and ulceration of the colon. Amoebae can invade the blood and are likely to be carried to the liver, where they cause amoebic hepatitis or an abscess. Usually only one abscess is present; it can become very large and rupture into the peritoneal cavity or through the diaphragm into the chest.

Clinical features
Amoebic dysentery is usually a mild infection with a long incubation period, in contrast to bacillary dysentery with its acute symptoms and short incubation period.

The incubation period is up to 8-9 weeks. Usually a mild enteritis is produced with slight fever, diarrhoea, a grumbling abdomen, nausea, vomiting and loss of weight. Recovery is usual, although recurrence is common; some patients pass into a chronic state with intermittent fever and abdominal symptoms.

Complications
Amoebic hepatitis and abscess: the patient has a tender enlarged liver, swinging temperature, sweating, raised diaphragm.

Special tests	*Faeces:* to discover the presence of the parasite. *Isotopic liver scanning* to discover amoebic abscesses.
Prevention	1. In countries where infection is common, unboiled water and raw vegetables should not be taken. 2. Carriers and people recovering from an attack should not handle food.
Treatment	1. Patient goes to bed and has a milk or low-residue diet. 2. Metronidazole 800 mg is given 3 times daily for 5-7 days to an adult. For children the dose is 50 mg/kilo 3 times daily. 3. Other drugs used are oxytetracycline, chlortetracycline, diloxanide furoate and chloroquine. 4. Any fluid or electrolyte disturbance is corrected. 5. Any anaemia is treated.
TRICHOMONIASIS	This is an infection by *Trichomonas vaginalis,* a uni-cellular organism with flagellae at one end and an 'undulating membrane' down one side and an ability to move in jerky movements. It is spread by sexual intercourse.

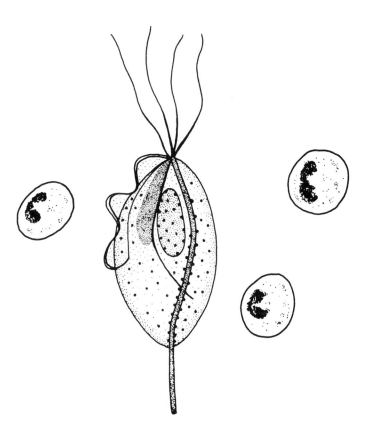

Fig. 99. Trichomonas vaginalis and pus cells.

In women the vagina is infected and a vaginal discharge is caused. It men it causes a low-grade urethritis and urethral discharge. It is commonly associated with gonorrhoea. In men there may be no symptoms.

Special test   The organism can be found on a smear or culture of the discharge.

Treatment   Metronidazole is given by mouth in doses of 200 mg three times a day for 7 days or 400 mg twice daily for 5 days; a second course can be given if necessary. The sexual partner should be investigated and treated simultaneously.

MALARIA   Malaria occurs throughout Africa (including Tunisia), South East Asia, South America, the Arabian peninsula and the Western Pacific islands. The number of cases in Europe has increased in recent years as a result of international travel and immigration. The parasite is a single-celled protozoon called *Plasmodium*, of which 4 species can cause the infection:

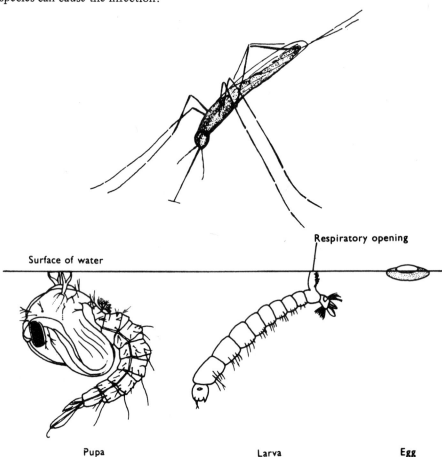

Respiratory opening

Surface of water

Fig. 100. An anopheles mosquito; its pupa, larva and egg are attached to the surface of water and can then be destroyed.

Pupa   Larva   Egg

Plasmodium falciparum, which causes malignant tertian malaria, a severe form common in Africa.

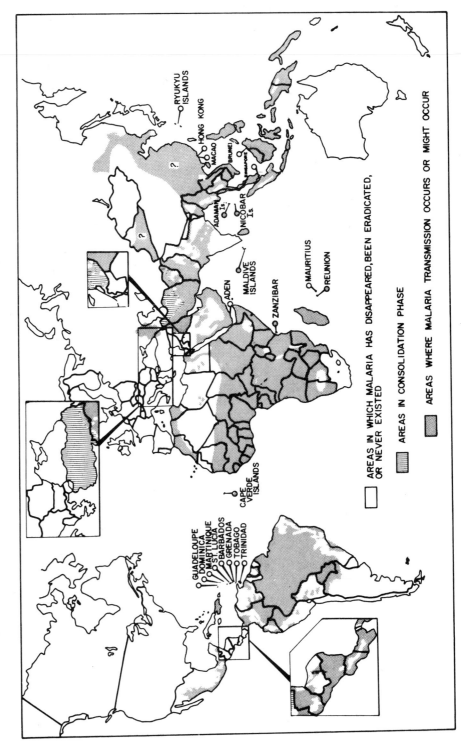

Fig. 103. Map showing malaria areas.

(by courtesy of the World Health Organisation)

AREAS IN WHICH MALARIA HAS DISAPPEARED, BEEN ERADICATED, OR NEVER EXISTED

AREAS IN CONSOLIDATION PHASE

AREAS WHERE MALARIA TRANSMISSION OCCURS OR MIGHT OCCUR

RYUKYU ISLANDS

HONG KONG

MACAO

BRUNEI

SINGAPORE

ANDAMAN Is.

NICOBAR I.s.

MAURITIUS

REUNION

MALDIVE ISLANDS

ADEN

ZANZIBAR

CAPE VERDE ISLANDS

GUADELOUPE

DOMINICA

MARTINIQUE

ST. LUCIA

BARBADOS

GRENADA

TOBAGO

TRINIDAD

Plasmodium vivax, which causes benign tertian malaria, common in India and
S.E. Asia.

Plasmodium malariae, which causes quartan malaria, mild and comparatively
rare.

Plasmodium ovale, causes a mild malaria, comparatively rare.

The malaria parasite has two hosts: man and the female of some kinds of
Anopheles mosquito, common in wet hot areas of the world. The parasite cannot
survive outside its hosts. In them the following cycle takes place:

1. An already infected female anopheline mosquito bites a man in order to suck
blood and in so doing discharges into the man a number of the organisms from its
salivary glands.

2. In the man the parasites have to pass through several stages. They invade the
liver and multiply and then pass out of the liver into the blood and invade the red
blood cells. The red cells are destroyed and thousands of new parasites liberated
from red cells invade new red cells.

3. If another female mosquito bites a man while he has these parasites circulating
in the blood it will infect itself; inside it the parasite goes through other stages to
arrive in the salivary glands ready for the next man bitten.

When the parasite is the *P. falciparum*, all the parasites are discharged from the
liver in stage 2; but with all the other kinds of parasite some of them are left in
the liver and go on re-infecting the man, being likely so to produce a chronic malaria
This difference affects treatment.

The infection is rare in young infants, but can become common after the first
few months of life. In childhood infections are usually severe; but if an affected
person continues to live in a malarious area, he builds up resistance and attacks in
later life are likely to become milder. Resistance to infection by one type of *Plasmodium* does not give resistance to the others. Travellers and holiday-makers in
countries where malaria occurs are at risk.

Clinical features
1. Vivax group

This group includes *P. vivax, P. malariae* and *P. ovale,* which can be considered
together because the clinical features are similar.

Incubation period: 12-15 days; up to 1 month for *P. malariae.*

An attack may begin with a paroxysm of fever or by a few days of malaise, loss
of appetite, nausea, vomiting and muscle-pain. Fever is at first irregular, rising to
40.5°C. (105°F.) for about a week, and then settling down to a rhythm of fever
on certain days and afebrility on others. Each invasion of the blood by parasites
from the liver or red cells produces a paroxysm.

A *paroxysm of fever* follows a pattern of:

(a) a cold stage: the temperature has started to rise but the patient feels very cold
and has a rigor, i.e. he shivers violently;

(b) a hot stage: the rigor stops, the patient feels and is very hot with his temperature
up to 40.5°C. and his pulse bounding;

(c) a sweating stage, in which the temperature falls to normal within an hour and he
sweats profusely.

An untreated attack of malaria of this kind lasts for about 6 weeks and is followed

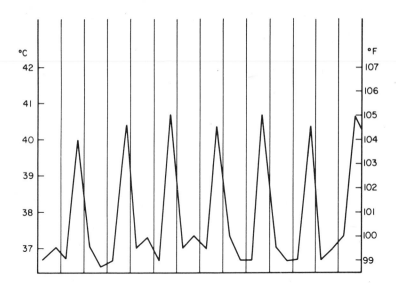

Fig. 102. Typical temperature chart in a *P. Vivax* malaria infection.

by a natural recovery. As however the parasite continues to live in the liver, recurrences are very common and may continue to occur for up to 3 years after a person has left a malarious district.

The destruction of red blood cells causes a moderate degree of anaemia. The spleen becomes enlarged during an attack and can be felt about the 10th-14th day. If the patient has recurrences of malaria, it can become enormous, filling a large part of the abdomen.

With *P. malariae* the incubation period is longer (up to 1 month), an attack can last longer, and relapses can occur over several years.

2. Infection with P. falciparum

This is a very acute form of malaria, very likely to be fatal.

Incubation period: usually 12 days.

The patient is acutely ill. The disease may present as an influenza-like illness, encephalitis, anaemia or hepatitis. Fever is often irregular. The patient may complain of headache, nausea, vomiting and joint-pains. The liver and spleen are usually enlarged.

Complications

Complications of *P. falciparum* can develop at any stage of the illness and can be fatal:

(a) *Cerebral malaria* is characterized by drowsiness, coma, twitching, mania, and incontinence of urine and faeces. Fits are common in children.

(b) *Renal failure:* the amount of urine passed is reduced; there may be complete suppression of kidney function and uraemia.

(c) *Algid malaria:* the patient goes quickly into a state of shock and coma.

(d) *Blackwater fever:* the urine becomes dark-brown or black due to haemoglobinuria; death can be due to uraemia, to vascular failure or to hepatic failure.

Special tests

Blood: the diagnosis of malaria is made by the identification of the parasite in red blood cells.

1. *Destruction of the mosquito.* National activities, often with the advice of the World Health Organization, are directed at the destruction of the mosquito, and some countries (e.g. Cyprus) have been cleared. Houses, other buildings, ships, cars, trains and aeroplanes are sprayed with insecticides; and as the larva of the mosquito has to live in still fresh water, marshes and pools are drained and oil is spread on water to prevent larvae getting oxygen and so kill them.

2. *Protection of man.* Houses are built away from marshes. Windows are screened with protective netting. People cover exposed parts of the body after nightfall, when the mosquito bites, and sleep under mosquito-netting.

3. *Prevention.* One of the following drugs must be taken (a) for one week before travelling to a malarious country, (b) continuously and regularly while there, and (c) for one month after leaving.

(i) Proguanil hydrochloride (Paludrine): 100 mg every day; 200 mg in areas where falciparum malaria is common.

(ii) Pyrimethamine (Daraprim): 25 mg once a week on the same day each week; 50 mg where falciparum malaria is common.

(iii) Chloroquine: 300 mg (base) once a week.

Travellers and holiday-makers in risk-countries (including those stopping for only a few hours) should be informed and provide themselves with one of these drugs.

Treatment

Treatment is by courses of anti-malarial drugs, such as chloroquine, mepacrine, quinine. The amount given and method of administration used depend upon (a) the type of infection – P. falciparum or Vivax group and (b) whether the patient is a resident in a district, has had previous attacks of malaria and has therefore some degree of immunity, or is a visitor and without immunity. Drug resistance can develop.

Cerebral malaria is treated by intravenous quinine, intravenous hydrocortisone, and the maintenance of fluid and electrolyte balance. Blood transfusion may be required for anaemia.

TOXOPLASMOSIS

This is an uncommon but widely spread disease of man and animals due to infection by a minute parasite *Toxoplasma gondii.* It appears to be on the increase; cases have occurred in Britain. The prevalence among adults in England, as judged by antibody tests, is about 30 per cent; but clinically evident infection is rare. There is little evidence about the way the parasite is transmitted; its life-cycle is unknown; it can infect any warm-blooded animal, including birds. Transmission is via the faeces. The organism produces an inflammatory reaction and ultimately small areas of calcification in many types of tissue.

In man the disease may be:

(a) *congenital:* an infected mother infects her child; the brain is affected and the child can die *in utero* or develop encephalitis, hydrocephalus, mental retardation and impaired vision.

(b) *acquired:* there may be no signs of infection; children can develop meningo-encephalitis; adults can develop enlarged lymph-nodes or a febrile illness with a rash, pneumonitis, myocarditis, or encephalitis.

The illness varies from mild to severe. After a severe attack convalescence can last up to 2 years.

The diagnosis is very difficult.

Special tests

Skin test: a small amount of toxoplasmin (a fluid obtained from the parasite) may produce a positive reaction.

X-ray: may show specks of calcification in tissues, especially the brain.

Organism: the parasite is sometimes identified in tissues, body fluids or by infection produced in laboratory animals by inocculation.

Treatment	The best method is thought to be a month-long course of pyrimethamine combined with sulphadiazine.
TOXOCARIASIS	This is a roundworm infection of dogs and cats (common in tropical countries, not so common elsewhere), which can be transmitted to man. The worms (*toxocara canis* and *toxocara cati*) live in the animals' intestines and produce eggs which if swallowed can infect man. The highest risk is an association of puppies with young children. About 2 per cent of people become infected, but few show clinical signs of infection.
Clinical features	These are: (a) eosinophilia, (b) eye infection, which can cause blindness, (c) liver infection, causing enlargement of the liver, (d) brain infection, causing epilepsy.
Prevention	Young children should not be in contact with puppies or kittens that have not been dewormed. Puppies and kittens should be dewormed at 3 weeks and at 3-week intervals until 2 months, then every month up to 6 months, and then every year up to 4 years. Hygienic measures should be carried out in the home — washing hands before meals, not allowing animals to come into contact with food, cleaning up animal faeces with strong disinfectant.
Treatment	Diethylcarbamazine 3 mg per kilo body-weight is given daily for 21 days.

Index